READER IN THE HISTORY OF APHASIA

AMSTERDAM STUDIES IN THE THEORY AND HISTORY OF LINGUISTIC SCIENCE

General Editor

E. F. KONRAD KOERNER

(University of Ottawa)

Series II - CLASSICS IN PSYCHOLINGUISTICS

Advisory Editorial Board

Volume 4

Paul Eling (ed.)

Reader in the History of Aphasia

READER IN THE HISTORY OF APHASIA

FROM [FRANZ] GALL TO [NORMAN] GESCHWIND

Edited by

PAUL ELING
University of Nijmegen

JOHN BENJAMINS PUBLISHING COMPANY
AMSTERDAM/PHILADELPHIA

The paper used in this publication meets the minimum requirements of American National Standard for Information Sciences — Permanence of Paper for Printed Library Materials, ANSI Z39.48-1984.

Library of Congress Cataloging-in-Publication Data

Reader in the history of aphasia : from Franz Gall to Norman Geschwind / edited by Paul Eling.

    p.   cm. -- (Amsterdam studies in the theory and history of linguistic science. Series II, Classics in psycholinguistics, ISSN 0165-716X; v. 4)

    Includes bibliographical references and index.

    1. Aphasia--History--Sources. I. Eling, Paul. II. Series.

RC425.R36   1994

616.85'52'009--dc20   94-20171

ISBN 90 272 1893 5 (alk. paper)   CIP

John Benjamins Publishing Co. • P.O.Box 75577 • 1070 AN Amsterdam • The Netherlands
John Benjamins North America • P.O.Box 27519 • Philadelphia, PA 19118 • USA

Table of Contents

Foreword

When the Max Planck Institute for Psycholinguistics was created in Nijmegen, Holland, it was decided that apart from fundamental research on normal language behavior, a project should also be devoted to the analysis of language behavior of aphasic patients, using theoretical views and methodologies developed within the field of psycholinguistics. Neurologists, linguists, and psychologists collaborated in this project. Several members of this group decided not only to investigate current views on aphasia, but also to study and discuss the views of the classic aphasiologists. The regular meetings were not only very instructive, but also great fun. Theories are not a set of dry statements; scientists believe in their theories and defend them from ruthless attacks from opponents. When one becomes more familiar with the scientific and social background of an influential scientist, it sometimes becomes clear that a particular theoretical point of view is a natural consequence of more general assumptions prevailing in the environment in which the author worked.

When we discovered in our meetings how important it can be to go back to the original aphasiological issues and to discover that the early aphasiologists were sensitive to important implications of their conceptions of language and the brain, we realized that every student should be able to read these texts in an early phase of their neurolinguistic training.

In order to make the original texts accessible to a greater public, it was decided to translate the French and German texts into English. Present-day specialists, often already well-acquainted with the work of a particular author (everybody has their favorite), prepared theoretical introductions, highlighting the most significant features of the views of a particular author. To complete the picture, short biographies and lists of references to other works of that author on aphasia were added. No attempt was made to be exhaustive or to refer to historical studies on a particular author. The aim of this book is to present the original text in a readable format, and not an historical analysis.

The project took a long time to come to completion, mainly due to the slowness with which the editorial operation progressed in order to enlarge the accessibility of the book. At first, I was very happy with the positive reaction of my colleagues towards the project and their willingness to contribute. Now, I am even more grateful for their patience. I would like to thank Stella Roomans, Kate and Patrick Hudson, and Peter Daniels for their work on the translations, and Joke Hermsen for compiling reference lists. Professor Eckart Scheerer, Antoine Keyser, and Marielle Gorissen helped me to trace references. I am grateful to Edith Sjoerdsma for typing the manuscripts, and to Pim Levelt for use of the facilities in his Institute. Konrad Koerner supported me enthusiastically and helped me to locate translations of classical aphasiological texts. Claire Benjamins and Yola de Lusenet suggested important improvements with respect to the structure and style of the book. These adaptations were surely worth the efforts they required, though any remaining blemishes must remain my responsibility. Finally, I want to thank all the contributing authors, old and new, for producing the materials for this book.

Paul Eling
Nijmegen
August 1994

Introduction

PAUL ELING

Language is an important function. This statement is true from many different points of view. Scientists investigating the functioning of the human brain will also recognize that we have gained much information from studying the relationship between language and the brain, or rather between language disorders and brain lesions. The tradition of this branch of science goes back to the beginnings of the 19th century. The observations, arguments, and opinions of these early papers are still crucially important, considering the frequency with which they are cited in current research papers.

Of course the techniques of studying the functioning of the brain have been much refined. In contrast to the pioneers, we do not have to wait until a patient dies to open the skull and examine the lesions. Today, we can visualize in detail not only the surface but also the inner parts of the brain, without harming the patient. We can even observe deviations in normal functioning of groups of nerve cells, as expressed in their metabolism. So why are these old papers still important, aside from historical curiosity? Like a piece of machinery, the brain not only consists of a set of components, but it also fulfills a function. Discovering the individual components and their mutual relationships is one thing, but describing what function they perform is a completely different matter. How should we conceive of the brain? Is it a single piece of machinery or does it house several independent functions or 'organs'? Looking at a box of loose parts may help a little, but in the end a particular view of the best way to describe the function(s) of the brain comes from the observer. The pioneers formulated particular views on mind–brain relationships and were convinced that what they observed in their patients supported their views, a way of working not unlike ours.

In the blank, scientifically unexplored area of the functioning of the brain, the pioneers drew the first boundaries. Of course the view expressed by one expert was countered by another, thus forming camps, schools. Undoubtedly the most controversial issue in that period was the principle of *localization of function*. The notion that the functioning of the mind was related to the brain — a heretical point of view in the 16th and 17th century — was accepted by students of the brain. Most of them also distinguished between perception, reasoning, and memory. The next step was to study in more detail the relationship between individual functions and parts of the brain. Many — not only researchers — believed this to be impossible in principle, not merely on empirical grounds. In the end the localizationists won the debate. Nevertheless, the discussion regularly flares up, using slightly different concepts. For instance, in the last decade the magic word was not localization but modularity. Today, as in the early days, the battle between proponents and opponents is conducted in the language area, which is considered to act as a model for other functions. That is one reason why the study of the psychology of language, including its psychological and biological basis, is so important and interesting.

Since the 1960s the interest in brain–behavior relationships has increased tremendously. This field is now designated neuropsychology. This development cannot be traced to a single event or person, but it is clear that Norman Geschwind played an outstanding role. He was a great connoisseur of the 19th-century neurologists who wrote about the functioning of the brain. Geschwind's views were largely determined by these predecessors. He not only studied these old papers but popularized the views expressed in them and applied them in his own research. He also stimulated people working in his environment, and out of this grew the Boston Aphasia Unit. This Unit became the preeminent center for aphasiology — the study of language disorders due to brain lesions. It is not only the center from which the most influential papers on aphasia originated, but it also attracted students from literally all over the world for training in aphasiology. This policy of the unit has recently led to an important new direction — the cross-linguistic description and comparison of aphasiological phenomena. Aphasiologists — or neurolinguists as they are called, since the emphasis now is more on linguistic peculiarities than neuroanatomical structures — who received their training in Boston and went back to their home countries can now exchange observations from aphasic patients speaking different languages, following different rules. The first fruits of this undertaking have appeared in three volumes edited by Menn and Obler (1990).

The study of language and the brain is important and fascinating. It is also heavily dependent on the work of the early aphasiologists. Whoever wants to get acquainted with this discipline will be confronted with frequent references to classic authors such as Broca, Wernicke, Dejerine, and Hughlings Jackson. Although these authors had limited means to empirically test their ideas, their theoretical views were not limited. On the contrary, in the periodicals of that time there was ample room for an author to elaborate on his position with respect to a particular issue, as well as on the philosophical implications. In general, characterizing the work of these classic aphasiologists with a few short statements and adjectives does not do justice to the careful analytic description and argumentation of these scientists. Textbooks are meant to provide structure to a student who is confronted with a chaotic congeries of names and theories. In doing so, it is often necessary or inevitable that matters are simplified and that subtle differences are deprived of the larger context in which they developed; the student then tends to read these descriptions with the current social and scientific context in the back of their mind. In this way, the risk of misinterpretation of the work of these classic aphasiologists is very great. Sometimes they are even erroneously credited with positions they have never defended. In the study of language and the brain it is therefore essential that one go back to the original sources, not only to check the wording of a particular statement, but also to get a feeling of the atmosphere in which the statement was produced and the specific meaning that was attached to certain concepts. This holds not only for specialists in neurolinguistics, but especially for beginning students. To provide easy access to the classics, we have compiled this book.

It will be obvious that it was necessary to make a selection with respect to both authors and texts that were to be included in this reader. Subjective impressions of who is to be regarded as important in the history of aphasiology play an important role here. A clearly disputable choice, for instance, is Gall. Franz Joseph Gall never wrote about aphasia, nor do we have any evidence that he was particularly interested in it, nor even in language in general. However, as I explained earlier, general issues of brain and mind have been studied in the language area. In this sense many papers on aphasiologic questions, certainly in the 19th century, deal with notions that were developed by Gall. Although his work was rejected and neglected because of the phrenological excesses that sprang from it, it has been fundamental to our current conception of the functioning of the brain. Broca, for instance, admits that his work on the localization of the articulatory function was inspired by the work of Gall and attests to the principle of localization of function in general.

Another surprising choice may be Geschwind. He died in 1984 — much too early and in the midst of a very productive phase in his rich academic career — and does not belong to the classic writers, long gone. However, it was he who revived the classics, especially in the area of aphasia. He put an important stamp on current discussions in neurolinguistics. We felt that an overview of authors who contributed significantly to the study of aphasia would not be complete without Geschwind.

Even more difficult than picking names is the selection of texts. It was clearly impossible to reproduce papers and chapters in their entirety. In selecting appropriate texts, the emphasis was placed on those parts that dealt explicitly with the opinion of an author on language processes as revealed by aphasic phenomena. This is not to say that no discussions about anatomical structures in the brain are included. These could hardly be avoided, since localization of the language function in the brain was the central issue in the 19th-century literature on aphasia. The reader will, therefore, regularly encounter neurological concepts. Within the scope of the book, it did not appear necessary to provide additional information about these technicalities. In most cases introductory textbooks on neuroanatomy will provide sufficient information. For those completely unfamiliar with the neurological terminology used to denominate specific parts of the brain, we have inserted two figures. Figure 1 represents 'directional' terms and Figure 2 gives the traditional side view and the parts of the cortex that are most frequently used. Of course, other selections might also have been suitable, but we do hope that we have picked passages that reveal how a particular author conceived of the representation of language processes in the brain. If this stimulates beginning students to read more of the classics, and specialists to be careful with their characterisations of them, we have reached our goal.

Since our main aim was to provide easy access to the most important passages of influential papers, rather than exact reproductions of the original texts, we had no feelings of remorse in changing the format of the texts and striving for uniformity. This has resulted in several adaptations, in particular with respect to references and footnotes. All chapters have the same structure. They start with a short biography, giving the reader an idea of where and how a particular author worked and lived. This is followed by a

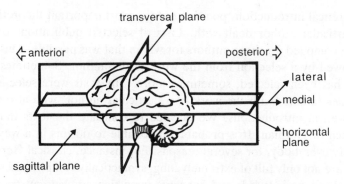

Figure 1. Illustration of the 'directional' terms, frequently used for describing localizations of lesions or directions of fiber tracts.

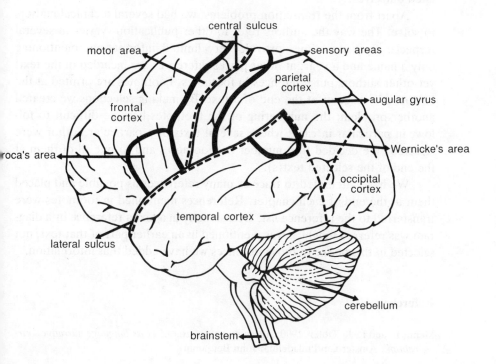

Figure 2. Areas of the brain that play an important role in the traditional aphasiology

theoretical introduction, pointing out the most important theoretical issues a particular author dealt with. Lists of selected publications on aphasia were compiled for those authors for whom that was possible. This in turn is followed by a selection from the work of the author. Sometimes only one text has been selected, sometimes more. The texts were selected by colleagues familiar with the work of a particular author, who also wrote the theoretical introductions. We decided to translate the texts that were in French or German. It is probably impossible to do this in a way that will satisfy everybody, for several reasons. For instance, classical German writings are not only full of extremely long, syntactically complicated sentences, but also contain words and concepts for which no clear-cut translation is available. For some texts we could make use of existing translations and checked these with the original papers. Several other pieces we have translated ourselves.

Apart from the translation problems, we had several technical matters to solve. The way the authors refer to other publications varies in several respects: they sometimes provide very limited information, mentioning only a name and a year; at other places references are included in the text; yet other authors put references in footnotes. Footnotes are printed at the bottom of a page or at the end of a text. By making selections we created another problem: the numbering of the footnotes became difficult to follow, in particular in cases where several texts of a particular author were selected. We decided to renumber the footnotes and to put all of them at the end of the selected text(s).

We have attempted to trace as many references as possible and placed them at the end of each chapter. References mentioned in footnotes were transferred to the reference list. Occasionally in a text a reference or a diagram was referred to which was mentioned in an earlier part of that text, not selected in this book. In those instances we have added that information.

Reference

Menn, L. and L. K. Obler. 1990. *Agrammatic Aphasia. A cross-language narrative sourcebook*. Amsterdam/Philadelhia: John Benjamins.

Franz Joseph Gall

Introduced by

CLAUS HEESCHEN
Max-Planck-Institut für Psycholinguistik
· Nijmegen, The Netherlands

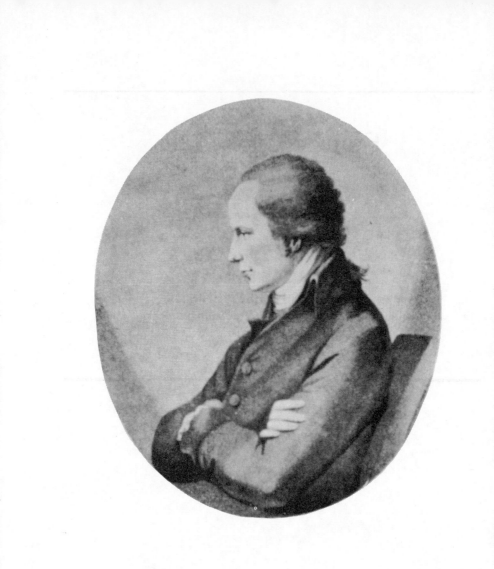

Franz Joseph Gall
1758-1828

Biography

Gall was born in Tiefenbrunn (southwest Germany) in 1758. He began his study of medicine in Strasbourg in 1777, continued and finished his study in Vienna (1781–1785). In Vienna, he worked as a neuroanatomist and as a practicing physician. There he developed his basic ideas concerning the relation between psychological faculties and the brain. He called his doctrine "Organology" or "Schedellehre". He wrote down his ideas in a letter to Retzer (1798). It is remarkable that Gall never modified his doctrine as outlined in this letter. In his later works, he only presented more data material, trying to adduce more evidence for his views. Gall's doctrine became popular among the higher social classes of Vienna. Nevertheless, the propagation of his ideas in Vienna came to a sudden halt in 1801 by a decree of the Holy Roman Emperor Franz II, which in turn was issued under pressure exerted by the church. Gall's views were banned by the church as "materialistic" and thus politically dangerous.

In 1805 he left Vienna and made a tour through several Middle European countries, where his lectures were always a success. In 1807, Gall settled in Paris. Although Gall was exposed to extreme hostility from the leading political powers in Paris, he was at least not forbidden to give private lessons. Furthermore, his doctrine quickly became as fashionable there as it had been in Vienna, especially among the women of the upper classes. Thus, Gall was successful in social and financial respects; nevertheless, he remained a scientific outsider, banned from the official scientific institutions. Two attempts (1808 and 1821) to gain admission to the Académie failed. In Paris, Gall wrote his most comprehensive works:

- *Anatomie et physiologie du système nerveux en général, et du cerveau en particulier, avec des observations sur la possibilité de reconnaître plusieurs dispositions intellectuelles et morales de l'homme et des animaux, par la configuration de leur têtes.* 4 vols. Paris 1810–1819.
- *Sur les fonctions du cerveau et sur celles de chacune de ses parties.* 6 vols. Paris 1822–1825.

The first two volumes of the Anatomie *were written together with his pupil Spurzheim. In 1813, they went their different ways and Spurzheim went to England, where he made Gall's doctrine popular under the name "phrenology". From England, phrenology was carried to the USA, where it really began flower. Gall remained in Paris, where he died in 1828 as a result of a stroke. Needless to say, he bequeathed his own skull to his pupils, who added it to his large collection of specimens. We can still see it in the Musée de l'Homme as number 19216.*

Introduction

Some Remarks on the Prehistory of Modularism in Modern Neuropsychology

> Immer steht jeder Wissenschaft eine
> Afterwissenschaft zur Seite
> (Lem 1984, p. 90)

Franz Joseph Gall and his doctrine — known as "phrenology" — have, for a long time, stood for utmost absurdity, scientific unrespectability, and charlatanry. In a sense, the relation between phrenology and serious brain research has been considered similar to that between alchemy and chemistry or between astrology and astrophysics: phrenology was the *Afterwissenschaft* of neuropsychology (*Afterwissenschaft* means something like pseudoscience, but the German term has much stronger connotations).

Thus it was quite a surprise, when recently a new Gall cult arose among serious neuropsychologists and cognitive psychologists, in particular among those who deal with language (most notably, Fodor, 1983). This rehabilitation of Gall is all the more puzzling as it occurred in a school of (psycho-)linguistics which located itself in a rationalist Cartesian tradition. As a matter of fact, one cannot conceive of two thinkers who are more opposed to each other than Gall and Descartes, and it requires a huge amount of sophistication to integrate Gall's thoughts into a Cartesian framework (cf. Schwartz and Schwartz, 1984).

In the following little essay I shall investigate whether this new invocation of Gall as the father of modern neuropsychology has some justification or whether it can only be viewed as a transient fashion which should not be taken too seriously. However, before discussing this matter I would like to point out that Gall's role cannot be reduced to that of a brain researcher alone: on the basis of his brain doctrine he developed several views concerning anthropological, ethical, sociological, and political issues, and these views were (although based on a dubious theory) undeniably reasonable, revolutionary, and outstandingly progressive. Just to mention one example: Gall attacked the atavistic principle of "crime and punishment" and postulated its replacement by the principle of disease and therapy: criminals are ill and should be treated or — as we would say nowadays — they should be resocialized. Note that Gall lived in the period of *Restauration* — a period of extremely restrictive reactionism in response to the French Revolution. Given these circumstances, Gall's clear and reasonable sociopolitical views, as well as his courage in provoking the whole of Europe with them, cannot be overestimated. In the following, I shall discuss Gall's doctrine only from the narrow perspective of its contribution to the rise of modern neuropsychology. Whatever one might think of Gall in this respect, one should never forget his merits with regard to the general stream of social and political ideas in Europe in the first half of the 19th century (for an excellent presentation of the sociopolitical implications of Gall's work see Lesky, 1979).

Let us now look at the essentials of Gall's doctrine (to repeat, only from the perspective of neuropsychology; readers who are interested in an evaluation of phrenology in the broader context of cultural history are referred to Lanteri-Laura, 1970). The essentials are:

(1) The human mind has its seat in the brain.
(2) The human mind can be divided into several individual components so that different components have different localizations in the brain.
(3) The seats of the mental components (Gall calls them faculties or propensities) are in the cortex; Gall speaks of cortical *organs*.
(4) The organs are autonomous and completely independent of each other in the sense that one given organ can work without any interaction with another component.
(5) The faculties are characterized by the *content* to which they are related; they cannot be characterized by the formal features of the mode of their operations. Thus, general reasoning and memory etc. do not rank among the localizable faculties, while, for instance, music, language, murderous instinct, veneration of God are localizable. Fodor (1983) refers to the general content-unspecific faculties such as reasoning as "central processes" and terms a division of the mind into such central processes a "horizontal" division. Opposed to this, Gall's components of the mind are *domain-specific*, and his division of the mind is termed by Fodor "vertical".

(6) All faculties are innate.

(7) A particularly well developed faculty requires an especially well developed cortical organ: the organ must be comparatively "big".

(8) Points (6) and (7) taken together lead to the conclusion that the particularly well developed organs should leave their traces in the formation of the skull because the infantile skull is still very malleable. Thus, a particularly well developed cortical organ can be "seen" as a bump on the skull. Conversely, somebody with a particularly poorly developed faculty or propensity may have a depression on the skull over the corresponding cortical organ. Therefore, palpation of the skull of a given individual can serve as a diagnostic means for the individual's specific gifts and personality features.

(9) The faculties which are candidates for localization in the cortex cannot be enumerated on the basis of a preestablished psycho-philosophical system, but only by empirical research. This enforces the following research methodology: Gall had to look for people with very one-sided talents, for instance people who showed only one extremely well developed faculty. If these people had an unusual bump at a given place on the skull, then it could be inferred that the cortical organ beneath that bump is the seat of the faculty at issue. As a consequence, Gall was looking for people in the extremes of society: geniuses (for instance outstandingly gifted composers), criminals with one outstandingly well developed propensity (such as murderers and prostitutes), and the so-called monomaniacs, that is, those lunatics who are obsessed by only one particular fixation.

Gall related that he became aware of the skull–mind relationships very early in his youth: he had a schoolmate who was especially language-gifted and had well-developed protuberances in the frontal parts of his skull. Gall at that time hypothesized that the language function can be located in the anterior parts of the brain. However, the involvement of the language function in Gall's first steps towards his "organology" did not reflect any particular interest in language; the possible reasons why the language function became so central in the localization debate after Gall will be commented on below.

Let us first consider Gall's methodology: As has been stated, it is a scientifically sound method — namely, the search for a correlation between the formation of the skull and the profiles of mental faculties. However, Gall ended up with a mental geography of the skull and thus a geography of the cortex which is simply, and without any doubt, wrong. We know for sure that particularly pious people do not necessarily have a bump at the vertex of their skulls, nor conversely that particularly unbelieving people have a depression there. We know for sure that people with a well-developed murderous instinct do not necessarily have a bump behind their ears, nor do non-aggressive people have a depression behind their ears. Since Gall came up with such a geography of the skull and claimed that it was established in a purely empirical way, only two conclusions are possible: either Gall simply cheated, or he followed a methodology which made his theory immune to falsification. I am inclined to choose the second possibility rather than the first. It was certainly impossible even for a man like Gall to cheat incessantly for more than 30 years of his life. Thus, he must have made his theory waterproof against falsification. However, hypotheses or theories which in principle cannot be falsified belong characteristically to what I have referred to as *Afterwissenschaften*. Thus, we have to accept that Gall really was a charlatan. However, let us be charitable and have a look at the remaining points of his theory.

Point (1) presents a view which I would like to call the weak localizationist position, while points (1) and (2) together constitute the strong localizationist position. In some publications (see Riese and Hoff, 1950) it is maintained that for the period of modern science (that is, the post-Renaissance period) it was Descartes who was the first localizationist and that it was he who opened the routes of research culminating in Broca and Wernicke and modern neuropsychological research. I feel, however, that this appraisal of Descartes as the founder of modern localizationist approaches is unwarranted and misleading. First of all, Descartes localized the mind as a *whole* in the pineal body; the idea of a compartmentalization of the mind is incompatible with Cartesianism. Thus, the best we can say about Descartes is that he presented a weak localizationist view. Nevertheless, I should like to call even this into question. As is well known, Descartes introduced the radical distinction between the 'res extensa' and the 'res cogitans' — this is the famous and notorious Cartesian dualism. In his discussion of the pineal body as the seat of the mind (or soul) he anticipated the possible counter-argument that such a huge thing as the human mind should not be located in such a tiny organ as the pineal body and suggested that the mind as a 'res nonextensa' is not dependent on the physical dimensions of its seat. Given this argument together with Cartesian dualism, it would be only logical to go one step further and claim that the mind does not need any localization at all. As a matter of fact, after a long development of idealistic philosophy Kant finally ended up with the conclusion that the soul has no bodily instantiation and does not need it, and that it is only the *activities* of the soul which have to be bound to certain corporeal loci. Thus, Cartesianism did not *open* the localizationist debate, but rather *blocked* it and did so quite effectively for approximately 200 years (for a brief outline of the dilemma of 18th-century psychologists due to dogmatic dualism, see the introduction of Young, 1970; see also Hécaen and Lanteri-Laura, 1977, for the extreme caution and scepticism of 18th-century brain anatomists with respect to the possibility of localization).

If not Descartes, then was it really Gall who was the first to formulate a localizationist theory? Definitely not! The strong(!) version of localizationism is at least as old as Plato, who divided the mind into three distinct components and assigned them to three different parts of the body. At the end of antiquity a system of localization had been developed which was taken over, with some modifications, by medieval thinkers (for an overview of this development see Clark and Dewhurst, 1972; Bruyn, 1982). The Middle Ages, so often supposed to be extremely antimaterialistic, really indulged in making brain– mind diagrams. Basically, they divided the mind into three parts, following the Aristotelian tradition: perception, reason, and memory. They were located in the three ventricles. This basic scheme, best known in the version of Albertus Magnus (ca. 1200-1280), was very often enriched and modified in the course of the Middle Ages, but never completely rejected. Thus the real forerunners of our modern 'boxologists' are Albertus Magnus and his successors rather than Gall and his followers.

Another point in the medieval approach is quite remarkable and indeed establishes a much closer relation between the Middle Ages and modern neuropsychology than there is between Gall and our contemporary neuropsychological activities. The main source of data for neuropsychological research comes from patients with focal brain damage. The underlying logic of modern research can be characterized in the following — admittedly oversimplified — way: given a circumscribed brain lesion, and given an observable behavioral deficit in the patient, then the defective function can be associated with the damaged part of the brain, and can furthermore be considered to be autonomous and independent of the remaining preserved functions.

It is quite surprising that Gall completely neglected evidence coming from brain-damaged patients (I shall discuss the possible reason for this neglect below), but it is all the more surprising that already in the Middle Ages, clinical observations were taken into consideration as relevant for the localizationist system. In Bruyn (1982) we find a reference to a medieval physician who connected the behavioral deficit of "melancholy" to a malfunctioning of the second ventricle; in the very last phase of the Middle Ages a physician attributed an apparently global aphasia to damage in the third ventricle.

What then is new in the Gallian localizationist approach? Certainly point (3): the detection of the significance of the cortex. As pointed out by Hécaen and Lanteri-Laura (1977), Gall was a gifted neuroanatomist, and by inventing a new way of doing sections he became aware of the fact that the cortex contained the end points of the major neuronal tracts and thus must be more than just a sort of degenerated crust covering the "really" important parts of the brain, a view dominating in the field before Gall. The discovery of the relevance of the cortex for higher functions can undeniably be credited to Gall.

Let us now briefly discuss Gall's neglect of clinical evidence for localizations. One should remember that in the three centuries before Gall entered the scene, a large number of careful, meticulous, and comprehensive descriptions of cases of aphasia after a stroke had been published (see Benton and Joynt, 1960; Benton, 1964). Quite obviously, the most important dissociations in language disturbances had been observed and described in the clinical world before 1800 — dissociations such as automatic speech versus propositional speech, speaking versus singing, comprehension problems versus output problems, and even the dissociation of word finding versus sentence formation problems. Together with what was known at that time about strokes and about the crossing of pathways from the hemispheres to the extremities, the observed aphasia cases could have led to an at least rough localization of the mental function "language". That this had not happened before 1800 is — in my view — due to the blocking effect of Cartesian dualism. The whole question of localization of mental functions was "suppressed", and even the leading neuroanatomists of that time simply did not dare to make any inferences with respect to localization of the mind.

What, though, what made Gall so blind to clinical evidence after he had already broken the taboo of dualism anyway? The answer is quite straightforward: Gallian psychology is what we now call individual or personality psychology rather than what is now termed general psychology. He was exclusively interested in individual personalities with some outstanding faculty. He was not interested in statements about human abilities shared by the whole species. When his great adversary Flourens presented evidence, by means of brain ablation experiments in birds, that the ability to move depended on the mass of ablated tissue and not on the locus of the ablation (thus advocating a classical antilocalizationist view), Gall replied that these data are of no relevance for his doctrine: he was not interested in what every "idiot" could do such as moving (and speaking?), but rather in what exceptional individuals can do (geniuses, criminals, prostitutes, monomaniacs). Consequently, patients having lost the power of speech due to brain damage, but without having been linguistic geniuses *before*, were of no interest to Gall.

It appears, therefore, that the subtitle of LeMay (1977: "... Phrenology revisited") is highly misleading. Although Gall's general idea that well-developed cortical organs are reflected in the formation of the skull gets some support from the recent finding that the asymmetry of the left and right planum temporale leaves its traces in an asymmetry of the two halves of the skull, nevertheless this has nothing to do with the essentials of Gall's approach. What LeMay (1977) and other authors found holds for the whole human species including the "idiots", or in other words, the "average human beings" so emphatically ignored by Gall. It was only Bouillaud who transformed Gall's individual-psychological approach into a general-psychological approach, and consequently he became aware of the significance of brain-damaged patients. However, concentration on the consequences of brain damage almost necessarily brought about a concentration on the language function. Why? Among the cognitive deficits following local brain damage, the loss of the power of speech and/or language is definitely the most conspicuous one. Other deficits could be easily misunderstood as dementia or simply not detected at all given the standards of testing in the early 19th century. Thus, it was quite natural that the localizationist debate after Gall focused on language. It is not without irony that Bouillaud, to whom we owe this important methodological shift, had no other pretension than to show that Gall was right (see the title of Bouillaud's paper of 1825).

Let us now turn to maybe the most important aspect of Gallianism — points (4) and (5) above, i.e. the assumption that the human mind is organized in a domain-specific way, that is, in terms of the type of information to be processed rather than in terms of the modes in which information is processed. This "vertical" division of the mind actually distinguishes Gall from the medieval divisions, and this "verticalism" is what Fodor (1983), Marshall (1984), and other modern modularists believe they owe to Gall. Fodor, however, makes a strong point which should temper the modern Gall fashion, and I feel that Marshall overinterpreted Gall a little bit. Fodor admits that the human species is not only endowed with "vertical" faculties, but in addition with "horizontal" faculties, as for instance making inferences over information stored in a "horizontal" memory. In Gall's geography of the mind, however, there is no space for these *domain-unspecific* components of the mind, the existence of which cannot be denied. If we take Gall seriously, then we would have to assume that for Gall every cortical organ representing a domain-specific faculty is computationally autonomous in the sense that each faculty has its own memory, its own reasoning capacity, etc. A *Gedankenexperiment* would thus yield the result that a gifted chess player remains a good chess player even if the whole cortex, except for the chess organ, is damaged, that is, even if he has become a complete idiot in every other respect than chess playing. Such a radical verticalism and such a radical view of the autonomy of the human faculties should be ruled out without any further argumentation. Consequently, Fodor replaces computational autonomy by the much more plausible notion of informational encapsulation.

In his explication of "horizontal" versus "vertical", Marshall (1984) also contrasts the Gallian and the medieval ways of breaking up the human mind. He writes that the Middle Ages took over the Aristotelian position according to which acoustic, tactile, visual, olfactory, and gustatory information is integrated in the sensus communis (localized in the first ventricle) and that from here on, percepts are presented in a common code, thus constituting a homogeneous class of objects over which the same formal operations can be carried out, independent of the modality via which the objects originally entered the mind. Marshall seems to sympathize with a view according to which there are multiple representations of objects in our minds, dependent on the modality via which the objects are perceived. However, be this view justified or not, it cannot be related to anything in Gall's organology. It is a sort of modularism which goes far beyond anything that is explicitly or implicitly argued for by Gall. Thus, once again there is no need for a new "Gall rush".

However, leaving aside Fodor's restrictions and the hyper-Gallianism of Marshall, must we not ascribe to Gall at least the merit of having been the first to introduce the idea of verticalism as such, i.e. the (at least partial) domain-specific compartmentalization of the mind? Isn't there a more respectable historical figure than just the charlatan Gall to whom we can appeal as the forerunner of modern modularism? As a matter of fact, I believe there is somebody else. Note that in Marshall's paper the Aristotelian tradition is mentioned, and Marshall is perfectly right in describing the main variants of medieval Aristotelianism as doctrines maintaining that the recognition of an object is considered to be the product of elementary sensations plus domain-unspecific central reasoning. It is, furthermore, true that nowadays we no longer accept such a model of object recognition given the findings of modern cognitive psychology and modern neuropsychology. We would prefer the assumption that we can recognize objects because we have the faculty to do so or because we have a special organ for object recognition. If we rephrase the idea of domain-specificity by emphasizing the aspect that the process of recognition cannot be *decomposed* into more elementary operations *plus* the recruitment of more central processes, then it becomes immediately clear that characterizing the approaches before Gall as exclusively horizontal ignores another whole rich and blossoming tradition of European thought which was as fruitful and influential as Aristotelianism was. Besides Aristotle there was Plato. The idea that we recognize something on the basis of elementary sensations plus reasoning is exactly the idea which is rejected by Platonism. Furthermore, just as modern modularism maintains that we can recognize objects because we have a special mental organ for this job, Platonism, likewise, assigns our object-recognizing faculty to a special preformation of our mind: the mind is a priori endowed with a store of Forms which enable the mind to recognize an individual object as belonging to a class of identical objects (i.e. as derived from the same Form). Nothing can be recognized that is not already in our mind in an abstract form. This idea has never been expressed more beautifully than by Goethe's famous dictum that our eye could not see the sun if it were not "sonnenhaft" (an untranslatable neologism by Goethe; its meaning is something like "having an ontological affinity to the sun"). We have an 'organ' to see the sun, and if this is not related to the modern idea of the domain-specific organization of the mind, I do not know what could be.

The element common to an infinitely large class of individual objects — the element enabling us to recognize the individual objects as members of one class — is in the Platonic tradition 'ante rem' and not 'in re' (Aristotle) and not 'post rem' (the Nominalists, and maybe modern researchers of Artificial Intelligence). That this Platonic view really foreshadows the idea of domain-specifity is underlined by the following two facts: In *Kratylos*, Plato discusses whether the words for objects are introduced *by nature* or *by convention*. Although he demands that in a philosophical language the names should be intrinsically related to the objects they refer to, he is aware of the fact that the verbal expressions in natural languages are not. That is, they are not part of the objects, but are arbitrarily and extraneously attached to them. The Form of an object in the human mind does not contain its verbal sign. Human beings are quite obviously able to understand (recognize) verbal signs — consequently the *faculty of word recognition is independent of object recognition and vice versa*. This modularistic view was — at least as an argument — present in all philosophical debates from Antiquity through the Middle Ages. Admittedly, domain-specificity or "verticalism" had not been stated very explicitly before Gall — not even in the Platonic tradition. However, verticalism exists potentially in almost every variant of Rationalism that (unlike the Cartesian variant) allows for a division of the mind.

Another point relevant to verticalism can be found in Aristotle. Aristotle was not so far away from Platonism as one normally assumes. He sympathized greatly with Plato's explanation of our faculty of recognizing objects, but in his *Metaphysics* he raises the question whether Plato's explanation could only hold for natural objects and not for artifacts. Whatever Aristotle's answer was, the raising of the question as such implies the idea that the human mind might be organized according to the *content* of the cognitive operations rather than according to the formal characteristics of the operations.

In short, every essential point in Gall's doctrine (except the emphasis on the cortex) either has its roots somewhere else in the tradition of European thought, or it is complete nonsense. So, then, what do we owe to Gall? Virtually nothing! However, although this is exactly the appropriate judgment a charlatan deserves, I shall not end with this condemnation. I feel that Gall's entering the stage around 1800 served its historical function. Remember that in the period before Gall the localization or even the problem of localization as such was blocked by Cartesian dualism. By taking ingredients from wherever, Gall concocted a spectacular and explosive mixture which brought inquietude into the intellectual world, broke down traditional thinking barriers, and provoked and initiated modern discussion on the relation between brain and mind. Gall's merit is that he set serious researchers like Bouillaud and Broca on the right track. And it might also be that the appearance of such an unscrupulous charlatan as Gall was actually necessary because only such a person could have audacity enough to ignore all the traditional severe restrictions on psychology (for the role of *agents provocateurs* in scientific innovations, cf. Kuhn, 1962 and 1977).

References

Benton, A.L. 1964. "Contributions to aphasia before Broca". *Cortex* 1:314-327.
―――. and R.J.Joynt. 1960. "Early descriptions of aphasia". *Archives of Neurology* 3:205-221.
Bouillaud, J.B. 1825. "Recherches cliniques propes à démontrer que la perte de la parole corresponds à la lésion des lobales antérieures en cerveau". *Archives Générales de Médecine* 8:25.45.
Bruyn, G.W. 1982. "The seat of the soul". *Historical Aspects of the Neurosciences*, ed. by F. Clifford Rose. New York: Raven Press.
Clark, E. and K. Dewhurst. 1972. *An Illustrated History of Brain Function*. Berkeley: University of California Press.
Fodor, J. 1983. *The Modularity of Mind*. Cambridge, Mass.: MIT Press.
Gall, F.J. 1798. "Das Programm". *Der Neue Teutsche Merkur* (Dec. 1798): 311-382 Reprinted in E. Lesky, 1979.
Hécaen, H. and G. Lanteri-Laura. 1977. *Evolution des connaissances et des doctrines sur les localisations cérébrales*. Paris: Desclé de Brouwer.
Kuhn, T.S. 1962. *The Structure of Scientific Revolutions*. Chicago: University of Chicago Press.
―――. 1977. *The Essential Tension: Selected Studies in Scientific Tradition*. Chicago: University of Chicago Press.
Lanteri-Laura, G. 1970. *Histoire de la phrénologie. L'homme et son cerveau*. Paris: Desclé de Brouwer.
Le May, M. 1977. "Assymetries of the skull and handedness". *Journal of the Neurological Sciences* 22:443-453.
Lem, S. 1984. *Solaris*. Berlin: Deutsche Taschenbuch Verlag.
Lesky, E. 1979. *Franz Joseph Gall: Naturforscher und Anthropologe*. Bern: Huber Verlag.
Marshall, J. 1984. "Multiple perspectives on modularity". *Cognition* 17:209-242.
Riese, W. and E.C. Hoff. 1950. "A history of the doctrine of cerebral localization". *Journal for the History of Medicine* 5:51-77.
Schwartz, M.F. and B. Schwartz. 1984. "In defense of organology". *Cognitive Neuropsychology* 1:25-42.
Young, R.M. 1970. *Mind, Brain and Adaptation in the Nineteenth Century*. Oxford: Clarendon.

Selection from the work of
Franz Joseph Gall

**Letter from Dr. F. J. Gall to Mr. Joseph F. von Retzer
on the prodromus he has completed on the functions
of the human and animal brain***

At last I have the pleasure of presenting to you a draft of my essay "On the faculties of the brain, and on the possibility of recognizing a number of skills and propensities from the form of the head and cranium". I have already noticed, much to my pleasure, that everywhere men of intelligence and education have patiently awaited the development of my efforts, while others saw only the fantast or the dangerous neologist.

Overall, I have the following intention: to determine the faculties of the brain, and in particular its parts; that indeed a number of abilities and propensities can be recognized from elevations and depressions on the head or cranium, and to give a lucid presentation of the most important facts and consequences for medical science, ethics, education, law, etc. and in general for a closer understanding of mankind. Of course, an extensive production of drawings and engravings should be included. Therefore of the special properties and their characteristics I will include only as much as is necessary for the establishment and elucidation of the main principles. So the specific purpose of this work is to indicate the point of view of my investigations, to establish principles, and to teach their use in further observations. You do understand that it is a hazardous enterprise to find the pure sources of human thinking and acting. Therefore, I may or may not have

---

* Translated from "Das Program" which originally appeared in *Der Neuen Teutsche Merkur*, Dec. 1798, pp. 311-382.

achieved anything, but the venture itself deserves your approval or your indulgence.

For now, please keep in mind that I mean by head or cranium only those bones of the head or cranium that constitute the brain cavity and even then only those parts that are in direct contact with the brain itself. Also, don't blame me for not using Kantian language. I have not yet carried my investigations far enough that I might have discovered special organs for mental acuity and profundity, for the principle of imagination, for the various kinds of judgment and so forth. I may sometimes even have been too careless about the exact definition of the concepts I have been using, because my intention was no more than to make myself understood by a large number of readers to begin with. The complete work is divided into two parts (together they amount to about 10 sheets). The first part contains the principles.

Therefore I will commence with my readers at the point where nature left off. After I had collected my careful observations, I formulated a construct of the laws governing their relationships. I would like to set forth the principles in brief for you.

I.   *Abilities and propensities are innate in men and animals.*

You are surely not among those who would disagree with me about this. But, as a son of Minerva, you are certainly equipped with the right weapons to wield for her. So if someone might object to you that because of this innateness, we are rather tools than masters of our own actions, that we are at the mercy of our inner impulses; what would become of freedom if that were true? How could good and evil be imputed to us? — so allow me to transcribe for you my answer verbatim from my prodromus. All the rest you can add from your own ethical and theological knowledge.

"Those who want to convince themselves that our qualities are not innate derive them from upbringing. But is it not so, that in either case we behave in a passive way, whether we are formed by innateness or by upbringing? This objection confounds the concepts of ability and proclivity, of pure predisposition, with behavior itself. Even animals are not absolutely, with no free will, subservient to their abilities and propensities. However powerful the urge is for the dog to hunt and for the cat to catch mice, after repeated punishments they will cease to act on this urge. Birds repair their smashed nest and bees cover with wax the offal that they cannot remove.

But man has, apart from the animal-like properties, the ability to speak and the most extensive capacity for education: two sources of inexhaustible knowledge and motivation. He has a sense of truth and error, of justice and injustice, of images of an independent being; the past and the future can guide his actions; he is gifted with a sense of morality and with evident consciousness, and so forth.

"With these weapons, man battles his propensities. They are still there as impulses that lead him into temptation, but not in such a way that they cannot be overcome, be suppressed by opposite or stronger impulses. You all have the impulse, the proclivity to debauchery: only morality, conjugal love, health, social propriety, religion, and so forth serve you as opposing impulses not to surrender to this debauchery. Only from this battle will spring virtue, vice, and temptation. What would be the significance of self-denial, which is so highly prized, were it not for the struggle with our inner selves? Therefore the more the opposing impulses are multiplied and strengthened, the more free will and moral freedom man obtains. The stronger the inner urges are, the stronger the opposing impulses must be. From this originates the necessity for and the usefulness of deeper knowledge of men, the doctrine of the origin of his capabilities and propensities, of upbringing, of laws, of rewards and punishments of religion. The temptation disappears, however, even according to the strictest theologians, in those cases where an individual is either not aroused at all, or completely unable to resist the overwhelming impulses. Would one praise the chastity of one who is born a eunuch from his mother's womb? Rush cites the example of a woman who could not resist the temptation to steal, despite the fact that all other moral virtues were present. Similar examples, including even an irresistible impulse to murder, are known. Although we maintain the right to put away these unfortunate people, in a way any punishment laid upon them is unjustified and useless and they deserve nothing but our compassion. I will one day acquaint judge and doctor with this rare but sad phenomenon".

Now that our opponents are reassured, I will ask them: In what way are the abilities and propensities of men and animals interconnected in their nature? Are they expressions of a purely spiritual, purely spontaneous force of the mind, or is the mind connected to some physical apparatus? And if so, to what kind of apparatus? This leads to the second principle.

II.   *The abilities and propensities are situated in the brain.*

I will provide the evidence. 1. Mental activities are crippled by injuries to the brain, not directly by injuries to other parts of the body. 2. The brain is not necessary for life. But since nature has not made anything without a purpose, the brain must have some other function. 3. The properties of the mind and the soul or the abilities and propensities of men and animals are both multiplied, and refined, proportional to the brain's gradual increase in volume in relation to the size of the body, particularly the size of the nerves. This we have in common with the boar, the bear, the horse and the ox, with the camel, the dolphin, the elephant, and a stupid old hag. Consequently, a man like you has more than twice as much brain as a stupid fanatic and at least two and a half times more than the wisest of all elephants. So everyone will eventually agree to accept the second principle.

III. IV. *Not only do the abilities differ essentially and independently from the propensities, but also the capabilities and propensities per se among themselves differ essentially and independently from each other; therefore they must be situated in different and independent parts of the brain.*

Evidence. 1. It is possible to put mental and emotional properties alternately in a state of rest and into action, so that the one, after being tired out, can rest and recover, while the other is quite active and gets tired. 2. Abilities and propensities relate to each other, in man as well as in animals of any kind, in widely varying ways. 3. Different abilities and propensities are completely separated from each other in different kinds of animals. 4. Abilities and propensities develop at different times, since some disappear without impairing others, which can even become stronger. 5. With diseases and injuries in separate parts of the brain, separate properties are injured, stimulated, suppressed, destroyed, and when healing takes place, they also return separately to the original state. I do not think of myself as so eminent a man that I can state something without proving it; therefore I have tried to validate all the evidence with facts. Nevertheless, many a soft-natured conscience makes the objection: If one establishes bodily tools, organs, for mental operations, is not then the spiritual nature and consequently the immortality of the soul challenged?

Please pay attention to the answer to this. The scientist investigates only the laws of the physical world, and presupposes that no natural truth could contradict any revealed truth. Further, he knows that neither mind nor body could be deranged without a direct sign from the Creator; that he cannot determine anything about spiritual life. He only watches and learns that in this life the mind is tied to the bodily apparatus. This in general.

In particular, however, I give the following reply: this objection confounds the active being with the tool by which it operates. What I have claimed about the inner senses, that is about the inner organs of the actions of the soul under nos. 1 2 3 4 5, all happens with the external senses. For example, while the tired eye is resting, one can hear attentively; the hearing can be destroyed without the least impairment to vision; some senses can be defective, others especially sensitive. Worms cannot see or hear, but they have a fine sense of touch; the newborn dog is deaf and blind for several days, yet his taste is completely developed. In aging, hearing usually deteriorates before vision, and taste often remains excellent. So, just those features of their independence and self-reliance that no one doubts! Has anybody for this reason ever concluded that because of the essential diversity of the senses the soul must be material or mortal? Is there then one soul to hear and another soul to see? I will carry the comparison somewhat further.

It is a mistake to believe that it is the eye that sees, the ear that hears, and so on. Each external sense-organ is connected by its nerves with the brain, where at the beginning of the nerve an appropriate amount of brain-matter constitutes the actual inner organ of this sense. Even if the eye itself is healthy, even if the optic nerve is undamaged: if the inner organ is ill or destroyed, eye and optic nerve are of no use any more. Consequently, the external sense-organs have their organs in the brain, and these external organs are no more than the means by which their inner organs connect or react to external objects.

For these reasons, it never occurred to Boerhave, Haller, Mayer, or even the good Lavater, who seeks the mental properties in the head and the spiritual ones in the trunk, that from the diversity and independence of the abilities and propensities, and from the diversity and independence of their inner organs, anything might be argued against the spirituality and immortality of the soul. This selfsame soul, which sees by means of the optical organ and smells by means of the olfactory organ, learns by means of the memory organ and does good by means of the organ of kind-heartedness. Always one and the same spring to drive fewer wheels in you and more in me. Now that we have settled the actions of the brain in a general sense, I will proceed to show you the evidence: that it is possible to determine the presence and condition of several abilities and propensities from the structure of the cranium, through which the actions of the specific parts of the brain can be determined directly.

V.   *Different forms of the brain develop from the different distributions of the different organs and their different development.*

Among the evidence that is appropriate here, I adduce the differences in the form of the brain between carnivorous, herbivorous, and omnivorous animals. Then I will adduce the origin of the different kinds of animals and the arbitrary differences of types and individuals.

VI.   *Out of the combination and the development of certain organs a certain form emerges, both of the entire brain and of its specific parts or their surroundings.*

Here I take the opportunity to prove that organs are even more active, when they are further developed, without excluding other stimuli. How does all this lead to the possibility of recognizing several abilities and propensities in the form of the cranium? Does this perhaps imply that the form of the cranium is a cast of the form of the brain?

VII.   *From the origin of the bones of the skull until old age, the form of the inner of the cranium is determined by the external form of the brain; consequently certain abilities and propensities can be concluded from the form of the outer surface of the cranium as long as it agrees with the inner form or does not diverge from the known deviations.*

Here I will explain the origin of the bones of the skull, from which it follows that they are shaped by the brain until the moment of birth. Further, I speak of the influences of various causes on the development of the head, which may lead to the consideration of other continuing pressures. Now I will demonstrate that the organs develop one after the other until full development is reached, in precisely those proportions and that order that we observe from earliest childhood on, according to the phases and the order of the abilities and propensities, and that the bones of the skull acquire their various forms in precisely the same proportions and in precisely the same order. Finally I will explain the decrease in our abilities in part by the fact that the organs shrink, and I will show how nature deposits new bone-material in the now empty space. These are all facts that have been hitherto unknown in the study of the bones of the skull. They constitute the first step in determining the particular functions of the separate parts of the brain.

PART TWO

Application of the general principles

On the establishment and determination of
the independent abilities and propensities.

As a consequence of the fact that I presume each independent quality to have its own organ, it is very important to decide which qualities are indeed independent in order to know what organs one would hope to discover. This has been causing me much difficulty for several years. In the end I have again, as so often, been convinced that the shortest and safest way to proceed is to skip the preliminary hair-splitting and let oneself simply be guided by the facts.

I will now present some of these difficulties to my readers. They may discover that they are cleverer than I was. Finally I will come to the resources that have served me best in determining the independence of the qualities. Now I will begin to speak more specifically of the site of the organ. First of all I must indicate and test those means by which the site of the organ is discovered. Among these I include: 1. The discovery of certain elevations and depressions that correspond to certain qualities. It will be noted in passing how examinations of this sort are to be performed. 2. Certain qualities corresponding to certain elevations. 3. A collection of plaster-casts. 4. A collection of skulls.

With respect to the human skull, this is going to be difficult for some of you. You know how everyone threw up their hands in desperation and how many tales were concocted against me when I first started dealing with this. Unfortunately everybody thinks so much of himself that they all think I am after their heads as one of the most important additions to my collection;

and yet I have gathered in the last three years no more than 20, aside from those I have taken from hospitals and the madhouse. Were it not for the support of a man who understands how to support the sciences and do away with prejudice, a man who is valued for his mental and spiritual qualities by every class and nation, I would, in spite of all my efforts, have achieved only a few pitiful fragments of work. Some even go so far as to reject the idea that their dogs and monkeys could have a part in my collection. I would be very pleased if the heads of animals would be sent to me, animals whose character had been observed closely, for example a dog who would not eat what he had not stolen, who found his way back to his master from a very long distance — heads of apes, parrots, or other rare animals with life histories that should, however, not be written until after their death, because otherwise I would fear that they would be too flattering.

If you could finally make it fashionable henceforth for any kind of genius to leave his head to me as a legacy, I would bet my own head that in 10 years time a wonderful system would be developed, for which I would meanwhile just provide the raw materials. It would certainly be dangerous to a Käster, Kant, Wieland and the like for me to be in command of David's angel of death. As a good Christian I will patiently wait for God's longsuffering mercy.

But, my dear Retzer, do have a look into the future with me. There the chosen of the human race throughout the centuries would stand together; how they thank each other for each little seed that each of them has planted for the benefit and pleasure of mankind. Why did nobody preserve the skull of a Homer, Ovid, Virgil, Cicero, Hippocrates, Boerhave, Alexander, Friedrich, Joseph, Catherine, Voltaire, Rousseau, Locke, Bacon, Newton, etc.? What a treasure for the magnificent temple of the Muses! I will return to the 5th resource.

5. Symptoms of illnesses and injuries of the brain: Again I have much to say. The most important is a completely new, unknown doctrine about the different kinds of madness and the methods of healing them, all of which will be supported by facts. If I had achieved only this in my investigations, I would have been amply repaid. So if there are no intelligent people to thank me, at least I would be sure of the gratitude of fools.

The 6th resource for discovering the site of the organs consists of examining the constituent parts of different brains and their behavior, always with consideration of their different capabilities and propensities. 7. Finally I come back to one of my favorite subjects, the scale of improvements.

With respect to this subject, I conceive of myself as a one-eyed Jove, who looks down from heaven on his swarming terrestrial animal kingdom. Imagine the enormous stretch I have to examine, from the starfish and the polyp all the way to the philosopher and the theosophist. Of course, like you respected poets, I will permit myself many a breakneck leap. In the beginning I will only create excitable fibres; by and by I will invent nerves and hermaphrodites. When one of these merits something more, it can mate with itself and observe the world through the sense organs. Only now will I call upon my supply of tools, distribute them discreetly, produce beetles, fish, birds, mammals, lap-dogs for the ladies, horses for the stud-farmers, and human beings for myself, including fools and wise men, Vestals and Sultans, poets and historians, theologians and scientists, etc. So I would have ended with man, as Moses told you long ago.

It has cost me many a new thought for you to have finally become kings of the earth. And in order for you to perform a pantomime, or if someone should become a deaf mute, another language is left for you: I have given you the language of signs. Although it has not occurred to any-one to thank me for that, I will reveal just this much: that I have achieved this only by relating in a special way your bodies, your muscles, to the organs of the brain. As a matter of fact you are to me but marionettes in a puppet-show. As certain organs begin to move, you must assume a position according to their sites, as if you were pulled by a string, so that you can dis-cover the site of the active organs only by means of this gesticulation. I know quite well that you are still short-sighted and that you will laugh about this; but if you make an effort to study this issue, you will be convinced that I have discovered more from my creation than you are actually worthy of. There you will find still other enigmas solved, such as why you fight so bravely for your wives; why you become miserly when getting older; why nobody sticks to his opinion more than the theologian; why many a bull has to sneeze when a Europa tickles him between the horns, etc.

Now I will return to you, my dear Retzer, a poor scribbler, to render a further account to you. This being the end of the first division of the second part, I should have asked my readers to compare everything that has been said so far, so that they will be even more convinced of the truth of the first principles, which I may have presented too casually. But my only thought was that he who is blind in daylight, won't see much with a torch.

The second main section includes a variety of topics.

1. On national heads. Here I agree somewhat with Helvetius, whom I have contradicted so far. Perhaps I will get a bit onto the bad side of highly esteemed men like Blumenbach, Camper, and Sömmering, although I am willing to admit that I do not know much about this. But maybe you will come to understand why some of our brothers cannot count over three; why others do not have a notion of private property; why eternal peace among mankind remains an eternal fantasy; etc.

2. The difference between the heads of men and women. Whatever I have to say about this will remain between us. We all know that women's heads are difficult to decipher.

3. About physiognomy. Here I will show that I am nothing less than a physiognomist. It has come to my attention that respected scientists have christened the child before it was born. They call me a cranioscopist and my proposed theory cranioscopy. As regards the first, I won't accept any fancy title; as for the second, it is not the title that fits me, nor is it justified for my trade. The object of my inquiries is the brain; the cranium is considered only insofar as it is a true cast of the outer surface of the brain, and consequently the cranium is only a part of the main topic. Therefore to call it cranioscopy is just as one-sided as to call a poet a rhymester. Finally I will adduce some examples in order to give my readers something to examine, so that they may judge not from principles alone, but also from facts, what to hope for in the course of these discoveries. Indeed you know, my dear reader, how strictly I proceed in comparison. If, for example, if I do not find the same feature in the good-natured donkey as in the good-natured dog, and in the good-natured dog I do not find the same feature as in the good-natured cock or philosopher, and if I do not find them at the same site, then a sign means nothing to me, because in the works of nature I accept no exceptions. To end with, I warn my insufficiently critical followers against the vile use of the doctrine presented here, by acquainting them with some obstacles. On the other hand, I will dispose of some obstinate opponents.

Please allow me to mention two important shortcomings of my work. First of all, it would have been my duty and to my advantage to have conformed to the taste of the age. I should have claimed unconditionally that one could recognize all abilities and all propensities from the head and the form of the cranium. I should have presented the individual experiences as if they were thousandfold, make them all object of one study, and not subjected them to so much probing and comparing, not demanding so much previous knowledge and perseverance, and moreover, I should not have mounted Parnassus on Pegasus, but on a tortoise. Where is the attraction, where hence the participation? The numerous anticipatory, clever or not so clever gibes about me, long before either my enterprise or its purpose was known, should have convinced me plainly of the fact that judgmental mankind is not holding its breath for results.

Second, I noted that I have not appreciated well enough the so-called a priori or 'in advance'-philosophy. I was so weak as to follow others. What I assumed to have been settled by my own acute reasoning would usually sooner or later turn out to be either defective or faulty. Even correctly judging the experiencing and the experienced has become more and more difficult for me, although I am convinced that it is the only way in which I can find the truth: by experience. But it is very well possible that other people possess a larger organ for a priori yielding insights. Therefore they will be reasonable enough not to demand of me that I should ever go into battle with weapons other than my own.

Vienna, October 1st, 1798

Paul Broca

Introduced by

PAUL ELING
Psychological Laboratory, University of Nijmegen
Nijmegen, The Netherlands

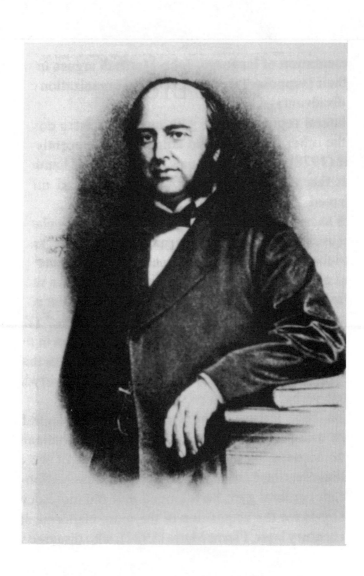

Paul Broca
1824-1880

Biography

Pierre Paul Broca was born on 28 June 1824 in Sainte-Foy-la-Grande, in the district of the Gironde. He started his career in Paris when he was only 17 years old. He was Professor of surgical pathology at the Medical Faculty in Paris, surgeon at the Hospitals of Saint-Antoine and the Pitié, and later professor at the 'Laboratoire d'Anthropologie des Hautes Etudes'. In 1859 he denied the immutability of race and species — a denial which is a cornerstone of Darwin's famous work On the Origin of Species, *which was published in the same year. As a consequence of the position taken by Broca, he founded the Anthropological Society, of which he became general secretary. Broca was also the founder and editor-in-chief of the* Revue d'Anthropologie. *He was one of the principal professors of the Anthropological Institute, founded in 1876. He married Augustine, the wealthy daughter of Dr. Lugol. They had two sons: Auguste, who later became a professor in pediatric surgery, and André, who later became professor in medical physics. In 1880 Broca was elected life senator for the left. In the Senate he suffered a ruptured aneurysm and died in Paris on 8 July 1880. Broca wrote over 500 papers on a wide variety of topics such as tumors, the order of primates, physical features of prehistoric man, the origin of the Basque language, and the localization of the faculty of speech.*

Selected Bibliography

Broca, P. 1861a. "Perte de la parole. Ramolissement chronique en destruction partielle de lobe antérieur gauche de cerveau". *Bulletin de la Société d'Anthropologie* 2:235-238.
———. 1861b. "Remarques sur le siège de la faculté de langage articulé, suivie d'une observation d'aphémie (perte de la parole)". *Bulletins de la Société Anatomique* 6:330-357.
———. 1861c. "Nouvelle observation d'aphemie produite par une lésion de la moitié postérieure des deuxièmes et troisième circonvolutions frontales". *Bulletins de la Société Anatomique* 6:398-407.
———. 1863. "Localisation des fonctions cérébrales: Siège de langage articulé". *Bulletin de la Société d'Anthropologie* 4:200-208.
———. 1865. "Sur le siège de la faculté de langage articulé". *Bulletin de la Société d'Anthropologie* 6:377-393.
———. 1875. "Sur les poids relatifs de deux hémisphères cérébraux et de leur lobes frontaux". *Bulletin de la Société d'Anthropologie* 10:534-536.

Introduction

Setting the Scene

Perhaps the best known name in aphasiology is that of Broca. Not only did Broca write certain papers which turned out to be very important; but also the most intensively studied type of language disorder is named after him, i.e., Broca's aphasia. In order to be able to understand Broca's view of aphasia, it is important to place his work in a larger historical context, namely that of the discussion, then current, on the (im)possibility of localization of function. It was not until the 19th century that the cortex of the cerebral hemispheres was considered to be the place where 'faculties' were localized. A second, more relevant, break with the classical writings concerns the classification of the functions. The traditional conception refers to general notions such as 'perception', 'imagery', and 'memory'. As can be seen in the preceding chapter by Heeschen, Gall set up a research program to find more specific faculties ranging from very ordinary functions such as 'musicality' to strange ones such as 'love of offspring' (situated in the back of the head).

Thus when Gall defended his insights in Paris, it was not so much the kind and number of functions described which were important, but the principle that the mind should be considered to be built up of independently operating functions. The inference that these functions can be located at demarcated areas of the cortex should be seen as the kind of evidence adduced to defend the principle. The debate on localization was not so much about the spatial arrangements of functions but rather about whether the localization of individual functions could be inferred from lesions: symptom localization vs. localization of function. (For a more detailed discussion of these and related issues the reader is referred to Young, 1970).

At the time Broca expressed his opinions on the loss of language after brain disorder, the issue mentioned above was very popular. In the first quarter of the 19th century the animal studies of Flourens in Paris apparently convinced most researchers that localization was not possible. Bouillaud, however, was not convinced, having received part of his training from Gall. He stated several times, starting in 1825, that language disorders only occur after frontal lesions. Retrospectively, we can say now that the debate entered its decisive phase in 1861, when Broca gave it a last push. Since then the principle of divisibility of the mind and the localization of functions seems to be the generally accepted position.

Broca's claims

The localization debate was reopened in 1861. Gratiolet presented a primitive skull to the Société d'Anthropologie in February. The topic was brought up again at meetings in March and April. In these meetings Broca expressed his admiration for the anatomical work of Gall and argued that the principle of cerebral localization "has been, one may say, the point of departure for all the discoveries of our century on the physiology of the brain". On April that year a man named Leborgne died in Broca's department, the surgical department of the Bicetre in Paris. He had been in that hospital for 21 years but Broca did not see him until 11 April 1861. By then Leborgne was in a very bad condition. However, it was known that apart from a severe speech problem this patient behaved like a perfectly sensible man. The only 'word' he could utter was: 'tan'. Broca presented his patient's brain on the 18th of April to the Anthropological Society as evidence in support of the thesis of Bouillaud. Four months later Broca's paper on the site of language was published, in which he gave a more detailed description of the patient's history and of his own interpretation of the speech disorder 'observed' in this patient.

Broca starts this 1861 paper by acknowledging that the originator of the notion of localization of language in the anterior part of the brain was Bouillaud, who in turn 'rescued' certain important aspects of the phrenological school. Bouillaud had also noted that only one of the essential elements of the complex phenomenon of language was represented in that part of the brain. Broca calls it the "faculté du langage articulé", which is not to be confounded with the "faculté génerale du langage". In the paper Broca elaborates on the different types of language, such as spoken language, mime, and writing. He defines *aphémie*, as he prefers to call it, as follows: there are cases where the general language faculty remains unaltered, where hearing is intact, where all the muscles, even those of the voice and articulation, obey the voluntary will and where a cerebral lesion abolishes 'articulated language' completely. What those patients lack is solely the faculty to articulate words. This description in itself seems clear. However, Broca goes on to explain this inability. Why can these patients not speak a single word (apart from the word that they use all day)? Broca's answer is, in fact, simultaneously the definition of the 'faculty of articulated speech'. Stated negatively, it has nothing to do with the general language ability, because these patients are normal in all other modalities. The memory for words is also intact. Not even the action of the nerves and muscles for phonation and articulation are involved. Stated positively, it is a special faculty, described by Bouillaud as the faculty to coordinate the individual movements in speech. Broca then asks himself whether this faculty should be considered a kind of memory, not of words but of the procedures which should be followed to articulate these words (perhaps we would call it a 'motor program'). According to Broca these procedures are learned in childhood.

In 1863 he made the following remarks on 'memory'. He considers memory not to be a simple faculty, not even a complex faculty, but conceives of it "as a state or if you wish a property inherent in each of our faculties and unequally developed in each of them". This formulation suggests that the memory of the procedures for pronouncing words is only part of the faculty. The consequence would be that the faculty consists of something else too: something not clearly described by Broca. Furthermore, if only the memory is lost, the complete faculty is not lost.

Yet another possible interpretation of the disorder remains, one which Broca does not believe in. This hypothesis refers to the notion of 'ataxie locomotrice'. Perhaps the disorder is the result of paralysis limited to that part of the central nervous system that 'governs the movements for the articulation of sounds'.

With respect to the localization of the faculty, Broca notices the following. Due to the old prejudice that the cerebral convolutions are not fixed, no system had yet been generally introduced for referring to particular places on the cortex. One of his colleagues, Gratiolet, developed such a system, which formed the basis for the classification of the sulci and gyri which is still used. In this context Broca notices that even the simple term 'anterior part' is not unanimously interpreted. For some authors it refers to the part of the hemispheres in front of the optic chiasm and the most forward point of the temporo-sphenoidal lobe. However, according to Broca, the anterior part continues over the Sylvian fissure as far as the Rolandic fissure on the sides of the hemispheres. Broca points out that this discrepancy has been the source of considerable misunderstanding, in that some cases have been presented as counterevidence where the patients could speak even though the 'entire' anterior part was destroyed.

Broca gives a quite detailed description of what he knew about the patient he refers to as Tan, who certainly had more deficiencies than only loss of speech. For instance, the man could not write when Broca saw him, nor was his comprehension intact. This suggests that the traditional account of 'Broca's aphasia' is not inspired by this particular patient. Perhaps the clinical picture was already known though perhaps not identified as a separate syndrome. In agreement with the clinical picture of Tan, the cerebral lesion Broca observed was rather large. He summarizes it thus: The destroyed organs (!) are the following: the small marginal inferior convolution (temporo-sphenoidal lobe); the small convolutions of the insula and the part subjacent to the corpus striatum; finally, on the frontal lobe, the inferior part of the transversal convolution and the posterior half of the two large convolutions, referred to as second and third frontal convolution. Keeping in mind the extended history of symptoms of the patient, Broca attempts to locate the starting point of the lesion. He designates that part where the destruction is most severe as the original locus which presumably was also the cause of Tan's speech problems. The site thus demarcated was the third frontal convolution. In his conclusions he argues that in this case the principal lesion was probably restricted to the third frontal convolution, but he is not certain whether this holds in general and whether localization on such a small scale was possible.

In 1863 a very interesting discussion took place following the presentation of an important case, seen by Dr. Parrot. The two main discussants were Broca and Laborde. The importance of the discussion lies in the restrictions Broca made before the counterevidence could be considered acceptable. Laborde provided a large number of objections to the position taken by Broca and referred to several cases as not being in line with Broca's theory. Broca was more or less forced to take the important step of claiming that only left-sided lesions result in aphasia. Broca thus eliminated all the cases where the right hemisphere is destroyed but no aphasia is observed. In fact, he eliminated all cases where language is retained as irrelevant. At that time Broca had seen 15 cases of aphasia. Together with the observations of colleagues, approximately 25 cases had been described. In this series Broca knew of one case of aphasia, studied by Charcot, which was in clear contrast to his position. Broca and Charcot together studied the brain at autopsy and found that there was a considerable posterior lesion. The third frontal convolution was intact.

In his 1865 paper he presented some observations which he had not yet interpreted. Studying the brains of aphasics, he had noted that the extension of the lesion is not always related to the impact on the language. He interpreted this as showing that in some cases (those where there is a huge lesion and only partial loss of speech) the right hemisphere can take over some functions and support the left hemisphere. Broca was uncertain of the extent to which the right hemisphere is capable of speech production and why this take-over does not occur in some patients with relatively small lesions in the left hemisphere.

Broca on language

There is no trace in his papers on aphasia to suggest that Broca was acquainted with linguistics. The reader looks in vain for concepts like 'grammar' or 'word formation'. What Broca described can, perhaps, best be referred to as a psychological model for language production. Broca distinguished three levels, on which functions or groups of functions operate. On the highest level ideas are developed (the general language faculty). On the second level that idea is mapped onto the conventional signs, the verbal forms of language. On this level different faculties operate. If one wants to express oneself in speech, the articulated language faculty will be called upon for this mapping function. If one prefers another mode of expression other faculties come into play. These two levels belong to the 'intellectual' part of the brain. He also considered these to be higher level functions because they are restricted to man. In the discussion which took place in 1863 Broca argues that animals, although deprived of speech, transmit their primitive ideas with signs that we do not comprehend but which he considers to be a particular type of language. (In my view Broca is inconsistent here.) The last layer belongs to the motoric part of the brain. At this level the faculties governing the action of muscles and nerves for the actual emitting of the message are represented. Broca is only slightly more specific about each of these three levels.

The general language faculty is described as the faculty to establish a constant relation between an idea and a sign. This general faculty presides over all modes of expression. With respect to the second-level faculties, Broca claimed that the faculty is used to coordinate the movements for speech. One property or aspect of the faculty is a memory of procedures for articulating the words. It is not a memory of the words themselves, because the aphasic still knows the words and their values. This memory is independent of other memories and is also not a part of a general memory for movement. What is not clear in this description of the faculty is how it uses the memory to relate ideas to the conventional verbal forms. One could look at it as a retrieval mechanism: on the basis of conceptual information, the right procedure is retrieved and this is passed on to the third-level functions. Thus little interesting work is left for these third-level functions. They pull the strings according to the program they receive from the faculties they serve, as Broca expressed it.

Evaluation of Broca's contribution

Considering the content of the papers Broca wrote on language and the brain, and the fact that almost every general introduction to aphasia (and also to laterality) refers to Broca, it seems that he has been credited with too much. This is even more obvious if one recalls that Broca himself stated on several occasions that his teacher, Bouillaud, formulated the essential ideas, and he in turn drew heavily on the work of Gall. Apart from the lack of originality, Broca's view on the process of language production is far from articulated. One would very much like to know how ideas are mapped onto language signs. This is exactly what is supposed to happen at the second level. However, all we know is that part of each of these functions is a memory with procedures for the emissive organs. Broca mentioned that he observed differences in severity of speech disturbances but failed to describe in what respect these patients differ from each other. The way in which Broca inferred from the brain of Leborgne that the third frontal convolution is the site of the faculty of articulated language would seem unacceptable to any scientifically oriented medical doctor. Therefore, his neuroanatomical work also seems to show severe shortcomings. Why then did Broca, or rather his work on aphasia, become so important? We can nowadays only speculate about the 'actual' reasons. It may be that he formulated some ideas which had been energetically suppressed a few decades before but which by 1860 had become acceptable to wider circles.

References

Broca, P. 1861b. "Remarques sur le siège de la faculté de langage articulé, suivie d'une observation d'aphémie (perte de la parole)". *Bulletins de la Société Anatomique* 6:330-357.

———. 1865. "Sur le siège de la faculté de langage articulé". *Bulletins de la Société d'Anthropologie* 6:377-393.

———. 1863. "Atrophie complète du lobule de l'insula et de la troisième circonvolution du lobule frontale avec conservation de l'intelligence et de la faculté du langage articulé. Observation par Dr. Parrot". *Bulletins de la Société d'Anthropologie* 8:393-399.

Young, R.M. 1970. *Mind, Brain and Adaptation in the Nineteenth Century*. Oxford: Clarendon.

Selection from the work of Paul Broca

Notes on the site of the faculty of articulated language, followed by an observation of aphemia*

The paper and observation that I present to the Anatomical Society are both supportive of ideas on the site of the faculty of language expressed by Mr. Bouillaud. This question, both physiological and psychological, deserves more attention than most physicians have accorded it so far, and the material is delicate enough, the subject obscure and complicated enough for me to think it useful that I should precede the account of what I have observed with some notes.

It is known that the phrenological school placed the site of the language faculty in the frontal part of the brain, in one of the convolutions that rest on the orbital vault. This opinion, which, like many others, admittedly lacks sufficient proof, and which was only based on a very imperfect analysis of the phenomena of language anyway, would doubtless have disappeared with the rest of the system, were it not that Mr. Bouillaud has saved it from shipwreck by submitting it to important modifications, and by surrounding it by a host of sound proofs, mostly having to do with pathology. Without considering language as a simple faculty depending on one single cerebral organ, and without trying to describe the site of this organ to within some millimeters, as was done by the school of Gall, this professor has been led by the analysis of a great number of clinical facts, followed by autopsies, to admit that certain lesions of the hemispheres damage speech

* Translated from "Remarques sur le siège de la faculté du langage articulé, suivier d'une observation d'aphémie (perte de la parole)", *Bulletins de la Société Anatomique*, 6, pp. 330-336 (1861)

without destroying the intelligence, and that these lesions always have their site in the frontal lobes of the brain. From this he concluded that somewhere in these lobes there must be one or more convolutions on which one of the essential elements of the complex phenomenon of speech depends, and so he placed the site of the faculty of articulated language, which should not be confused with the general faculty of language, less precisely than the school of Gall did, in these anterior lobes, without further specification.

There are, as a matter of fact, several kinds of language. Every system of signs which makes it possible to express ideas in a more or less intelligible, complete, and rapid way is a language in the most general sense of the word: thus speech, mime, typing, picture writing, phonetic writing, etc. are all equally kinds of language. There is a general language faculty that oversees all these ways of expressing thought, and that can be defined as the faculty of establishing a constant relationship between an idea and a sign, no matter if this is a sound, a gesture, a picture or any other record. Moreover, each kind of language requires the working of certain *emissive* and certain *receptive* organs. The receptive organs are hearing, sight, and sometimes even touch. As for the emissive organs, they work via the voluntary muscles, including those of the larynx, the tongue, the palate, the face, the upper limbs, etc. Each structured language thus supposes the integrity of 1. a certain number of muscles, the motor nerves which lead to them, and that part of the central nervous system where these nerves originate; 2. a certain peripheral sensory apparatus, a sensory nerve emerging from it, and that part of the central nervous system where the nerve ends; 3. finally, that part of the brain which the general language faculty depends upon, as we have just defined it.

Absence or destruction of this faculty renders impossible any kind of language. Congenital or accidental lesions in the receptive or emissive organs can deprive us of the particular kind of language that these organs contribute to; but if the general language faculty persists in us with a sufficient degree of intelligence, we are still capable of substituting another kind of language for the one we have lost.

The pathological causes that deprive us of a mode of communication usually make us lose just half, because it is quite rare that both the emissive and the receptive organs are affected at the same time. For example, the adult who becomes deaf continues to express himself in speech, but in order to transmit an idea to him one uses a different language, such as gestures or writing. It is the other way round when paralysis affects the muscles of speech; the patient we address in articulated language replies to us in another language. It is in this way that the different systems of communication can be substituted for each other.

This is no more than elementary physiology; but pathology has made it possible to advance in the analysis of spoken language, which is the most important and probably the most complex of all.

In some cases the general language faculty remains unaltered; the auditory apparatus is intact; all muscles, including those of the voice and articulation, function properly, and nevertheless a cerebral lesion destroys spoken language. This loss of speech in individuals who are neither paralyzed nor idiots constitutes a very specific symptom for which I consider it useful to invent a special name. So I will name it *aphemia* (alpha-privative, φημι = I speak, I pronounce); for it is only the faculty of articulating words that these patients lack. They hear and understand everything that is said to them; they are in full possession of their senses; they produce vocal sounds without difficulty; they execute with their tongue and lips movements that are far more elaborate and energetic than is required for the articulation of sounds; and yet the perfectly sensible answer that they would like to give is reduced to a very small number of articulated sounds, always the same ones and always arranged in the same way; their vocabulary, if one may call it that, consists of a short series of syllables, sometimes of one monosyllable expressing everything, or rather expressing nothing, for this single word is most of the time unknown to any existing vocabulary. For some patients not even this bit of articulated language is left; in vain they struggle without pronouncing a single syllable. Others have, in a way, two degrees of articulation. Under ordinary circumstances they invariably pronounce their preferred word; but when they get angry, they become capable of articulating a second word, usually a coarse swearword, that they probably knew before their illness, and then they stop after this last effort. Mr. Auburtin has observed a patient who is still alive and who needs no stimulus to pronounce his stereotyped swearword. All his responses begin with a bizarre word of six syllables and invariably end with this supreme invocation: "*Sacré nom de D...*".

Those who first studied these strange facts may have believed, for lack of sufficient analysis, that in such a case the language faculty is damaged; but it evidently is completely intact, because the patients understand spoken and written language perfectly well; because those who cannot or do not know how to write are intelligent enough (and in such a case one has to be quite intelligent) to find a way to communicate their thoughts; and finally, because those who are educated, and who can use their hands freely, write their ideas down clearly. So they know the meaning and value of words, in aural as well as graphic form. The language that they spoke before is still familiar to them, but they are no longer able to execute the series of systematic and coordinated movements that correspond to the syllable they are looking for. What has vanished is not the language faculty, nor word memory, neither is it the action of the nerves or muscles of phonation and articulation; it is something else, a particular faculty, considered by Mr. Bouillaud to be *the faculty of coordinating the movements necessary for spoken language*, or more simply, *the faculty of spoken language*, because without it, speech is not possible.

The nature of this faculty and the place it should be assigned to in the cerebral hierarchy may give rise to some hesitation. Is it not just a kind of memory, and did not the individuals who have lost it lose not the memory of words, but only the memory of the procedure to follow in order to articulate these words? Have they thus returned to a condition comparable to that of the young child who already comprehends the language of its relatives, who is sensitive to rebuke and praise, who points at all the objects named, who has acquired a host of simple ideas, and who, in order to express them, can only babble a single syllable? Little by little, after innumerable efforts, he succeeds in articulating some new syllables. Yet it still often happens that he is mistaken and says, for example, *papa*, when he wants to say *mama*, because at the moment he utters this last word, he no longer remembers the position of his tongue and lips. Soon he will know the mechanism of some simple and easy syllables well enough to pronounce them at once without error or hesitation; but he still hesitates and makes mistakes on more complicated and difficult syllables, and when he is finally well acquainted with a number of monosyllables, he has to acquire new experience in order to learn to pass from one syllable to another at once, and to pronounce, instead of the repeated monosyllables of which his first vocabulary consisted, words composed of two or three different syllables. This gradual perfecting of spoken language among children is due to the development of a particular kind of memory, which is not the memory of words but the memory of the movements necessary to articulate words. And this particular memory has no relation whatsoever to other memories, nor to the rest of intelligence. I have known a child of three years with an intelligence and a will beyond his age, with a well-formed tongue, who nevertheless could not talk. I know another very intelligent child who at the age of twenty-one months understands two languages perfectly, who consequently has a high degree of word memory, and who has not been able to lift himself beyond the pronunciation of monosyllables to this very day.

If the adults who lose their speech have only lost the art of articulation, if they have simply gone back to the condition they were in before having learned to pronounce words, the faculty of which the illness has deprived them should be ranked among the intellectual faculties. This hypothesis appears to me quite probable. However, it could be possible that it is otherwise, and that aphemia is the result of a *locomotor ataxia*, limited to that part of the central nervous system which presides over the movements of the articulation of sounds. One might object, indeed, that these patients are capable of freely executing all movements of their tongue and lips other than those of articulation; that they are capable of immediately raising the tip of their tongue when asked, of lowering it, of shifting it to the left, to the right, etc.; but these movements, however precise they appear to us, are infinitely less precise than the extremely delicate movements required by speech. With locomotor ataxia of the limbs, one can observe patients execute at will all the large movements: if they are told to raise their hand, open it, close it, they will do so almost without hesitating; but when they want to execute more precise movements, for instance to grasp a small object in a certain way, they overreach or fall short of their goal; they cannot coordinate the contraction of their muscles in such a way as to obtain a particular result, and they are mistaken less as to the direction of their movements than as to the amount of force required and the order of the sub-movements of which grasping is composed. One could therefore ask whether aphemia is not a kind of locomotor ataxia limited to the muscles for the articulation of sound, and, if this is so, whether the faculty lost by the patients is not an intellectual faculty — a part of the thinking section of the brain — whether it is nothing but a specific case of the general faculty of coordinating muscle action, a faculty that depends on the motor part of the nerve centers.

At least two hypotheses, then, may be suggested on the nature of the special faculty of *spoken* language. On the first hypothesis, it would be a superior faculty, and aphemia would be an intellectual disorder; on the second hypothesis, it would be a faculty of much lower order, and aphemia would only be a disorder of locomotion. Although the second interpretation seems much less probable to me than the first, I would nonetheless not presume to express a categorical opinion if I had nothing to go on but clinical observation.

However that may be, in conformity with the functional analysis the existence of a special faculty of articulated language as I have defined it cannot be questioned, because a faculty that can fail independently, without neighboring faculties being altered, is clearly a faculty distinct from all others, in other words a special faculty.

[Same text, pp. 343-346]

Aphemia, lasting twenty-one years, produced by chronic and progressive softening of the second and third convolutions of the superior layer of the left frontal lobe.

On 11 April 1861, a fifty-one-year old man, named Leborgne, who was stricken by a diffuse gangrenal inflammation of the complete right lower limb, from the instep up to the buttock, was brought to the general infirmary of Bicêtre, to the surgical ward. To the questions I asked him the next day about the origin of his condition, he answered only with the monosyllable *tan*, repeated twice in succession, and accompanied by a gesture of the left hand. I inquired about the history of this man, who had been at Bicêtre for twenty-one years. In turn the caretakers, his fellow patients on the ward, and relatives who came to visit him were interrogated, and the following was the result of this inquiry.

From childhood on he had suffered epileptic attacks, but he had been able to work as a farmer until the age of thirty. At that time he lost the use of speech, and that was the reason he had been sent to the hospital of Bicêtre as a patient. I could not find out whether the loss of speech came upon him slowly or rapidly, nor if any other symptom had accompanied the onset of the condition.

When he arrived at Bicêtre he had already been without speech for two or three months. He was in perfect health and intelligent and showed no difference from a healthy person except for the loss of speech. He came and went about the hospital, where he was known by the name of *Tan*. He understood everything that was said to him; he even had very fine hearing;

but whatever question was posed to him, he always answered *tan, tan*, accompanied by very diverse gestures, by means of which he managed to express most of his thoughts. When the people who questioned him did not understand his miming, he easily became outraged and added a rude swear-word to his vocabulary, only one and exactly the same as I pointed out above, discussing the patient observed by Mr. Auburtin. *Tan* was considered selfish, vindictive, ill-natured, and his fellow patients, who detested him, even accused him of being a thief. These flaws could be largely due to the cerebral lesion; however, they were not significant enough to seem pathological, and although the patient was in Bicêtre, nobody ever thought of putting him in a psychiatric ward. On the contrary, he was considered to be fully responsible for his actions.

Ten years after he lost his speech, a new symptom appeared: the muscles of his right arm gradually weakened and finally were completely paralyzed. *Tan* continued to walk without difficulty, but the paralysis gradually took over the lower right limb, and, after dragging his leg for some time, the patient was confined to bed. Four years passed from the beginning of the paralysis of the arm until the paralysis of the leg was so advanced as to make standing completely impossible. So *Tan* had been bedridden about seven years when he was brought to the infirmary. This last period of his life is the one about which we have the least information. As he had become incapable of harming anyone, his fellow patients took no more notice of him, except sometimes to amuse themselves at his expense (which made him lose his temper very easily), and he lost what little celebrity his unusual malady had previously given him in the hospital. It was observed that his sight had deteriorated markedly over about two years. This was the only worsening of his condition observed during his confinement to bed. Furthermore, he did not become senile; his sheets were changed only once a week, so the extended inflammation for which he had been taken to the infirmary on 11 April 1861 had not been recognized by the caretakers until it had progressed considerably and had spread all over the lower right limb, from the foot to the buttock.

The study of this unfortunate man, who could neither talk nor write, as his right hand was paralyzed, presented quite a problem. Indeed, he was generally in such bad shape that it would have been cruel to torment him with lengthy investigations.

However, I noted that his general sensitivity had been preserved everywhere, albeit unevenly. The right side of his body was less sensitive than the other side, and this doubtless helped relieve the pain of the extended inflammation. The patient was not in much pain when untouched, but palpation was painful, and some incisions that I had to make provoked flinching and screams.

The two right limbs were completely paralyzed; the other two limbs obeyed the will, and, although weakened, could perform all movements without hesitation. Urination and defecation were performed naturally, but swallowing presented some difficulty; chewing, on the other hand, went quite well. The face was not contorted; in the act of blowing, however, the left cheek appeared to be a bit more inflated than the right one, indicating that the muscles on that side of the face were a little weaker. There was no tendency to squint at all. The tongue was perfectly free; it was in no way out of shape; the patient could move it in any direction and stick it out of his mouth. The two sides of this organ were the same thickness. The difficulty with swallowing I just mentioned was due to the onset of paralysis of the pharynx, and not to paralysis of the tongue, because it was only the third phase of swallowing that was laborious. The muscles of the larynx did not seem impaired at all, the timbre of the voice was natural, and the sounds the patient made in pronouncing his monosyllable were perfectly pure.

His hearing was as sharp as ever: *Tan* could hear the sound of a watch quite well; but his sight had grown worse; when he wanted to see what time it was, he had to take the watch itself with his left hand and place it in a certain position about 20 centimeters from his right eye, which seemed to be better than his left eye.

The state of his intelligence could not be determined exactly. It was certain that *Tan* understood almost everything that was said to him; but, being unable to express his thoughts or desires other than by moving his left hand, our dying patient could not make himself understood as well as he could understand the others. Numerical answers were the ones he managed best, by opening or closing his fingers. I asked him several times how many days he had been ill. He sometimes answered five days, sometimes six. How many years had he been at Bicêtre? He opened his hand four times and then added one finger; this made twenty-one years and, as mentioned above, this information was exactly right. The next day I repeated the question and received the same answer, but when I tried a third time *Tan* understood that I was having him do an exercise; he became outraged and produced the afore-mentioned swearword that I had only heard once before from his mouth. Two days later I showed him my watch. The second hand was not working, so he could not distinguish the three hands except by their shape or length; nevertheless, after he had examined the watch for a few moments, he could tell the right time every time. So it is indisputable that this man was intelligent, that he could think, and that he had preserved to a certain extent the memory of past things. He could even understand quite complicated ideas: I asked him in what order his paralyses had come upon him; first he made a small horizontal gesture with the index finger of his left hand meaning: "I get it!", then he indicated successively his tongue, his right arm, and his left arm. This was perfectly correct, except that he attributed his loss of speech to paralysis of the tongue, which was only natural.

However, several questions which a man of ordinary intelligence would have found a way to answer with a gesture, even with only one hand, remaine unanswered. In other cases, it was not possible to understand the meaning of certain answers, which seemed to try the patience of the patient; finally, in still other cases, the answer was clear but wrong: although he had no children, he claimed that he did. So it is beyond doubt that the intelligence of this man had suffered extreme damage, caused either by his cerebral illness or by the fever which consumed him; but he was evidently much more intelligent than is required for speaking.

Complete atrophy of the insular lobe and of the third convolution of the frontal lobe with preservation of the intelligence and the faculty of articulated language.*
– Observations by Dr. Parrot, hospital physician –

Mr. Broca — I believe that in my first lecture on the site of the language faculty (*Bull.*, 1861, p. 330) I answered some of the questions raised today by Mr. Laborde. Our colleague extends the meaning of the word aphemia too far; moreover, I clearly want to establish the meaning that I myself give this expression. By aphemia I mean a state in which the patient cannot speak, even though he is more intelligent than is required for speaking and the organs of phonation and articulation are functioning. One can observe speech being blocked, diminished, or having disappeared altogether in people suffering from idiocy, dementia, imbecility, senile dementia, softening of the brain, general paralysis, apoplexy, etc. These people do not suffer from aphemia as a result. Speech depends on three different conditions; it depends on three functions or rather on three groups of functions which are not of equal value. To speak, you have to conceive a thought; this is the highest ranking faculty. Second, you have to establish a relationship between that thought and the conventional signs constituting the verbal forms of language; this is still a very elevated faculty, because it is peculiar to mankind, but quite inferior to the first, because every day one sees inviduals of very low intelligence who nonetheless speak very easily and distinctly. Finally, the performance of speech puts into operation a third group of functions which are not of an intellectual order: once the thought is conceived, once the verbal form is found, the muscles of phonation and articulation must obey the will. Language can thus be impaired or destroyed by three very different kinds of causes, affecting either thought itself, or the special faculty of the coordination of words, or, finally, the mechanism for the articulation of sounds. The individual who does not speak for lack of ideas, or who only pronounces words without order, is no more aphemic

---

* Translated from "Atrophie complète du lobule de l'insular et de la troisième circonvolution du lobe frontale avec conservation de l'intelligence et de la faculté du langage articulé". *Bulletins de la Société Anatomique*, 8, pp. 393-399 (1863)

than one who has a paralyzed tongue. But he who is unable to put his thoughts into speech, without having lost his intelligence or movements of the tongue, lips, and palate, is deprived of a particular faculty, which in the functional hierarchy is subordinated to thought, while this faculty itself governs the mechanical function of the articulation of sounds; and it is the loss or impairment of this particular faculty that constitutes aphemia.

Theoretically, nothing is more clear and simple than identifying aphemia, and cases where this is completely evident are found in practice. There are patients without any paralysis, whose full intelligence is preserved, and who can express without hesitation the most complicated thoughts in written words, but who nevertheless have lost the faculty of expressing themselves by spoken language; these people are aphemic, and the nature of their illness makes it absolutely certain. These examples prove that one can become aphemic via cerebral lesions that are fairly shallow and relatively unimportant. But a more serious and more extended lesion can occupy a large number of convolutions, spread over the corpus striatum and the optic layer, and affect intelligence, the faculty of language, and articulation all at the same time. These cases are manifold and give rise to immense difficulties of diagnosis. Most often, it can quite easily be ascertained that impairment of speech is not due to paralysis of the muscles of phonation and articulation. But when the issue is to know whether it does or does not depend on impairment of intelligence, the question becomes particularly complicated. The diagnosis of aphemia cannot be established unless it is properly stated that the patient still possesses a measure of intelligence equal or superior to what is needed for speaking. But intelligence cannot be measured, and if it is already very difficult to rate the intelligence of a man who can speak, it is even more difficult to rate it in a man who has only completely defective means of expressing his ideas. One may admit that an individual who is deprived of speech is intelligent enough to talk, since he understands the questions addressed to him, and since he finds a way to answer them by signs, gestures, attitudes, or by judicious use of those few articulated sounds that constitute his entire vocabulary. Once we have the proof that he understands the language of another person, we can conclude that he is aphemic, which means that the only thing that fails him is the special faculty of spoken language. In many cases this proof is acquired only after much trial and error, and sometimes, in spite of the deepest inquiry, one is still uncertain. This would not be the case if the patient had preserved his full intelligence, all his senses, all his movements.

He would still find a way to make clear his principal thoughts, for example by writing or by miming. But here we are considering the case of a man whose intelligence is very enfeebled; where half of the body, namely the right half, is paralyzed. It is the hand, specifically the right hand, which is, after speech, the principal means of communication. An ordinary hemiplegic who is deprived of the use of his right hand can exercise his left hand and will eventually learn to use it adroitly, even to write. But things are different when the cause of the paralysis at the same time has degraded his intelligence: the aphemics we are talking about belong to the latter category.

There is something else even more distressing. Spoken language is just one kind of language; there are several other kinds of language, spontaneous ones or conventional ones. Animals, although lacking speech, communicate their rudimentary ideas in signs we do not understand, but which are a kind of language. All languages are based on a common foundation, which is the relation established between an idea and a sign, whether verbal, vocal, graphic, or mimetic. The fact that they depend on several different faculties is irrefutably demonstrated in that one of them, spoken language, can perish on its own; but that these faculties are very close to one another, be it on the mental or the anatomical level, appears extremely probable; and that is why lesions that damage or destroy spoken language often affect other kinds of language as well. Therefore many aphemics who are neither blind nor paralyzed can no longer read or write. Some of them still can read but can no longer assemble the signs of writing. With perseverance, it is possible to teach them to read a certain number of words, as well as to write them, and even to pronounce them. But the normal process of decomposing words into syllables and letters is no longer within their capabilities. They learn to recognize a word by its form, its physiognomy, in the way they recognize a watch or a face, without being aware of the elements of which it is composed. I have been able to study these curious phenomena with an aphemic in Bicêtre, whom I have kept in the infirmary for a whole year and whom we have more or less re-educated. Aphemic patients who have lost spoken and written language at the same time can also lose the language of gesture and expression, and these complications can make it impossible for them to make themselves understood. One may believe that they do not comprehend any questions, that they have no thoughts to express, and the aphemia could be unrecognized.

One can see how many causes combine to make the assessment of aphemia quite difficult. So one has to pose more questions, interrogate the patient in a thousand ways, asking him first about simple things, those he can answer comprehensibly in the gestures of universal language. One should particularly stress notions of immediate concern to him, things he could not forget without having forgotten everything; and in the most serious cases, one has to phrase the questions in such a way that the patient can answer yes or no or with equivalent gestures. Finally, I strongly recommend questions that can be answered by a number. Sometimes the notion of numbers survives with aphemia patients whose intelligence has profoundly deteriorated. I have known several patients who could tell time with their fingers and were never mistaken with numbers under ten. I knew another patient — but she was very intelligent for an aphemic — who could count by digits of the second and first places, raising first eight and then four fingers in order to say eighty-four.

It has been asked whether aphemics have lost a special faculty, or whether they have simply lost the memory of words. This opinion has been uttered mostly by those who, acknowledging the unity of intelligence, refuse to accept the existence of faculties that can be isolated from and are independent of one another. But first I would like to point out that aphemics have not lost the memory of words, since they understand what is said to them. Many make vain efforts to repeat a simple monosyllable that is emphatically asked again and again, while every morning when they wake up, they are able to recall the few words that constitute their small vocabulary. Next I would like to note that, if the memory of words could perish by itself, it would be a completely separate faculty from all the others; aphemia resulting from such a deficit would not be the loss of general memory either, but the loss of a particular memory, a memory independent of other kinds of memory and other kinds of faculties; and this point of view would be inconsistent with the doctrine I have adopted.

As for me, I do not consider memory to be a simple faculty, nor even a complex faculty, but rather a state or, if you will, a property belonging to each of our faculties and unevenly developed in each. Each faculty has its memory, which is more or less complete and has nothing to do with the other memories. I do not know whether there are brains that are well enough balanced to remember everything equally well. I quite doubt that, and I must say I have never known one. Many a one who can sing an opera score from beginning to end without missing a single note, after a single hearing, is unable to learn by heart ten lines of prose. Many another who has never been able to remember a date or a formula can recite half a volume word by word after a single reading. A painter who is gifted with what is called memory of sight could paint from memory the portrait of a person he merely chatted with for a few hours, and whom he would not even recognize if he ran into him the next day. When it is said that a person has a good memory, what is meant is a person who remembers a great many facts for a long time. But memory for facts can be well developed in individuals who have no ability whatsoever to learn by heart and who have never been able to succeed in reciting fifty lines. By virtue of rhyme and rythm, poetry comes close to music; therefore one sees people who, gifted with music memory, learn verse quite easily but cannot retain prose. There is one kind of memory very different from the others, memory for location; one is almost tempted to consider it a special instinct. Those who possess it are able to remember after 30 years a small path they have walked only once, a rock on which they sat, insignificant objects to which they paid no attention when passing by. I know a physician who has done quite a lot of botany who never remembers the specific names but who, on seeing a plant whose name eludes him, can immediately indicate all the places where he has encountered it; and it is by remembering the location where he first saw it that he comes to retrieve the name of the species after a moment's reflection. Note that he knows the distinctive characteristics of the species very well. With him, it is only the names he forgets, while other botanists, gifted with the memory of names, immediately recall the name of any species, but are often quite blocked from telling how it differs from others. This memory for names is one of the most unusual, one which is allocated most unequally; it is compatible with the dullest of intellects, it exists even in considerable degree in some idiots, and it is lacking in very eminent minds. Consequently, there are many kinds of memory, independent of one another, and mnemonic techniques aim precisely at making up for those memories one is more or less devoid of, and helping those one is luckily endowed with.

Such different phenomena as can be observed in aphemic patients could thus, if necessary, be attributed to a defect in the memory for words, accompanied in certain cases by a defect in the memory for written signs or a defect in the memory for facts. In order to explain how an aphemic understands spoken language without, however, being able to repeat the words he has just heard, one could say that he has lost not the memory for words, but the memory for the means of coordinating used in articulating words.

But this analysis would be a bit too clever. It is much simpler merely to state that the faculty of articulated language has been damaged, without trying to find out whether the damage affects the entire faculty, or only the particular kind of memory which forms an integral part of this faculty.

On the site of the faculty of articulated language*

Finally, our late colleague Gratiolet reported a fact that was recalled by Mr. Bertillon a few months ago, and quite recently by Mr. Baillarger in his address to the Academy: the fact that in the development of the brain the convolutions of the left hemisphere are ahead of those of the right hemisphere. The former already take shape when the latter are not yet apparent. So the left hemisphere, which governs the movements of the right limbs, is earlier in its development than the opposite hemisphere. That is why the young child prefers to use from the start those limbs whose innervation is the most complete, why, in other words, he becomes right-handed. The upper right limb, being stronger and more skillful than the left from the start, is called upon more often for exactly that reason; and thereafter it cannot but acquire more and more strength and skill with age.

Up to now I have called "right-handed" those who prefer to use their right hand and "left-handed" those who prefer to use their left hand. These expressions come from the external manifestation of the phenomenon; but if we consider the phenomenon with respect to the brain, and not with respect to its mechanical agents, we would say that most people naturally are lefties according to the brain; and that exceptionally some people, those called left-handed, are on the contrary, actually right-brained.

Now I will proceed with the much more complex phenomena of spoken language. I will leave aside all that is related to articulation itself as a purely muscular phenomenon, and to the motor action that in going from the relevant cerebral organs to movement is transmitted by the motor nerves to the muscles of the tongue, lips, palate, and so on. Articulation depends on both cerebral hemispheres equally, because it is produced simultaneously and uniformly by the muscles of both sides, with their movements coordinated.

But neither in the muscles, nor in the motor nerves, nor in the motoric cerebral organs, nor in the optic layers or the corpora striata does the essential phenomenon of spoken language have its residence. If one had no more

---

* Translated from "Sur le siège de la faculté du langage articulé", *Bulletin de la Société d'Anthropologie*, 6, pp. 383-387 (1865)

than these organs, one could not speak. Sometimes these organs do exist, perfectly healthy and as they should be, in individuals who have become completely aphemic, or in idiots who have never been capable of either learning or understanding any language. Spoken language thus depends on the part of the encephalon that is relevant to intellectual phenomena and for which the motor organs of the brain are only a sort of agent. This function on the intellectual level, which dominates the dynamic as well as the mechanical aspects of articulation, is apparently a more or less constant property of the convolutions of the left hemisphere, inasmuch as the lesions that produce aphemia are found to occupy this hemisphere almost exclusively.

It comes down to the fact that, for language as well as for the much less complicated and refined actions about which I will speak later, we are left-brained. In the same way that we direct our movements in writing, drawing, embroidering, etc., with our left hemisphere, we talk with our left hemisphere. It is a habit we have had since our earliest infancy. Of all the things we have to learn, spoken language is perhaps the most difficult. Our other faculties, our other actions exist at least in a rudimentary form in animals; but although these certainly have thoughts and know how to communicate them in a genuine language, spoken language is not within their means. It is this complex and difficult thing that the child must learn in infancy, and at which he arrives after much trial and error and after cerebral work of the highest order. Indeed! This cerebral work is brought to the infant at a point very near to the embryonic periods when the development of the left hemisphere is ahead of the development of the right hemisphere. From there on, we can safely admit that it is the hemisphere which is more developed and more precocious, rather than the other, that directs the execution and the coordination of those simultaneously intellectual and muscular acts which constitute spoken language. This is how the habit of talking with the left hemisphere comes about, and this habit finally becomes so much a part of our nature that, if we lose the functions of this hemisphere, we also lose the faculty of making ourselves understood through speech. This does not mean that the left hemisphere is the exclusive site of the general language faculty, which consists of establishing a particular relation between an idea and a sign, or even of the special faculty of spoken language, which consists of establishing a particular relation between an idea and an articulated word. The right hemisphere does not belong any less to this special faculty than the left hemisphere. What proves this is that an individual who has become aphemic by a deep and extended lesion of the left hemisphere is generally deprived only of the faculty of his own production of the articulated sounds of language; he continues to understand what is said to him, and obviously knows perfectly well the relationship between ideas and words. In other words, the faculty of conceiving these relationships, belongs simultaneously to both hemispheres, since they can in case of damage mutually compensate for each other; but the faculty of expressing these ideas via coordinated movements, attained only after much practice, seems to belong only to one hemisphere, which is almost always the left hemisphere.

Now, as there are left-handed individuals to whom the native pre-eminence of motoric forces of the right hemisphere gives a natural and unalterable pre-eminence of the functions of the left hand, so one understands that there is a certain number of individuals in whom the native pre-eminence of the convolutions of the right hemisphere will reverse the order of the phenomena I have just described, in whom therefore the faculty of coordinating the movements of spoken language will become the distinctive property of the right hemisphere, by virtue of a habit taken up since early childhood.

Where language is concerned, these exceptional invididuals will be comparable to those who are left-handed. Both are right-brained. But from this I would not conclude that these two exceptional categories must coincide; because it does not seem at all necessary to me that the motor part and the intellectual part of each hemisphere need to be interdependent with regard to the timetable of their respective development in the two hemispheres.

The existence of a small number of individuals who, exceptionally, speak with their right hemisphere would explain very well those exceptional cases where aphemia is a consequence of a lesion of that hemisphere.

From the preceding it follows that a subject whose third convolution of the *left* frontal lobe, normally the seat of spoken language, has been atrophied since birth would learn to speak and would indeed speak with the third convolution of the *right* frontal lobe, as a child born without a right hand becomes as skillful with its left hand as one normally is with the right.

Carl Wernicke

Introduced by

ANTOINE KEYSER
*Institute of Neurology, Catholic University of Nijmegen,
Nijmegen, The Netherlands*

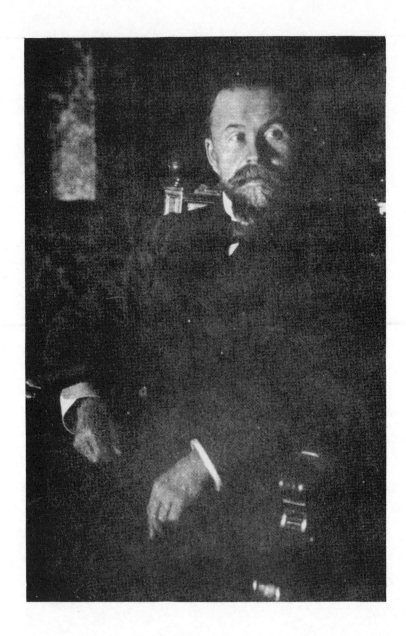

Carl Wernicke
1848-1905

Biography

Carl Wernicke was born in a small town in Upper Silesia on 15 May, 1848.
He received his secondary education at the gymnasium in Oppeln, near Bres-
lau. With great difficulty his mother managed to enable her son to study
medicine at Breslau University. After graduation Wernicke took a position as
assistant in the Ophthalmology Department of Professor Foerster for six
months. Then he served in the Franco-Prussian war of 1870 as an army sur-
geon. He became assistant of the "Allerheiligen Hospital" at Breslau once
again, this time in the Psychiatric Department under the direction of Profes-
sor Neumann. Neumann sent Wernicke to Vienna for a period of six months
to study neuro-anatomy under the supervision of Meynert. In 1866 Meynert
had written an article on language disturbances in which he discussed five
patients in whom autopsy revealed brain lesions at the level of the insula of
Reyl. This study may have influenced Wernicke; shortly after his stay in Vie-
nna, at the age of 26, he published his first important work on aphasia, Der
aphasische Symptomencomplex *(1874). Its subtitle* A psychological study on
an anatomical basis *directly points to both the method according to which*
Wernicke operated and the scientific program he was going to pursue in the
years to come.

In 1875 Wernicke was appointed assistant in the Berlin Charité clinic
under Westphal, where he stayed until 1878. From 1878 to 1881 he practiced
medicine and, more particularly, neurology in private practice. During that
period Wernicke prepared a number of publications. At the same time, he
maintained a vivid interest in psychophysiology and aphasiology. Wernicke's
name as an expert in the field of neurology and psychiatry was definitively
established by the authoritative Lehrbuch der Gehirnkrankheiten *(1881 and*
1883), in which a classification of the multitude of brain diseases was attemp-
ted, and the neurological method of localizing lesions was strongly furthered.
In 1885 Wernicke agreed to take over the position of Neumann in the
Allerheiligen Hospital and in addition he became head of the Department of
Neurology and Psychiatry of the University Hospital in 1890. In the next
twenty years the Breslau clinic became a center of neuropsychological investi-
gations, where a number of eminent scientists such as Liepmann, Goldstein,
Kleist, and Foerster developed basic concepts, such as the apraxias, the
agnosias, and the asymbolias. At the turn of the century Wernicke faced a
number of problems in his relationship with the municipal and university
authorities. In 1904 the course of events finally made him accept an offer to

succeed Ziehen as the head of the Klinik für Psychiatrie und Neurologie in Halle. In 1905, Wernicke was killed in a road accident, which ended the life of one of the most outstanding neuroscientists of his time.

Selected Bibliography

Wernicke, C. 1874. *Der aphasische Symptomencomplex. Eine psychologische Studie auf anatomischer Basis.* Breslau: Cohn & Weigert.

———. 1882. "Aphasie und Anarthie". *Deutsche Medische Wochenschrift* 8: 163.

———. 1875. "Das Urwindungssytem des menslichen Gehirns". *Archiv für Psychiatrie und Neurologie* 6: 298-326.

———. 1884. "Uber die motorische Sprachbahn und das Verhältnis der Aphasie zur Anarthia". *Fortschritte der Medizin* 2: 1,405.

———. 1885. "Einige neuere Arbeiten über Aphasie". *Fortschritte der Medizin* 3:824-830; 4 (1886) 371-377, 463-469. Reprinted in C. Wernicke. *Gesammelte Aufsätze und kritische Referate zur Pathologie des Nervensystems.* Berlin: Fischer, 1983.

———. 1903. "Ein Fall von isolierter Agraphie". *Monatschrift für Psychiatrie und Neurologie* 12: 241-265.

———. 1906. "Der Aphasie Symptomenkomplex". *Die Deutsche Klinik am Eingange des 20 Jahrhunderts*, Bd. 6, Abt. 1:487-556. Berlin: Urban & Schwarzenberg.

Introduction

One should realize that at the beginning of Wernicke's career as an "Assistenzarzt" in the psychiatric and neurological department, knowledge of the structure and function of the brain was very spotty when compared to our present-day insights. As an example, it may be mentioned that even the central course and innervation of the eighth or acoustic cranial nerve was essentially unknown. As far as cerebral cortex function was concerned, different opinions were expressed at that time as to the possibility of localizing functions at particular sites. Holistic views were defended by the Flourens school. Followers of this school denied the possibility of any type of localization on the basis of animal experimental studies. Clinicians, on the other hand, on the basis of data from daily practice that were correlated with examination of the brain at autopsy, claimed the correspondence of localized cortical lesions with circumscribed behavioral disturbances in the patient or with neurological function losses. Broca's (1861) description of "aphemia" in relation to a lowermost left frontal gyrus lesion in one of his patients constituted such an attempt to establish a correlation between brain lesion and function. This new development met with strong opposition, as is apparent from the famous debate between Broca and Trousseau in 1864 in the Académie de Médecine. The latter advanced the term "aphasia", thus indicating a wide variety of language disturbances. On autopsy of the patient, these aphasias were found to relate to brain lesions at sites different from those described in Broca's patient, and Trousseau concluded from this observation that Broca's notion of a language center could not possibly be right. It is against this intellectual background that Wernicke worked in Meynert's laboratory in Vienna in the early 1870s.

In Meynert's opinion, the cerebral cortex could be subdivided into a posterior sensory part and an anterior motor part, both parts being interconnected by numerous fiber bundles. A meticulous analysis of the fiber connections of the brain was performed by means of teasing out preparations and by microscopic observation. The fibers were supposed by

Meynert to be the substrate of functional connections between different parts of the brain. On the basis of these studies Meynert distinguished between projection fibers, association fibers, and commissural fibers.

The system of "projection fibers" consisted of centrifugal ones that connect the anterior lobes with the cranial nerve nuclei and the spinal cord, and the centripetal sensory fibers that project the various streams of stimuli from the sense organ receptors towards the posterior lobes of the brain. One should realize that a definite terminal site for the auditory system within the cerebral cortex was not yet established at that time.

A second system of intrahemispheric fibers connects the primary projection cortex with the large surface of cortex that is located between these primary areas. These "association fibers" may consist of large bundles of fibers connecting rather remote cortical areas (as for instance the arcuate fascicle, the uncinate fascicle, and the cingulum) and of fibers connecting neighboring parts of cerebral cortex (fibrae arcuatae, U-fibers) or even intracortical fibers (fibrae propriae). The "commissural fibers" of the corpus callosum, anterior commissure, and commissura hippocampi that interconnect homonymous brain areas constitute the third category.

Apart from data obtained from human pathology, Meynert also referred to data from comparative neuro-anatomy. He pointed to the disproportionate development in man of that part of the cerebral cortex that borders the lateral Sylvian fissure. Wernicke later on clearly followed this lead in his publication "Das Urwindungssystem des menschlichen Gehirns" (1875). The reconsideration of the question of the relationship between dysphasic phenomena and the location of cerebral cortical lesions against the background of the knowledge obtained in Meynert's laboratory resulted in Wernicke's concept of the "aphasic symptom-complex", consisting of on one extreme the pure aphemia and the motor aphasia, and on the other extreme the sensory aphasia, with a bewildering variety of dysphasic syndromes in between.

Another important concept contributed to the development of Wernicke's theory of aphasia; this was the hypothesis that stimuli affecting a particular cortical area may cause a lasting change in the organization of the local circuitry of that cortex, thus providing a "memory-image" of the pertinent stimulus. In Wernicke's opinion this applied both to the primary sensory and to the primary motor cortex regions. In addition, he ventured, motor activity *ipso facto* was always accompanied by a simultaneous sensory stimulation and, therefore, the memory-image of motor activity at the same time was to be fixed both in the motor and in the sensory cortex. Association fibers between motor and sensory cortices automatically aroused the memory-images in the associated field when the cerebral cortex is stimulated at one particular site.

Broca's description of motor aphasia and Wernicke's own observation of a number of patients with what he called "sensory aphasia" provided the cornerstones of Wernicke's language model. This model eventually consisted of a three-story edifice. The two lowermost stories together constituted the substrate of verbal language and speech, named by Wernicke the "word-concept" faculty of the brain. If a lesion occurred in one of the anatomical structures that mediate this "word-concept" function, a language disturbance of a more or less instrumental character results, as will be explained later on.

The uppermost story of the language model possessed a different function. This level comprises the whole of the telencephalic cortex, furnishes the drive to communicate orally, and also determines the content of the spoken word. The word-concept of the lower stories serves as the infrastructure of the top of Wernicke's hierarchical model.

The term "word-concept" is used by Wernicke to indicate the capacity of the brain to produce formal oral language; this capacity is acquired only gradually during the first years of life. Important constituent structures that contribute to this function are the primary motor cortex, which influences the bulbar and spinal motor organization through descending fiber tracts, and the primary acoustic cortex, which receives its input through the ascending acoustic system. The casual and spontaneous production of vocalization sounds and the imitation of language sounds heard from the environment is instrumental in developing the child's ability to produce language. The recognition of a sound as pertaining to "language" rests on the analysis of the signal arriving on the primary acoustic cortex by the nearby association cortex, where "memory-images" of earlier acoustic experiences are stored. The acoustic association cortex (nowadays we would say "Wernicke's sensory language center") is connected to the motor type association cortex by means of the arcuate fascicle. In this motor association cortex "memory-images" of motor patterns are stored. This motor association cortex is often designated "Broca's motor language center" and may be said to play the primary motor cortex like an instrument, thereby producing the motor pattern of oral language. The endless repetition of inummerable language experiences during the early years of life supplies an enormous store of memory-images as the basis of language production by means of the circuit that is formed in the way described above. Lesions at different sites in this circuit result in a variety of dysphasic syndromes. "Subcortical sensory aphasia" was the term used by Wernicke to describe the consequence of a lesion in the connections between the primary acoustic cortex and the surrounding association cortex. Often this type of disturbance is also called "pure word deafness". The patient may hear the sounds but is unable to interpret the sounds as language expressions. A lesion in the association cortex itself was called "cortical sensory aphasia" and resulted in the well-known symptoms of auditory comprehension impairment, fluent paraphasic aphasia with word-finding difficulty. Analogous to the previous syndromes, a lesion in the connections between the primary motor cortex and Broca's "motor language center" resulted in a "subcortical motor aphasia", according to Wernicke. Another designation of the same disturbance is "pure word mutism". A lesion in Broca's motor language center results in a "cortical motor aphasia". In addition to the four types of aphasia enumerated above, Wernicke postulated the existence of a "conduction aphasia" in patients with a lesion in the arcuate fascicle; this conduction aphasia consisted of the inability to repeat a word or sentence which had been spoken, the sensory and motor language functions otherwise being intact. The word-concept function as the infrastructure of Wernicke's hierarchical language model was considered by him as a basic faculty of the brain, necessary for the production and comprehension of language; later investigators amplified this subject of study to the exploration of the areas of "inner-language" and the existence of a "language programmer". The superstructure of Wernicke's language model consisted of the connections of the functional structures of the lower levels with all the various cortical areas elsewhere in the hemisphere. A disconnection of these relationships between the so-called sensory and motor language centers on the one hand and the other cortical areas elsewhere results in what Wernicke refers to as "transcortical aphasia". He discerns a sensory transcortical aphasia and a motor transcortical aphasia.

As far as this uppermost level of the language model is concerned, Wernicke is inclined to point to the fact that he considers the cerebral cortex with its manifold local differences and variations to be an undivided whole. In this respect Wernicke is quite a bit less of a localizationist than many an author wants us to believe he is. The transcortical function activates the language patterns that are associated with a particular content of consciousness. These language patterns are worked out by the "word-concept" infrastructure, which may be compared to a language programmer. The emphasis of Wernicke's theory of language is on the existence of a limited number of localizable functions and on the importance of the fiber connections of these centers with other areas of the brain cortex. The cerebral cortex figures as the organ of consciousness, the various parts of which are interrelated and coactivated by means of the associative fiber connections. Wernicke, therefore, should be considered neither a localizationist, nor a wholist. The view held by Wernicke on brain functions in relation to language might be characterized most appropriately by the term "connectionism".

Wernicke incorporated his language model in a comprehensive theory on the relations of psychic life and the functioning of the brain. In the later years of his career Wernicke endeavored to apply the psychophysic parallelism that is intrinsic to his aphasia theory to the explanation and classification of the signs and symptoms of psychiatric disease.

Analysis of the life and work of the man reveals a scientist interested in the formulation of a theory of psychic life and in the unraveling of the relationships between psychological phenomena and the facts known about the functioning of the central nervous system. His study of disturbed language sprang from this same source; he considered language to be a mere particularized form of human behavior. By education and training Wernicke was one of the great German "Nervenärzte", being equally eager to study both neurology and psychiatry. A lifelong quest for the correlation between those phenomena that can be observed in disturbed human behavior and those that can be observed at the level of the structural-functional organization of the central nervous system resulted in a wealth of publications on most of the main topics of neuro-psychiatry of the day. A number of them, even nowadays, stand out as fundamental contributions to medicine and indicated the opening of new avenues for research in the neurosciences.

Wernicke on Aphasia

Wernicke's three most important contributions to the study of aphasia appeared in 1874, 1885, and 1906. They cover only a small part of his voluminous scientific productivity. Here the second chapter of Wernicke's thesis *Der aphasische Symptomencomplex: Eine psychologische Studie auf anatomischer Basis* (1874) is reproduced. In this chapter Wernicke applies Meynert's ideas to the functions of speech and language, and he develops his aphasia theory. In the third and final chapter of his thesis Wernicke reports on ten case studies of aphasic patients, two of them with a typical pure sensory type of aphasia. Wernicke concludes, "The great variability of the clinical picture of aphasia moves between the two extremes of pure motor aphasia and the pure sensory form. The demonstration of these two types must be regarded as conclusive proof of the existence of two anatomically separate language centers".

Wernicke's second main contribution on aphasia was his publication "Einige neuere Arbeiten über Aphasie" in 1885 and 1886. Here he showed the elaboration of a number of notions already present implicitly in his 1874 work. Part of it is reproduced here because it gives a comprehensive overview of the ideas of Wernicke on the various types of aphasia. This overview (chapter II of the work) is preceded by another quotation from the same publication. Here Wernicke made it very clear that he maintains his localizationist ideas only with respect to a very restricted part of the cerebral cortex, i.e., the part that corresponds with the effector functions and their sensory counterparts. He refrained from any attempt to localize the "higher" part of the psychophysiologic process leading to communication by means of language. As such Wernicke's view holds a rather differentiated position between the holistic and the localizationist approach of cerebral cortex functioning.

References

Broca, P. 1861b. "Remarques sur le siège de la faculté de langage articulé, suivie d'une observation d'aphémie (perte de la parole)". *Bulletins de la Société Anatomique* 6:330-357.

Wernicke, C. 1874. *Der aphasische Symptomencomplex. Eine psychologische Studie auf anatomischer Basis*. Breslau: Cohn & Weigert.

———. 1875. "Das Urwindungssytem des menslichen Gehirns". *Archiv für Psychiatrie und Neurololgie* 6: 298-326.

———. 1885. "Einige neuere Arbeiten über Aphasie". *Fortschritte der Medizin* 3:824-830; 4 (1886) 371-377, 463-469.

Reprinted in C. Wernicke. *Gesammelte Aufsätze und kritische Referate zur Pathologie des Nervensystems*. Berlin: Fischer, 1983.

———. 1906. "Der Aphasie Symptomenkomplex". *Die Deutsche Klinik am Eingange des 20 Jahrhunderts*, Bd. 6, Abt. 1:487-556. Berlin: Urban & Schwarzenberg.

Selection from the work of Carl Wernicke

The Aphasia Symptom-Complex:
A Psychological Study on an Anatomical Basis*

PART II

This initial review has attempted to illustrate certain general principles based on current anatomical and physiological evidence, which may be applied to the lawful generation of spontaneous movement. All spontaneous motor action, including that of speech, is based on such principles. The fact that speech movement must be classified as conscious voluntary action needs no detailed elucidation. The evidence clearly shows that speech production must be laboriously acquired during childhood. This is true of all spontaneous movement. Speech acquisition coincides so closely with the development of consciousness that it may be considered as a gauge thereof. Motor speech production emerges only after the child has perfected many other conscious motor actions.

The primary speech movements, enacted before the development of consciousness, are reflexive and mimicking in nature[1] and are discharged to the same areas of the pons and medulla oblongata along the inner half of the cerebral peduncle tegmentum, which constitutes the origin of the acoustic nerve. Numerous large, many-tailed cells may be found there, which apparently may be regarded as excrescences of the facial, vagal, and hypoglossal nuclei. Meynert maintains that these cells are anatomically connected

* Reprinted with permission from G. Eggert "Wernicke's Works on Aphasia", The Hague: Mouton, pp. 92-117 (1977)

with the arcuate fibers associated with the origin of the acoustic nerve. Experimental evidence indicates that the respiratory center is located within this extensive area containing the origin of the acoustic nerve. The advantage of such a location can readily be seen in the newborn child, in that the medulla itself can produce the unarticulated cry, a unitary muscular response which in spite of its simplicity requires the combined action of expiration and adduction of the vocal folds.[2] Probably even the complicated patterns of muscle action involved in the formation of monosyllabic words may first be produced reflexively, although possibly in a more complex organ, the cerebellum. Because its functions are still incompletely known, we often try to use it as a convenient solution to fill all of the gaps in our knowledge. However, let us rather merely draw general conclusions from this notion and admit the difficulty of explaining the production of entire words by means of the reflex apparatus of the medulla oblongata. Whether the situation is such that complete words or merely word fragments are formed reflexively in the medulla, in any event, it appears that an acoustic image of the word or syllable is transmitted from the site of the reflex process to a sensory area of the brain, and the innervatory sensation of the movement produced is transmitted as a motor speech image to the frontal area. The association of acoustic and motor images is then maintained by means of myelinated fibers. Production of the spontaneous movement, that is, the consciously formulated word, would be brought about by the rearousal of the motor image through the associated memory image of the sound. The stimulus is then transmitted along the tract within the foot of the cerebral peduncle, as is true of all other voluntary actions, until it reaches the speech musculature.

Before we try to suggest an anatomic basis for this interpretation of the speech process, let us pause and review some of the past attempts to localize a specific speech center within a definite anatomic cerebral region.

I shall pass over the host of older works regarding this problem, summaries of which may easily be found in detailed references, and shall turn immediately to Broca. This author was the first to reject broad, indefinite expanses of the cortex as sites of speech areas and instead ventured to designate a very circumscribed, anatomically specific region as the seat of this function. As is well known, he localized the faculty of speech to the posterior portion of the so-called third frontal gyrus, — or the first, according to Leuret's principle, in which counting proceeds from the Sylvian fissure. That is that portion of the most inferior and external part of the operculum, located in the frontal part of the central gyrus, just anterior to its juncture. In spite of the opposition to this view, which was very strong at the outset, such a large number of case studies of speech impairment have been reported in its support, and the contradictory cases have furnished so little new positive evidence, that this theory continues to pave a constantly broader path and now boasts many followers.

In the meantime Meynert published a work which caused a great stir. In this study he demonstrated the connection of the acoustic nerve to the cortex of the Sylvian fissure by means of a fiber path which he called the acoustic tract ('Acousticusstrang'). This entire tract surrounding the origin of the acoustic nerve coincides to some extent with the region of the claustrum, which was named by Meynert an "acoustic field". He supported his hypothesis by a large number of post-mortem findings in aphasic patients demonstrating pathological changes either within the insular area itself or in the circumscribed portion of the Sylvian fissure.

Many well-known physicians who were involved in the controversy were inclined toward Meynert's view, particularly because it served to resolve the vaguely felt need to relate the acoustic nerve to the speech process. Strangely enough, many continued to recognize the entire area of cortex surrounding the Sylvian fissure as a speech center, in spite of the fact that Meynert himself disclaimed such a function of the acoustic tract. He, indeed, expressed the view that the acoustic nerve was not connected directly to the cerebrum, but first coursed through the cerebellum.[3] This can be explained from pathological-anatomical findings. Most cases of aphasia in which Broca's area was not found to have changed showed changes in the area claimed by Meynert. Recently this fact has been especially put forward again by Sander and Finkelnburg. Meynert too maintains his former point of view concerning the significance of this area. In advocating this point of view he advances as an argument the composition of the claustrum out of association cells, meaning spindle-shaped cells, and the intimate relationships of the claustrum to the other association systems of the cerebrum.

The fact that destruction of Broca's area is responsible for aphasia seems to me beyond doubt, considering cases like the striking one of Simon, which really is so much like an experiment. But I would doubt no less the confirming result of what other scrupulous and capable investigators have observed: the fact that focal lesions in the area surrounding the Sylvian fissure and its close environment cause aphasia as well; so

Broca's area is not the only one that functions as a speech center.

Which areas, then, make up the immediate neighborhood of the Sylvian fissure? In answering this question we must call attention to that particular gyrus on the convexity of the cerebral surface which extends in an arc directly upward and backward, enclosing the Sylvian fissure, and which continues as the first frontal gyrus (according to Leuret's terminology) anterior to the central sulcus, terminating longitudinally in a clear line formed by the first temporal gyrus. Comparison with the animal brain, such as that of the dog family, suggests that this entire region might be regarded as a single gyrus. A review of comparative anatomy reveals that this feature is also common to the embryological brain structure in man. Thus an arc is traced by the gyri around the Sylvian fissure, with its summit facing the occipital pole and its two limbs extending to the frontal and temporal area in a more or less parallel course.

The summit of the first frontal gyrus in Leuret's terminology must be differentiated from its two side surfaces. Only the summit lies completely exposed on the convex cerebral surface. One of the two sides is turned medially, facing the sulcus of the second frontal cortex. The other side forms the direct continuation of the insular cortex and, projecting over the island, adheres flatly to it on all sides. Comparative anatomy thus reveals the entire first primordial gyrus to be unitary in structure. Its internal structure reveals a characteristic which Meynert had described earlier. He observed that the island-facing surface of the claustrum extended from the island, projecting a considerable distance to the summit of the gyrus. The entire region of the first primordial gyrus shares in the peculiar characteristic of the insular cortex in that the innermost cortical layer, that of the fusiform cells, is concentrated into a single gray mass.

Moreover, by fiber dissections, I have been able to demonstrate a typical feature of this area, namely the presence of white fiber tracts just under the cortex on the surface of the first primordial gyrus, facing the Sylvian fissure. This same tract forms a continuous sheet of radiating fibers extending together with the medullary lamina of the first primordial gyrus to the floor of the deep fissure, which divides the first primordial gyrus from the island (by means of the anterior superior and inferior sulci of Burdach). From this point it spans the fissure and ends in the insular cortex. The island resembles a large spider, whose fiber radiations from all parts of the first primordial gyrus converge within its core, presenting the picture of a mighty control center, reserved for special functions.

The presence of the fibrae propriae, the arcuate lamina (Arnold), has also been demonstrated between the insular cortex and the gyral system of the cerebral convexity. As far as I know, these fibers have not been previously described. Because they provide such significant evidence in support of the unitary nature of the entire first primordial gyral arc in association with the insular cortex, they deserve a fairly detailed study.

The fibrae propriae are readily visible between the gyri of the cortical convexity and its medial surface. Therefore, one must question whether the Rolandic central sulcus, which bisects the primordial gyral system vertically, is bridged by these fibers. The results of fiber dissection in this area are still very unclear. However, a different situation prevails in regard to the deep fissure which appears to tie off the insular region from the encircling first gyral arc. Embryologically, the island is known to be an organizational midpoint of the entire convex surface of the hemisphere, its cortex forming a portion of the side of the ventricle of the hemisphere. Within, it merges with the basal ganglia, and its growth has been checked externally in such a way that a deep depression, the Sylvian fissure, has been formed on the convex surface of the ventricle.

Because of their location, a study of the fibers in this region is extremely difficult. Successful tracing of their course can be carried out only in alcohol-fixed brains. But in such specimens, deflecting the overhanging portions of the hemisphere, which completely cover the island itself, is extremely difficult. If such dissection is not successful, one must work blindly and assume the most awkward and tiring postures to admit adequate light for visualization of the area. The region most easily dissected is that portion coursing vertically, spanned by the fissure (Burdach's superior sulcus) first superiorly and then inferiorly, between the operculum and the island. This layer is also of considerable thickness, extending over one-half cm. in cross-section. Following this, the dissection can be best carried out in the anterior sulcus, between the frontal area of the brain and the island. The deep section which extends between this part of the frontal area and the operculum from front to back and above is completely covered with the same type of fibers. The dissection of the temporal lobe presents the greatest difficulty of all, not only because of the deep position of the inferior sulcus which is spanned, but also because of the very narrow diameter of the arcuate lamina. This applies particularly to the deep sinus into which the rear terminations of the superior and inferior sulci converge.

In carrying out this dissection, it is recommended that the scalpel

handle be first placed in the semi-elevation of the inner surface of the operculum. From that point, the cortex may be removed from above and
towards the island. At the summit of the gyrus, the fibrae propriae branch
out and can no longer be dissected. Moreover, the fibers cannot be traced
within the insular cortex either, because they tend to interweave and lie
deeply embedded within the claustrum.

In harmony with the preceding review, which considers the development of a speech act from the standpoint of conscious movement, *a priori*
reasoning would view restriction of the speech center to a single area,
namely, Broca's gyrus, as highly improbable. A consideration of the
anatomic structure as described above, the support of numerous necropsy
findings, and finally, the variability in the clinical picture of aphasia all
strongly lead us to the following interpretation of the data. The entire region of the first primordial convolution, the gyrus surrounding the Sylvian
fissure in association with the insular cortex, serves as a speech center. The
first frontal gyrus (Leuret), which has motor function, acts as a center of
motor imagery; the first temporal gyrus, which is sensory in nature, may be
regarded as the center of acoustic images; the fibrae propriae, converging
into the insular cortex, form the mediating reflex arc. Therefore, the first
temporal gyrus may be regarded as the central terminal of the acoustic
nerve, and the first frontal gyrus (including Broca's area) as the central terminal of the nerves controlling the speech musculature.

In Figure 1, the letter *F* represents the frontal area of the brain; the
occipital terminal is designated by *O*, the temporal terminal by *T*, and the
central sulcus by *C*. The first primordial gyrus extends around the Sylvian
fissure *S*. Within this schema *a1* is the central terminal of the acoustic nerve
(whose origin is in the medulla oblongata). The motor images associated
with speech-sound production in the frontal brain area are designated by *b*.
The association fibers *a1-b*, coursing through the insular cortex, are connected with the motor images *b*. The centrifugal pathway of the cranial
motor nerves concerned with speech production extends from *b* to the
medulla, where a large portion of the fibers terminate. (The accessory and
phrenic nerves continue downwards.)

Aphasia may be caused by any disruption of the pathway *a-a1 — b-b1*.
The clinical picture, however, may vary considerably and is related to the
specific segment of the pathway involved.

I. Let us assume that pathway *a-a1* is disrupted by some pathological
process resulting in the destruction of the acoustic nerve at some site along

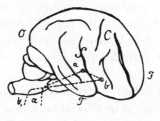

Figure 1.

its central course. Clinical experience shows that this would result in primary deafness with no trace of aphasia. However, this would hold only for adults already in possession of an extensive store of earlier-acquired acoustic images which may be revived at will. Should this disrupting process occur during some period of childhood, before this store of acoustic images has been accumulated within the cortex, muteness would be an inevitable consequence. This is the common cause of deaf-muteness. The child has not yet developed the acoustic imagery from which the motor images may be activated.

The inevitable occurrence of muteness in congenital or early-acquired deafness throws an interesting sidelight on the significance of auditory sensation for normal speech development. There is a common, widespread misconception, championed especially by philosophers and speech investigators (such as Steinthal), that the formation of the concept, the sum of sensory impressions of an object, is the most critical factor in speech development. The concept would then breed speech from an inner need, and its development would follow the same laws today as were originally operative in primitive man.

Speech then would not be regarded as mere mimicry but as an event which is self-activated, a process in which all sensory areas contribute essential elements necessary for development of the concept which is the fundamental prerequisite. An internal connection to a sensory area such as hearing would then not be considered relevant. If this were the case, muteness would occur more readily in the congenitally blind than in the congenitally deaf, since the eye, of all sensory structures, is unquestionably the most essential organ providing information regarding objects in the environment and hence by far the most important for the formation of concepts. All sensory areas associated with the tactile organs and those of vision and olfaction — in short, all areas essential to formation of the concept

— would then need to be regarded as bound up with the motor imagery activated during speech by means of a segment of the association system.[4] However, the pathway *a-a1-b* alone is most critical of all for speech development because it provides the means by which the child learns speech.

The major task of the child in speech acquisition is mimicry of the spoken word. This is first learned in association with a specific meaning after the child has long been in possession of the word. The word is essentially a reproduction of the auditory image and not that of vision or the tactile sense; therefore, the learning of speech by the congenitally deaf is as hard to achieve as is drawing by the congenitally blind.

A typical example might be mentioned here. What is the effect of unilateral deafness on the child's development? Muteness may follow only if one makes the thoroughly improbable assumption that the left speech center alone[5] is capable of development, and that the right center atrophies perhaps because of constitutional causes or at least on the basis of functional disuse. Although we must concede that the child with right-sided deafness, who is therefore dependent on the right hemisphere for speech learning, may have more difficulty in speech development than the child with left-sided deafness, yet one may definitely assume that the presence of the acoustic pathway coursing to the right temporal lobe will in itself be adequate to support speech development in childhood.

For purposes of comparison, a review of necropsy findings of this condition would be very important to provide an adequate explanation of the causative processes in many cases of aphasia with right-side lesions. This question sharply points up the critical gaps in our knowledge regarding the definitive localization of the course of the acoustic nerve within the cerebrum. The termination of the left acoustic nerve within the right hemisphere is a tentative educated guess.

The symptom-complex of deaf-muteness is so well known that the coexistence of its two components is self-explanatory but has not yet been specifically studied in relation to the problem of aphasia. In contrast, the condition described by some as congenital aphasia, which may occur in children with intact hearing and good intelligence but who do not develop language, is a rare finding.

II. Let us now consider the condition caused by destruction of the area containing the acoustic imagery *a1*. This area is not identical with the broad central radiation of the acoustic nerve itself, since complete loss of acoustic imagery with intact bilateral hearing has been observed in aphasia. Probably the same situation applies to the central endings of the sensory cranial nerves as is true of the motor nerves, namely that their dispersion and termination in different areas of the cortex is consistent with their various functions. Thus, in spite of destruction of the central acoustic radiation, which carries the sounds of words, perception of noise and musical tone would still be intact.

Loss of area *a1*, the cortex of the first temporal gyrus, would result in obliteration of the names [acoustic imagery] of all objects from memory. The concept itself, however, would remain fully clear, for in most cases, the acoustic image of a name is of secondary importance in relationship to the concept, while touch and tactile imagery, in contrast, are intrinsic components of the same. Disturbances of the visual and tactile imagery of the concept (Finkelnburg's asymbolia) are therefore not regarded as speech disorders, but as disturbances of the concept, that is, of the intellect. However, one must admit that such conceptual impairment may be divided into clearly differentiated subgroups.

It is obvious that integrity of the pathway *a1-b* in itself is of little value if the acoustic imagery is lost. In that event the word can no longer be activated by the acoustic image. Moreover, let us assume destruction of the path which connects the acoustic image with other sensory images of the object, i.e., the association fibers leading from the first temporal convolution to the other sensory regions of the temporo-occipital area. *In this event the patient would be able neither to repeat the spoken word, for that is the unique function of the pathway (a-a1-b-b1), nor would he be able to comprehend it.* The spoken word would be heard merely as meaningless noise. In cases presenting milder involvement, the word may be heard like a completely foreign language, with intact perception of individual sounds and gradual recovery of comprehension.

However, one possible means of activation of the motor speech images may still be available to the patient. Intellectual impairment is not a primary feature of this condition. The patient's ability to comprehend signs and gesture indicates intact recognition of sensory images of objects and of the concepts themselves. The associations of acoustic and motor imagery are so essential because they furnish the means by which speech is acquired. Shortly after the learning of oral production of the word, the desire to merely mimic and repeat sounds disappears and is replaced by the need to communicate a specific meaning. That is, the actual sensory image of an object is now able to activate the motor image directly. The capacity for speech production is maintained but with certain limitations. Observations of daily speech usage and the process of speech development indicate the presence of an unconscious, repeated activation and simultaneous mental reverberation of the acoustic image which exercises a continuous monitoring of the motor images. This monitoring device also functions in the deaf who demonstrate damage to the acoustic nerve alone.

The situation may be described schematically as follows. In Figure 2, which is similar to that previously presented, the tactile image c is associated with $a1$ and with d, the associated visual memory trace. The concept itself is represented by none other than the pathway c-d. The child initially learns speech through utilization of pathway $a1$-b, whose thousandfold use maintains a continuing significant control over the choice of the correct motor image. Later, the predominant use of this pathway is replaced by the shorter paths c-b and d-b, and the mere presence of $a1$-b, without its specific innervation, is adequate to assure choice of the correct motor image.

Therefore, the sum total of $d+c+a1$ always functions in harmony with the appropriate intensity necessary for correct selection of the word. However, if $a1$ should be absent, the sum of $d+c$ alone would be effective for such innervation with simultaneous suppression of the strong control of pathway $a1$-b.

Apart from impairment in comprehension, the patient also presents aphasic symptoms in speech produced by absence of the unconscious monitoring of the imagery of the spoken sound. This lack is reflected in frequent word-confusion. The ability to name objects is retained, but this control tends to be very labile and it is readily influenced by disposition and mood. There is no consistency of correct use of the word. The patient does not possess a vocabulary of specific words which are always used correctly. Furthermore, he seems unaware of the accuracy of his word-usage. Intense emotion may activate an explosion of words without the involvement of the associated memory image. Under such conditions, the monitoring device is missed least of all.

The severity of the symptoms will be dependent upon the degree and extent of the pathologic process involving the first temporal lobe. Diagnosis of the more severe forms, presenting loss of not only the acoustic imagery of concrete objects and actions but also the connecting words necessary for sentence formulation, is dependent upon two factors, *the availability of*

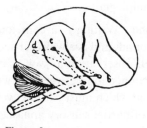

Figure 2.

words and impairment in comprehension. Such cases have not been observed up to the present, or at least have not been described in the literature. Apart from the infrequent occurrence of the condition, this lack stems from the erroneous interpretation of such symptoms as dementia by experienced and intelligent physicians, an error into which I myself have fallen in the past. The diagnosis, however, presents no difficulty at all to the psychiatrically oriented, who are familiar with this specific form of confusion.

This diagnosis may be confirmed by the use of suggestion-questions in mild types of the disturbance, which present preservation of the form-elements necessary for sentence formulation, and in cases in which comprehension of questions succeeds merely by retained understanding of certain isolated words. For example, a glass may be presented to the patient with the question "Is this a glass?" His response is usually not immediate. Frequently he may hesitate and reflect for a while and finally force a doubtful "yes" or "no". Such behavior would place him in this category of aphasia.

The following points deserve attention.

1. In partial lesions of the sensory speech center a residual fund of consistently and correctly produced and comprehended words will be retained. The extent of this word-store may be determined by the use of suggestion-questions. However, a tedious and lengthy period of observation is necessary to confirm the diagnosis in this partial form of sensory aphasia.

2. The primary feature of this particular form of aphasia is the retention of a sizeable fund of words. Cases whose word-store is restricted to a few simple words always belong to the category of motor aphasia discussed under section IV.

3. No evidence of hemiplegia.

4. Presence of agraphia. Writing is a conscious action, learned with close dependence on the sound, and is always carried out under such acoustic control. Analysis by self-observation as well as clinical experience indicate an absence of direct connection between the written response and the concept itself, similar to that which must exist between the speech response and the concept. In cases of partial sensory aphasia a partial agraphia may also be anticipated.

5. Comprehension of written or printed letters of the alphabet presents an entirely different matter. This is related to the level of educational achievement and is independent of the presence of auditory imagery. The individual who has been exposed to minimal training in reading may comprehend the written word only after it has been heard. But the educated person, trained in this skill from early childhood, may be able to grasp the general meaning after a glance at the page without awareness of the individual words. The first case presents symptoms of an alexia apart from his aphasia. The second, on the other hand, reveals intact comprehension of all written material in striking contrast to his lack of comprehension of the spoken word. Nevertheless, in oral reading the latter demonstrates as much aphasia as is evident in spontaneous speech.

Both conditions, agraphia as well as alexia, may also be caused by involvement of an entirely different area, that of the visual cortex, since the memory images of written signs are as indispensable to the writing process as to that of reading. However, one cannot deny the possibility that the images of written signs occupy a unique and specific cortical region through their intimate connections with the entire speech area. Therefore, the symptoms of a localized alexia with agraphia may occur on the basis of a very circumscribed cortical lesion. In such cases one would rather anticipate involvement of the entire visual sensory area. The symptom-complex would be complete if object recognition were also lost. However, this disorder is intrinsically not concerned with aphasia.

III. Now let us consider the condition characterized by involvement of the association fiber tracts, i.e., pathways *a1-b*, connecting the acoustic imagery to the associated motor imagery. In this condition the acoustic image *a1* and the motor image *b* itself are intact.

This patient presents a picture of *good comprehension in marked contrast to that which is typical of the form* of aphasia previously described. He speaks a great deal but shows a disturbance in his choice of words very much like the other type. The auditory image is intact. It is activated by the residual sensory imagery forming the concept. However, since pathway *al-b* is disrupted, it cannot make its own unique contribution to the appropriate selection of the motor images, or it contributes but minimally. While in the previous cases the total effect of *c+d* alone was active for motor innervation from *b*, in this situation *c+d+al* is operative. The latter, however, since it is designated as a part of the pathway *c-b*, is normally of minimal signficance. Word-confusion is also observed in these cases. While this symptom is not as marked as in the preceding form, it is still very much in evidence. Nevertheless, in this case another monitoring device may be operative which is little used in normal speech, namely, the gradual substitution of an unconscious process for one which is conscious. The acoustic nerve is intact and permits transfer of the sound of the spoken word to the undamaged area containing acoustic imagery. The spoken word can therefore be heard and its accuracy assessed. The patient has definite awareness of his error and therefore often becomes emotionally upset. If given a choice of words he usually chooses successfully, just as suggestion-questions are correctly answered. Such a patient is able to rehearse what he wishes to say by first quietly repeating the word to himself. If he is a strong-willed individual, capable of intense and keen vigilance, compensation may eventually develop by a conscious but laborious and time-consuming monitoring mechanism.

In pure and complete forms the patient presents a picture which is very similar to that of sensory aphasia. He comprehends correctly, answers suggestion-questions accurately, and so appears more intelligent than he actually is. Hemiplegia of the opposite side is almost always present.

A moderate circulatory disorder may be the assumed cause of decreased neural transmission in milder cases. The symptoms of word-finding difficulty in these patients who show no signs of hemiplegia is more striking than the confusion of words. Their speech is very hesitant and is characterized by long pauses in which the patient gropes for expression. After a long period of search, he may give up and attempt a new sentence. The beginning of the sentence may be fluent, then follow the same hesitation, the same laborious effort. This experience also occurs in normal speech when a word suddenly cannot be found in the midst of conversation. One then tries to substitute another and must finally be satisfied with a word which may be only partly adequate. I have sometimes observed even in intelligent individuals the sudden occurrence of startling combinations of sounds in the midst of speech, as if they were speaking in an abbreviated manner during intense mental absorption. If Steinthal in his *Abriss der Sprachwissenschaft* ("Outline of Linguistics") found the process of thought to be highly complex in itself, how much more difficult would be simultaneous thought and speech. The functional hyperemia which causes facilitation in conduction between the continuously newly aroused sensory imagery results in a corresponding anemia in the speech areas.[6]

The disturbance in reading and writing produced by aphasia of the insular region can only be understood by a detailed study of the means by which both are acquired (Figure 3).

Reading is learned in the following way during childhood. The visual image located in area a (a portion of the entire visual sensory area) is brought into relationship with its acoustic image, thus forming a strong association. In this way the child learns to read aloud, since the sum of $a+a1$ by means of the path $a1-b$ activates the motor image b. The union of the acoustic and visual imagery constitutes the entire concept of the letter. It is not endowed with other qualities.

In the event of disruption of pathway $a-b$, the same process does not apply to letters as applies to all other concrete object-representation, namely the activation of the motor speech image by the concept itself. Patients are therefore unable to read individual letters. To this extent alexia always accompanies the forms of aphasia just discussed. The patient's level of education determines whether such an alexia will also extend to entire words. If earlier reading achievement has been limited to the reading of individual letters, and words are formed letter-by-letter, the aphasia would cause complete loss of reading ability. If, on the other hand, this early reading achievement has been equal to that of educated classes, the concept can be revived by means of the written word. Under optimal conditions the word might then be comprehended and retrieved orally. Single letters, however, could not be read aloud by such a patient, because oral reading requires integrity of the pathway $a-b$. Nevertheless, if a choice of names of a number of letters are given to such a patient, he would be able to select the name of the letter he is attempting to read and reject all others offered. In this way he demonstrates complete comprehension of the meaning of the letter.

The educated individual with aphasia of the insular region therefore does not sustain impairment of comprehension of the written word. Unfor-

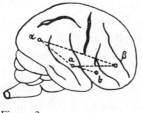

Figure 3.

tunately, this statement must be modified by the fact that in this form of aphasia, a right hemianopsia is a frequent complication.[7]

Writing is learned in the following way. The visual association image of the letter is copied by means of the path α-β (β is the center of graphic motor imagery.) Only through intensive drill is association between the acoustic and motor imagery $a1$-β achieved, permitting us to write in the absence of a model. The original pathway α-β, by means of which we learned to write, maintains the same control of discharge of the written response as is exercised by the path $a1$-b in discharge of speech movements. Because the motor center β is located in the frontal area of the brain, and the pathway $a1$-β is consequently a close neighbor to the path $a1$-b, damage to this general area affects both simultaneously. This circuit provides the most direct route between the complex of sensory imagery constituting the concept and the motor writing center which activates graphic movements by means of the acoustic imagery. For this reason, aphasia of the insular region is frequently accompanied by agraphia. Nevertheless, the copying of letters and words may still be possible, since the pathway α-β is yet intact.

IV. A completely different picture is presented in aphasia of the frontal lobe, caused by destruction of the motor speech images in area b. *The patient presenting this condition comprehends all but is suddenly mute or has only a few simple words at his disposal.* These same words are used repetitively in reference to all objects, not because the patient lacks comprehension of their significance, but because they alone are available to him. This situation is similar to the dog's use of barking as a response to all commands. A single sound must serve to convey many meanings. The strong neural stimulation passing from $a1$ and c-d to center b can find expression only in this single movement.

The absence of word-confusion in the pure motor form may be verified by means of suggestion-questions. These are always answered accurately by means of gesture. There is no difficulty in carrying out commands. The great majority of cases which have been reported up to this time belong to this category, i.e., Broca's aphasia.

If the pathological event is extensive, the neighboring central area of motor imagery involved in written motor imagery may also be involved, thus producing agraphia. One may well ask whether assumption of such a center is justified. The movements involved in writing are learned at a period after which the child has already developed significant and gross control of movement patterns. Therefore, the acquisition of new combinations of the motor images already present and refinement of muscular control alone is necessary. For that reason, one may not conclude that the graphic motor images are located only in the left hemisphere, since normal individuals are also able to write with the left hand, and not more awkwardly than is true of carrying out other actions with the left hand.

However, an event involving a large area of the frontal lobe would consequently also implicate the motor imagery of the opposite side, resulting in paralysis and a mechanically produced agraphia. If a patient can place a pen with his intact left hand into his tightly contracted, paralyzed right hand, and guide the right hand, the writing would really be carried out by the left hand and not the right. This situation would in no way prove the presence of a left center for the movements involved in writing.

One who is accustomed to rehearse aloud what he is writing may be compared to the one who forcefully guides his pen with the intact hand. He would become agraphic because of the close association between the speech and graphic motor imagery, apart from the actual localization of the pathological process.

If the event disrupts those fiber tracts which emerge from the first temporal gyrus and connect the area of acoustic imagery with that of the graphic motor images, the patient would still be able to copy by means of the pathway α-β but would fail in spontaneous writing. He would be partially agraphic.

Aphasia of the frontal lobe can never, except in the case described on page 25, abolish comprehension of written or printed letters.

V. Interruption of the pathway b-$b1$ as presented in Figure 3, which primarily involves fibers from the first frontal gyrus converging into the great ganglion, would create an effect similar to the destruction of the specific cortical area itself. *Therefore, it would produce the same motor aphasia which has just been described.* One would hardly anticipate an event to destroy only this portion of the fibers radiating to the lenticular nucleus and corpus striatum alone, without damage to the remainder. In other words, this would produce a pure aphasia without any further paralysis. Such a situation would apply even more strongly to the fibers coursing throughout the lenticular nucleus and striatum. Destruction of but a very small area within the lenticular nucleus produces a dramatic change in the organization of the fibers. It is very probable that the various fibers concerned with different motor representations enter the lenticular nucleus from different cortical areas of the frontal area of the brain. Their arrangement there may be such that the area of one of the peripheral nerves is already represented in an adjoining circumscribed region by means of a specific quantity of gray ganglionic substance.

For example, it has definitely been established that the facial nerve in the lenticular nucleus is represented by two circumscribed but widely separated nuclei. One of these contains fibers of the mouth area which possibly originate from the first frontal gyrus and serve in production of speech movements. Or they might originate from some other region of the frontal area of the brain containing the motor images of mimicry. The other nucleus contains fibers concerned with the orbital region of the facial nerve regardless of the motor images to which they are related. In the same way, the tongue musculature has its own nucleus into which fibers from different cortical areas converge, concerned with production of speech movements as well as other consciously executed movements involved in chewing and swallowing. Therefore, it follows that circumscribed lesions within the lenticular nucleus need not affect all speech movements simultaneously, but could produce a partial aphasia. Such an episode would present the appearance of a paralytic type of attack with involvement of innervation of the speech musculature, such as the branch of the facial nerve serving the oral region. Production of movements of the tongue and larynx used in the speech act would be intact and the word would continue to be intelligible.

It is very definite therefore that the difference between aphasia and alalia in regard to lenticular nuclear involvement is not one of kind but of degree. *Complete destruction of the left lenticular nucleus would therefore cause aphasia as well as paralysis.* This may be called "aphasia of the lenticular nucleus". This form deserves specific attention in contrast to the prevailing view, which I must emphasize is based on a very naive interpretation of the anatomic facts of this condition.

It should be clear from our discussion that disruption of the left cerebral peduncle must cause an aphasia. In fact, destruction of the inferior portion of the peduncle in itself can cause this condition, since the movements of speech are consciously learned, as has been discussed above.

It is self-evident that cases presenting two or three symptom-pictures in combination occur more frequently than the pure clinical forms caused by more or less isolated damage because the pathological event is generally very extensive. Undoubtedly, the typical pictures described, which adequately justify our formulation of a new clinical classification, actually do exist (see the section describing clinical studies below). I believe that the mere drawing of attention to such cases will result in the publication of many case histories supported by pathological findings. The mixed forms may readily be understood from the preceding discussion. If the psychic symptoms associated with aphasia of the temporal lobe are complicated by a right hemiplegia, one may predict involvement of both temporal lobe and the insular region. Combined lesions of the frontal area of the brain and the insular region are difficult to differentiate from those of the frontal area alone. Lesions of the entire first primordial gyrus arc result in complete speech loss with impairment in comprehension, together with agraphia and alexia.

A correct diagnosis of aphasia requires a very detailed history of a specific period in the course of the illness. On the one hand, such diagnosis rests on remission of the generalized brain symptoms which accompany the onset of aphasia as well as other focal brain lesions. On the other hand, the duration of the condition must not have been of such length as to allow substitution of function by the other hemisphere. Fortunately, both of these sources of error can be avoided, since substitution by the opposite hemisphere in aphasia of the frontal area generally occurs late. This form of aphasia produces the most severe generalized symptoms. Compensation in sensory aphasia, however, occurs early, and the generalized symptoms are relatively mild. Unfortunately, only experienced examiners record the precise time of onset of the various symptoms, and then only if they have observed the case from onset of the condition. I need not stress the significance of this point in evaluating the pathological findings.

This newly formulated theory of aphasia requires further elaboration lest one judge as inadequate the treatment of the valuable previous material on which it is based.

I must now return to that hypothesis confirmed by clinical experience which offers a clear basis for a fruitful interpretation of the symptomatology of aphasia. Speech is bred in mimicry of the spoken word. Speech is not identical with achievement of a specific level of mental development. Thought and speech are two independent processes which may be individually delayed. Daily observation supports this view. All children in the process of learning speech go through a stage in which they typically reveal "Romberg's echolalia". They repeat questions put to them instead of answering. They play with words, experimenting with word-distortion in the process of achieving stable control of the production of sounds. The meaning of the word at this stage is of secondary importance to them.

Caspar Hauser, who grew up without human contact, did not develop speech although his brain development was normal. He showed much cunning and mental keenness in his struggles with animals. However, speech was learned rapidly when he eventually came into contact with other men.

Another pertinent example of this is supplied by the deaf-mute. Man normally learns speech by means of the acoustic nerve. Deprived of this pathway, he remains mute, regardless of his level of intellectual achievement. One must assume that the same factors as exist in normal speech development are operative in pathological speech changes .

Let us consider what occurs in deaf-mutes who may acquire articulate and clear speech by means of complicated training methods. These cases merely confirm the existence of direct connections between the visual and tactile sensory areas and the region of motor speech-representation and prove that such connections are eventually adequate to support normal speech function. The fact that such cases can produce some speech and even learn entire sentences, in spite of loss of acoustic imagery, can be explained in no other way.

The speech learning process in other deaf-mutes who may achieve some limited speech by specific methods of training differs from that of the normal individual. In such cases visual and tactile association-images rather than the acoustic imagery may act as the initial links in the chain of the psychic reflex-arc. If such a deaf-mute achieves fairly adequate speech, even he may later become the victim of aphasia. Such an aphasia might be motor, sensory, or conduction in form, depending upon the location of the involvement.

But only in motor aphasia is the location of the lesion in the deaf-mute identical with that in normals, namely in the frontal area of the brain. This is well supported by the available evidence. In sensory aphasia the tactile and visual imagery areas c and d, as designated in Figure 4, may be lost.

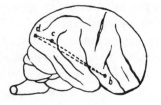

Figure 4.

Their anatomic locations are not yet well defined but are definitely not identical with the imagery of the first temporal lobe.

In conduction aphasia there must be disruption of the fiber tracts connecting the frontal lobe with the temporo-occipital area in the medullary tract of the hemisphere, particularly the superior longitudinal fasciculus of Burdach.

Further description of these three situations which may occur in deaf-muteness would be redundant. One might just point out that in deaf-muteness with sensory aphasia, an asymbolia (Finkelnburg) is inevitably present, and therefore the picture may become more complex and difficult to recognize. Pathological studies of such deaf-mutes as well as of those previously described would be of great value in formulating a model of aphasia.

Let us now consider the concept of asymbolia, not from the standpoint of our rather limited definition, but as Finkelnburg has described it. One of Finkelnburg's patients was no longer able to recognize familiar persons or places. The other presented impairment in comprehension of the spoken word. She confused various actions and no longer crossed herself during table-prayer. The third patient suffered tactile confusion and was no longer able to read music. The fourth, as frequently occurs in aphasia, no longer recognized different coins. In the fifth case, the symbols of worship, of state service, and forms of social convention were no longer familiar. Asymbolia, based on such case studies, might be defined as failure in recognition of the significance of objects and actions. Cases 4 and 5 are not particularly striking, since a large percentage of the mentally ill demonstrate these same symptoms in their confused condition. Such symptoms may also accompany defects of intelligence.

The interpretation which is most damaging to the doctrine of aphasia is that which emphasizes the secondary intellectual deficits which often accompany aphasia as the primary feature of the symptom-picture. This type of error might be compared to the mistake of relating loss of consciousness occurring in an apoplectic attack to destruction of the lenticular nucleus. If our consideration of asymbolia is restricted to Finkelnburg's first example, we may formulate a suitable definition of this syndrome.[8] Asymbolia might then be described as a reduction or loss of the visual memory images of an object, or as the loss of a memory image essential for the conceptualization of the object. We cannot completely rule out the possibility of intellectual disturbance, but we have observed at least one form of circumscribed intellectual defect, the diagnosis of which — just like that of aphasia — was based on a focal brain lesion. In order to express myself even more clearly, I must take up a related topic which was mentioned earlier.

The spoken or written name of an object does not impart new qualities to the object. Therefore, it must be clearly differentiated from the unique sensory memory images of the object. The concept is fashioned only from the latter.

The concept of a "bell", for example, is formed by the associated memory images of visual, tactile and auditory perceptions. These memory images represent the essential characteristic features of the object, bell. The spoken word "bell" is not the same as the auditory perception which calls up the picture of a bell, and there is even less similarity between the written characters and the picture of a bell. Only the most primitive writing systems, such as hieroglyphics, might provide an exception to this. The importance of preserving a distinction between the two is therefore clear. Impairments of the concept, of the elements involved in thought processes, are always impairments of the intellect. Impairments of speech, on the other hand, reflect only an interference in the use of the conventional tools used in communicating ideas.

Some new studies on aphasia*

In my first work on aphasia I took pains to show that in such an interpretation of the speech process as has been reviewed above, we had probably found the scheme of cortical function as a whole, that memory images were the psychic elements populating the cortex in a mosaic-like arrangement as functional development, which may very well be localized according to the regions of the nerve-endings, so that the acoustic images find their abode within the cortical terminals of the acoustic nerve; the visual images, within the cortical endings of the optic nerve; and the olfactory images in that of the olfactory nerve; and so on. Likewise, the motor memory images or movement-representation could be located in the cortical sites of the motor nerve origins. For example, the images of speech movements would then be found in Broca's gyrus and those of writing within the cortical area serving arm movements, etc. Apart from that I assumed only that the discharge-sites of voluntary movements and the depository of motor images were identical. Any higher psychic process, exceeding these mere primary assumptions, could not, I reasoned, be localized, but rested on the mutual interaction of these fundamental psychic elements mediated by means of their manifold connections via the association fibers. Since that time I have become even more strongly convinced, particularly on the basis of clinical studies of aphasia, that nothing warrants our going beyond this elementary hypothesis.

Now, before undertaking a discussion of the work of Lichtheim, the author who has been the most consistent in his support of our own theory, and who has, as I am bound to recognize, carried it further with great perspicacity, I must first explain to the reader my interpretation of the term "concept".

It can be readily seen that our interest in the speech mechanism, at least in the light of present knowledge, lies particularly in its role as an

---

* Translated from "Einige neuere Arbeiten über Aphasie", *Fortschritte der Medizin* 3 (1885); 824-830; 4 (1886) 371, 463. Reprinted in "*C. Wernicke Gesammelte Aufsätze und kritische Referate zur Pathologie des Nervenssysteme.*", Berlin: Fischer, pp. 96-97 (1893)

agent of consciousness. As was indicated at the conclusion of my last discussion, the cerebral hemispheres *in toto*, as the organ of consciousness, function as the foreman of the motor speech center *b* in spontaneous speech production. Likewise, the organ of consciousness *in toto* receives the message which is first transmitted to the sensory speech center at *a*, functioning as a receiving station for acoustic messages. Therefore, it would seem that further localization within this single organ of consciousness is not the issue here. But as soon as we wish to point to a concrete example as a test of our schema, we can find other, more comforting results. For example, how might the process involved in comprehension and spontaneous expression of the word "bell" be explained? If we are to comprehend this word, the concept of a bell must be aroused within us by the telegram which has reached center *a*. The acoustic message must stimulate the memory images of a bell which are deposited in the cortex and located according to the sensory organs. These would then include the acoustic imagery aroused by the sound of the bell, visual imagery established by means of form and color, tactile imagery acquired by cutaneous sensation, and finally, motor imagery gained by exploratory movements of the fingers and eyes. Close association between these various memory images has been established by repeated experience of the essential features of bells. As a final result, arousal of each individual image is adequate for awakening the concept as a whole. In this way a functional unit is achieved. Such units form the concept of the object, in this case a bell. Thus when a spoken word is understood and provokes thought, these units are in a sense a second station, accessible to our own recognition, in the total activity of the hemispheres, a station which must be passed through if the spoken word is not to die away in our ears without having been understood. Moreover, our consciousness makes uses of this same station when the word "bell" is to be articulated spontaneously, i.e., as the result of what may be highly complex processes within our consciousness.

The first stage in this process then consists of the arousal of the concept of the object, "bell", and the second, the process of transmission to the pertinent motor memory images in *b*, the site involved in dispatch of the message. A schematic illustration of this process is indicated in the diagram in Figure 5, in which *B* represents the concept of the object bell. The reader may find a very similar diagram in Lichtheim's work.

In the same way, if we attempt to construct the concept of the word or "symbol" as the name of an object is often called, such as that of the word

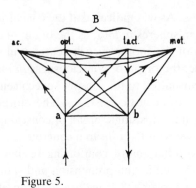

Figure 5.

"bell", we find that, completely analogous to the object itself, it consists of the relevant firmly associated memory images in *a* and *b*. These speculations then may suggest differentiation of speech comprehension into two stages, namely, 1) the arousal of the concept of the word and 2) arousal of the concept of the corresponding object. The same process occurs in spontaneous speech, but in the reverse order, with the concept of the object emerging first, followed by that of the word.

The brief digression in regard to the concept of the word or symbol might seem unnecessary. However, we have an immediate need to use it. For we shall have to examine the extent to which such word-concepts are indivisible unities. Pathological research yields two lines of evidence relevant to this problem. If center *b* is destroyed, speech comprehension may remain completely intact; in other words, the acoustic imagery of the word is adequate for arousal of the concept of the object. If, however, center *a* is damaged, the independence of center *b* can be seen in the continued production of spontaneous speech. The latter, however, is characterized by inconsistent word-choice, with symptoms of word-transposition or paraphasia. Therefore, preservation of the word-concept is of greater significance in the active phase of the speech process than in the passive. Or, translated into terms of our schema, the association between the acoustic word image and the concrete object is firm and independent, but that between the object-concept and the pertinent motor word image is more fragile and not adequate to ensure accurate speech production. Presence of the word-concept in its entirety is necessary for production of spontaneous speech. This finding, gleaned from pathological studies, is comprehensible if understood in the light of the mechanisms involved in speech acquisition.

Undoubtedly the first knowledge of language which the child acquires consists of the comprehension of words, the association of acoustic images with concepts of concrete objects, while in many cases a further period of years is necessary for the development of the faculty of active speech. A preliminary stage of the latter is the ability, by using the association pathway a-b, to imitate the speech sounds heard. On this basis I hypothesize that centrifugal innervation of the word-concept from the area (of sensory perception) of the concrete object follows a double path, namely the simple path B-b and the more complicated route B-a-b. If a portion of the latter is disrupted in any place, incomplete activation of the word-concept will be reflected in the transposition of words. In this matter I differ with Lichtheim, who explains these facts in another way.

According to his interpretation, arousal of the acoustic images is effected by the pathway B-b-a, but the influence of acoustic imagery on correct activation of speech production is first effected by the circuitous route a-B-b. In this interpretation Lichtheim assumes loss of the voluntary internal hearing of words experienced by patients who have sustained damage to center b, so that the voluntary innervation of a would have to pass through b. And, in fact, although good comprehension is evident, such patients are unable to indicate the number of syllables contained in the names of objects presented. This procedure is recommended by Lichtheim for testing the ability to voluntarily activate the acoustic imagery in aphasic patients. However, I do not regard this as decisive evidence for acceptance of his interpretation. These facts may be satisfactorily explained by recognition of the significance of pathway B-b and the inadequacy of path B-a for voluntary innervation of the word-concept itself. I believe that the later-acquired ability of analysis of words into syllables can probably occur only by means of the word-concept itself. Therefore, under certain conditions, it seems quite plausible that the pathway B-a may transmit centrifugally, i.e., bidirectionally, as is true of most association tracts, since voluntary mimicry is still intact in certain pathological cases demonstrating loss of spontaneous speech. And how shall the voluntary impulse reach center b if not by way of B-a-b? Later we shall offer still further applications of these preliminary observations.

If we now return to our original diagram and consider it in relation to a concept center, which for the sake of simplicity we shall reduce to point B, and if we also restrict the scope of aphasic symptoms to all such cases of speech disturbance in which the concept of the object itself is preserved,

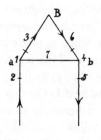

Figure 6.

damage to the centers under question and their various conduction paths would yield seven different forms of aphasia.

Let us enumerate the causes of these, using Lichtheim's model but changing the order.

1. Damage to center *a*.
2. Disruption of the acoustic path ending in *a*.
3. Disruption of the centripetal pathway between *a* and the concept center.

Forms 1-3 constitute the group of sensory aphasias.

4. Damage to center *b*.
5. Disruption of the motor speech pathway.
6. Disruption of the centrifugal pathway *B-b*.

Forms 4-6 constitute the group of motor aphasias.

7. Conduction aphasia (Previously recognized by us).

For the sake of facilitating scientific understanding, I now should like to settle the problem of nomenclature. Lichtheim, who earlier supported use of the original terms, sensory and motor aphasia, has abandoned them in his present work and recommends application of the term aphasia to forms 4, 5, and 6 only, with the following subclassifications.

4. Nuclear aphasia.
5. Peripheral conduction aphasia.
6. Central conduction aphasia.

He would apply the name speech deafness or logokophosis to the forms 1-3, again including subgroups:

1. Nuclear speech deafness.
2. Peripheral conduction speech deafness.
3. Central conduction speech deafness.

He proposes the term conduction paraphasia for type 7.

It is my feeling that the appropriateness of this nomenclature must certainly be questioned. It seems ill-advised to impose a new, narrower meaning on the well-established, widely accepted concept of aphasia, which already embraces all of these forms. Moreover, the application to the cortex of a term like "nuclear" — a term which should be limited to the nuclei of the cranial nerves and their analogues — seems inappropriate to me and is moreover anatomically incorrect. Finally, it seems to me misleading to draw a single symptom such as paraphasia into the nomenclature of distinct forms, since it belongs to several forms at once.

For these reasons, I would propose preserving the older terms motor, sensory, and conduction aphasia, and choosing relevant additions according to whether the cortical centers *a* and *b* themselves, or the conduction pathways on either side of them are destroyed. The adjectives *cortical* and *subcortical* have been in use for a long time, and the only new word needed is *transcortical*, a word that must be created anyway.

The following nomenclature of aphasia may then be formulated.

1. Cortical sensory aphasia.
2. Subcortical sensory aphasia.
3. Transcortical sensory aphasia.
4. Cortical motor aphasia.
5. Subcortical motor aphasia.
6. Transcortical motor aphasia.
7. Conduction aphasia.

Later I shall return to the objection which Lichtheim has raised in regard to preservation of the old terminology.

The critical point of Lichtheim's work lies in proof of the actual existence of his seven forms. I can only agree with that writer's comment that the general validity of my original simple diagram has yet to be subjected to such a test. I am also in complete agreement with him as regards the didactic value of the diagram when completed this way.

In regard to the delineation and clinical description of the individual forms, Lichtheim considers inclusion of the associated disturbances in written language to be necessary to a study of the entire clinical picture. In my opinion, this hinders agreement on the main argument, namely, recognition of the seven different types of speech disturbance. For the present I shall disregard the area of written language and return to it later in greater detail.

1.   Cortical sensory aphasia is characterized by lack of comprehension of speech and inability to repeat it. However, the patient is able to speak spontaneously, and while vocabulary is unmlimited, it is characterized by frequent word-transposition, that is, paraphasia. See Figure 6.

2.   Subcortical sensory aphasia presents the same lack of comprehension of the spoken word and the same impairment in word mimicry. Spontaneous speech, however, is fully maintained, because the word-concept remains intact.

This type of aphasia forms the basis of Lichtheim's chief argument against retention of the current nomenclature, as strictly speaking it is not aphasia inasmuch as speech is totally unimpaired. However, if one regards comprehension as a part of the speech process, constituting its passive stage — a view which seems valid to me and is held by the *French authorities* — and furthermore, if comprehension is regarded as a stage which can only be separated from the total process artificially, then one certainly cannot challenge this use of the term aphasia. Moreover, each clinical symptom-complex may include certain borderline cases, which can be accommodated under the nomenclature only with great difficulty. And exactly the same objection applies, as I shall demonstrate, to Lichtheim's nomenclature when it is used for another form.

A second point which must be raised here is of a purely personal nature. In my controversy with Kussmaul,[9] I did not condone use of the term "speech deafness" to designate that same clinical picture which I had earlier named "sensory aphasia". The usage of this term was based on the clinical material available. At that time I knew of no adequately studied case presenting isolated speech deafness without the symptom of word-confusion or paraphasia. Nor did Kussmaul at the time have one at hand, and I regard it as greatly to Lichtheim's credit that he has examined such a case more closely and put it in the proper light. Since that time I myself have had the opportunity to study a very clear-cut case of this kind, which shall soon be reported in the journal of my clinic. Thus, I now recognize that in certain rare cases isolated speech deafness does indeed occur; I have never doubted the theoretical possibility of its occurrence.

3. Transcortical sensory aphasia. Impairment in comprehension of speech with preservation of the ability to repeat it. Symptoms of paraphasia are evident in spontaneous speech. See Figure 6.

It will be agreed that the features of forms 1-3 are complete without having to consider disorders of written language. The assumption in all cases of sensory aphasia is that common deafness is not the basis of the lack of comprehension.

4. Cortical motor aphasia. Speech comprehension is intact, but the patient presents either muteness or a vocabulary limited to a few words. Spontaneous speech and repeating as well as the voluntary mental sounding out of the word are not possible.

5. Subcortical motor aphasia. This form is differentiated from the preceding type by the complete integrity of the word-concept. See Figure 6. The muteness is the same as that found in type 4. The patient is able to indicate the number of syllables [contained in a word corresponding to an object presented to him].

6. Transcortical motor aphasia. This is the form on which Lichtheim's nomenclature founders. He interprets this type as aphasia in spite of retained ability to speak, which, however, is restricted to repeating. There is loss of spontaneous speech but no evidence of impairment in speech comprehension.

Of these three forms of motor aphasia, only the differentiation between forms 4 and 5, i.e., cortical and subcortical motor aphasia, presents problems which demand a critical discussion of written language. This function, writing, to anticipate a bit, is impaired in the first form, cortical motor aphasia, and is intact in the second, subcortical motor aphasia. Transcortical motor aphasia, however, may be identified without this feature. The cause of muteness in motor aphasia does not lie in paralysis of the speech musculature, just as common deafness is not the basis for impaired comprehension in sensory aphasia.

7. Conduction aphasia is primarily characterized by negative symptoms. If motor or sensory aphasia is not evident, but speech is paraphasic, presenting word-transposition, one may predict a disturbance in conduction between centers *a* and *b*.

I shall return later to the problem of so-called amnesic aphasia. This type is not related to the aphasia forms just reviewed, but is rather concerned with an actual disturbance of memory.

Notes

1.   Should not mimicry, originating as a reflex process culminating in perfected performance by man, reflect the same innate, refined reflex capacity characteristic of all sensory areas? This feature differentiates us from all other animals, especially the closely related ape. Actually many imitative movements of an involuntary nature are also present in adults. In how much greater measure would one expect to find this in adulthood, by which time the intellect has strongly developed its controlling effect on reflex activity.

2.   Two such cases, in which the perforation had been made in the living child, have been reported by Dr. Grossmann, assistant in the Obstetric Clinic. The autopsy studies were carried out by Dr. Waldeyer.

3.   I am convinced that Meynert's error is justifiable, having reviewed his dissections. But many who reproach him for the error would not support him so openly.

4.   This point shall be demonstrated later.

5.   The question concerning the unilateral position of the speech center will not be considered any further here. See Simon, Wilks, and Broadbent (the latter two after Canstadt's *Jahresbericht*, 1872).

6.   See Meynert's ingenious interpretation of cerebral circulation in his "Bau der Grosshirnrinde" (1867).

7.   See below the cases of Beckmann and Kunschkel. Of all areas under consideration, the left optic tract lies closest to the island.

8.   In order that we may correctly utilize Finkelnburg's case study, we assume the right of applying the term asymbolia also to the essential tactile, auditory, images, etc.

9.   Wernicke, 1885 (see selected bibliography)

References

Lichtheim, L. 1885. "Über Aphasie". *Deutsches Archiv für Klinische Medizin* 36: 204-268.

Lichtheim, L. 1885. "On Aphasia". *Brain* 7:433-484.

Meynert, Th. 1867. "Die Bau der Gross-Hirnrinde und seine örtlichen Verschiedenheiten, nebst einem pathologisch-anatomischen Corollarium. *Vierteljahrschrift für Psychiatrie* 1: 77-93.

Wernicke, C. 1885. "Einige neuere Arbeiten über Aphasie". *Fortschritte der Medizin* 3:824-830; 4 (1886) 371-377; 463-469. Reprinted in C. Wernicke. *Gesammelte Aufsätze und kritische Referate zur Pathologie des Nervensystems*. Berlin: Fischer, 1983.

Henry Charlton Bastian

Introduced by

JOHN C. MARSHALL
*Neuropsychology Unit, The Radcliffe Infirmary,
Oxford, Great Britain*

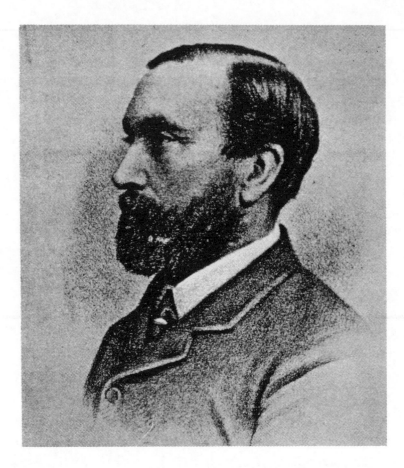

Henry Charlton Bastian
1837-1915

Biography

Born in 1837, in Truro, Cornwall, Henry Charlton Bastian studied medicine at University College, London, where he was awarded his M.B. in 1863 and his M.D. in 1866. Bastian briefly held the positions of assistant physician and lecturer in pathology at St. Mary's Hospital until, in 1867, he was appointed professor of pathologic anatomy at University College. A year later he was elected a Fellow of the Royal Society, albeit not for his neurological studies. Bastian had published numerous papers and monographs on parasitology; he had described a hundred new species of free nematodes and investigated their anatomy and physiology. It was this work that led to his election to F.R.S. in 1868 at the age of 31.

1868 also marks the beginning of Bastian's long association as physician with the National Hospital, Queen Square. In 1887 he vacated the chair of pathology at University College in order to take up the chair of clinical medicine there. He retired from the latter position in 1893, but retained his appointment as full physician at University College Hospital until 1897 and at Queen Square until 1902. As a physician and teacher, Bastian devoted his attention primarily to neurology, and attained early, and lasting, prominence for his contributions to the clinical neurology of higher mental functioning. Yet, during his lifetime, his greatest fame (some would say infamy) was the result of his studies of the origin of life. Bastian was a firm believer in abiogenesis, the spontaneous creation of life from non-living materials. He denied categorically the then current doctrine of Omne vivum ex vivo. *During the heyday of Tyndall, Pasteur, and Lister, these views, combined with a belief in heterogenesis (the theory that, in lower organisms, one life form can appear as the offspring of another quite distinct type) did little to further Bastian's reputation in general biology. On one notable occasion at the first International Congress of Medicine in London in 1881, he suffered an honourable defeat, his lecture flanked by those of Lord Lister and Louis Pasteur. Until his death, Bastian continued to publish extensive monographs on his experiments in which, in sealed glass tubes, ammonium phosphate, phosphoric acid and sodium silicate, under varying light and temperature conditions, would purportedly give rise to micro-organisms. Bastian's obituary in* The British Medical Journal *(November 27, 1915) reports that, in the opinion of many, "there was something pathetic in the persistence" with which Bastian clung to his views after the success of the bacteriological theory. But the obituary concludes "... for himself there was nothing of pathos in his*

*position; he deeply resented, as was natural, the indifference or ridicule
which his opinions encountered, but he never for a moment indulged in self-
pity. His intellect burned with too clear a flame".*

Selected Bibliography

Bastian, H.C. 1869a. "On the various forms of loss of speech in cerebral disease".
British and Foreign Medical and Chirurgical Review 43: 209-236; 470-492.
———. 1869b. "The physiology of thinking". *Fortnightly Review* 5: 57-71
———. 1880. *The Brain as an Organ of Mind.* London: Kegan Paul.
———. 1887. "On different kinds of aphasia, with special reference to their classification and ultimate pathology". *British Medical Journal* 2: 931-936; 985-990.
———. 1897a. "On some problems in connexion with aphasia and other speech
defects". *The Lancet* 1: 933-942; 1005-1017; 1131-1137; 1187-1194.
———. 1897b. "On a case of amnesia and other speech defects of eighteen years' duration with autopsy". *Medical and Chirurgical Transactions* 80: 61-86.
———. 1898. *Aphasia and Other Speech Defects.* London: H.K. Lewis.

Introduction

After his death, Bastian's reputation in neurology was assailed by scepticism. Bastian was, of course, a localisationist. He argued, as Head writes, that

> all high-grade disorders of speech are due either to the destruction of the auditory and visual centres, or to some affection of the fibres transmitting impressions between them and the lower motor mechanism for the tongue and lips, or for the hand in writing. (Head, 1926, Vol. 1, p. 56)

Head's scathing view of this enterprise that "inevitably led to the production of a diagram" is well known:

> As each case arose, it was lopped and trimmed to correspond with a lesion of some cortical centre or hypothetical path. (Head, 1926, Vol. 1, p. 56)

The accuracy of Head's judgement should be assessed against the detailed reports of patients with aphasia that Bastian presents in the text in which he summed up some thirty years of clinical experience (Bastian, 1898). The unprejudiced reader will, I think, be impressed by Bastian's careful testing and his openness to the range of individual variation shown from patient to patient, an openness that had earlier resulted in the first convincing descriptions of "word-deafness" and "word-blindness" (Bastian, 1869a). Likewise, his willingness to admit to error and publish a full report of a patient who did not fit his theory (Bastian, 1879b) scarcely merits the sarcasm with which Head greets the case. And, on the whole, the passage of time has vindicated Bastian's position while leaving Head as an isolated eccentric in the history of aphasiology.

Thus, rather than dismissing the diagram-makers wholesale, it might be more profitable to consider how Bastian, from his earliest writings on aphasia (Bastian, 1869 a and b), was led to formulate the *general* picture of central nervous system functioning that Head found so objectionable.

Although the influence of Gall is denied by Zangwill (1971), there can still be little doubt that *part* of the diagram-makers' paradigm is derived from the phrenologists' postulate of distinct mental organs located in discrete cortical areas. We should not forget the *full* title of Bouillaud's influential paper of 1825: "Recherches cliniques propres à démontrer que la perte de la parole correspond à la lésion des lobules antérieurs du cerveau, et à confirmer l'opinion de M. Gall sur le siège de l'organe du langage articulé". Nor should we forget that Broca always spoke of 'a phrenology of the convolutions', and specifically credited Gall as the prime mover of the "scientific revolution" that proclaimed "the great principle of cerebral localization" (Riese, 1936).

Bastian's admiration for Broca's role is considerable:

> The modern interest in, and development concerning aphasia and other speech defects dates from the publication of certain memoirs by Broca, some six and thirty years since .... The publication of his cases and conclusions formed the starting point for a whole new series of investigations, whose result has been a remarkable development in our knowledge of the localization of functions in the cerebral cortex. (Bastian, 1897a, p. 933)

His attitude to Gall and Spurzheim, however, is that they "were enthusiasts who attempted to systematize an extremely complex subject prematurely" (Bastian, 1880, p. 517). The price they paid for being premature antiholists, Bastian thought, was that:

> The 'system of Phrenology' of Gall and Spurzheim was, therefore, fallacious in almost every respect. It was altogether defective in its psychological analysis, eminently unsatisfactory in its localizations, and was, in short, as unreliable in its methods as it was inconclusive in its results. (Bastian, 1880, p. 520)

Yet neither Bastian's clinical experience of the patterns of impaired and preserved performance after focal lesion of the brain, nor his theoretical analysis of cerebral anatomy, would permit Bastian to espouse an anti-localizationist position. "Are we", he asks rhetorically, "to run into the opposite extreme, and subscribe to such doctrines as those put forth by Flourens?" (Bastian, 1880, p. 520). His answer is a clear 'No!':

> We know that the Olfactory, the Optic, and the Auditory Nerves, each go to different parts of the Brain, so that the primary processes in relation with the exercise of the corresponding Senses are distinct from one another. Can we believe that in their later or higher phases the tracts for such impressions lose their distinctness? Again, I touch the table at which I am now writing, with my forefinger: the impression thus produced travels by means of nerve fibres along a perfectly definite route from the part touched to my Spinal Cord. Can I doubt that the route by which it reaches

the Brain is just as definite (though not so well known), and that a similar impression would always follow the same route, so long as the conducting channels remained uninjured? In some such sense as this 'localization' would seem to be a simple à priori necessity. But if it holds good for Sensorial Operations it will be equally likely to obtain for Intellectual Operations and Emotions. Order and regularity could scarcely be absent in the carrying on of the functions of those parts of the Brain alone, where, from the subtle nature and multiplicity of the molecular actions involved in myriads of cells and fibres, these particular characteristics of lower Brain-actions would seem to be so prominently needful. (Bastian, 1880, pp. 521-522)

The passage is an interesting prefiguring of Geschwind's reflection that the concept of disconnection is "une idée banale mais importante" (Geschwind, 1974). And it echoes, without acknowledgment, Gall's original argument against the holists:

Most philosophers, it is true, find it ridiculous that the various psychic talents and concepts should be thought to have their seat in different parts of the brain. But if this is ridiculous, then it is ridiculous also that the different senses are located in different parts of the body, that our several parts feel in different ways ... for sight and hearing are just as much psychic talents as are the different kinds of ideas. (Gall, 1791)

Nonetheless, Zangwill has argued that the influence of Gallist ideas upon the early English diagram-makers was minimal:

The concept of a 'centre' arose from the altogether more respectable concept of reflex action, as it had been developed in 19th century neurology. At bottom, a 'centre' is simply "what is central" — the C. in C.N.S. Ferrier (1876) for example, refers to the brain and spinal cord as the 'cerebro-spinal centres' and points out that both the spinal cord as a whole and also its component segments are capable of a degree of independent action entirely comparable to that of a primitive invertebrate nervous system. These activities, of course, are wholly reflex and their central sectors may be defined as the 'centres' for the corresponding acts. (Zangwill, 1971, p. 54)

Zangwill's remarks have considerable validity. Certainly, Bastian's emphasis upon cell-circuit physiology enabled him to formulate the distinction between "punctate", "topographical" localization and distributed localization in a remarkably lucid fashion:

The fundamental question of the existence, or not, of real 'localizations' of function (after some fashion) in the brain must be kept altogether apart from another secondary question, which, though usually not so much

> attended to, is no less real and worthy of our separate attention. It is this: Whether, in the event of 'localization' being a reality, the several mental operations or faculties are dependent (a) upon separate areas of brain-substance, or (b) whether the 'localization' is one characterized by mere distinctness of cells and fibres which, however, so far as position is concerned, may be interblended with others having different functions. Have we, in fact, to do with *topographically separate areas of brain-tissue* or merely with *distinct cell and fibre mechanisms existing in a more or less diffuse and mutually interblended manner?* (Bastian, 1880, p. 522)

It is consistent with Bastian's belief in "diffuse and mutually interblended" localization ("the latter kind of arrangement seems, on the whole, to be an even more probable one than the former...") that his most famous aphasia-diagram (Bastian, 1887) is presented as an abstract psychological model without commitment as to the anatomic loci where the functions of the centres and tracts are realized. That is, the diagram is *not* drawn on a schematic representation of the left hemisphere (see Morton, 1984 for an acute analysis of such models).

A representative diagram illustrating the relative positions of the different word-centres and the mode in which they are connected by commissures is shown in Figure 1 (p. 118). The connections indicated by dotted lines indicate possible but less habitual routes for the passage of stimuli.

In other works (e.g., Bastian, 1897a, 1898), Bastian *did* draw small, punctate, unifunctional centres and thin commissures across pictures of the human brain. How he reconciled *these* diagrams with his beliefs about functional neuroanatomy is a mystery that aphasia scholarship has not yet solved.

If Bastian's underlying assumptions are indeed derived from sensory–motor physiology and from reflexology, the question arises of how 'higher', 'mental' functions will fare within this framework. As Zangwill phrases the problem:

> It is when we turn to the activities of the cerebral hemispheres, however, that the concept of a centre ceases to be governed by purely physiological conceptions, and becomes, so to speak, contaminated by psychology. (Zangwill, 1971, p. 54)

And somewhat earlier, Freud has puzzled over the same issue:

> Is it justified to immerse a nerve fibre, which over the whole length of its course has been only a physiological structure subject to physiological

> modifications, with its end in the psyche and furnish this end with an idea or memory? (Freud, 1891)

Bastian, in common with practically all the nineteenth-century diagram-makers (English, French, and German), took the bull by the horns. He argued that "we think in words" and that "these words become nascent in consciousness primarily and perhaps principally as revived auditory impressions" (Bastian, 1869a).

This 'proto-behaviourist' position is not unique to diagram-makers. It can be found in exceptionally explicit form in Hughlings Jackson but with greater emphasis upon the reduction of ideas to motoric processes:

> It is asserted by some that the cerebrum is the organ of mind, and that it is not a *motor* organ. Some think that the cerebrum is to be likened to an instrumentalist, and the motor centres to the instrument; one part is for ideas, and the other for movements. It may then be asked, how can discharge of part of a *mental* organ produce *motor* symptoms only? [...] But of what 'substance' can the organ of mind be composed, unless of processes representing movements and impressions; and how can the convolutions differ from the inferior centres, except as parts representing more intricate co-ordinations of impressions and movements in time and space than they do? [...] What can an 'idea' say of a ball be, except a process representing certain impressions of surface and particular muscular adjustments? [...] Surely the conclusion is irresistible, that 'mental' symptoms from disease of the hemisphere are fundamentally like hemiplegia, chorea, and convulsions, however specially different. They must all be due to lack, or to disorderly development, of sensori-motor processes. (Jackson, 1870, p. 163)

Indeed, until very recently, the only neuropsychologist who did not subscribe to this view was Gall.

The behaviourist position derives, of course, from the English empiricist and associationist tradition, with which Bastian was extremely familiar (see chapter 26 of Bastian, 1880), but shorn, as it were, of Ideas with a capital I. As William James was quick to spot, the theoretical apparatus of associationism was ideally (perhaps too ideally) suited for grafting onto cells and axons:

> If we make a symbolic diagram on the blackboard of the laws of association between ideas, we are inevitably led to draw circles, or closed figures of some kind, and to connect them by lines. When we hear that the nerve centres contain cells which send off fibres, we say that Nature has realized our diagram for us, and that the mechanical substratum of thought is plain. In some way, it is true our diagram must be realized in the brain, but surely in no such visible and palpable way as we at first suppose. (James, 1891, p. 81)

I am accordingly inclined to believe that it was associationism that determined the structure of Bastian's diagram-making to a far greater extent than did either Gall's theories or reflexology *per se*. Buckingham (1984) provides an excellent review of the relationships between association theory and connection theory in the development of early models of the aphasias. Certainly, the account of language acquisition that Bastian gives in *The physiology of thinking* is pure Watson:

> The young infant first begins to distinguish natural objects from one another by differences in shape, colour, touch, odour, etc., which these may present to its different senses; it is then taught (slowly and with difficulty) to associate some object possessing certain combined attributes by which it is remembered, with a certain articulate *sound* which has been often repeated whilst the object is pointed at, till by dint of continual repetition this sound (or word) becomes to be identified with the various attributes of the object that, when heard, it invariably recalls to memory the object of which it may now be said to form a kind of additional attribute, just as the sight or touch of the object will in turn call up the memory of the *sound* which has first been employed as its designation. (Bastian, 1869b)

Indeed, so firmly does Bastian seem to be located within the associationist tradition that it comes as a very considerable shock to read his views on the role of the developing nervous system in language acquisition:

> Speech has now become a truly automatic act for human beings, and that if children do not speak at birth this is in the main due to the fact that their nervous systems are still too immature. (Bastian, 1880, p. 607)

What, one wonders, would be the language spoken by an overdue baby? But then, developmental psycholinguistics has rarely been overconcerned with logical consistency.

Associationism had, of course, loomed large in English works on aphasia ever since the eighteenth century. Thus, for example, Crichton's discussion of word-finding difficulties concludes that:

> this very singular defect of memory ought rather to be considered as a defect of that principle, by which ideas, and their proper expressions, are associated. (Crichton, 1789)

Later, one of Bastian's contemporaries, William Ogle, began to classify the agraphias into "amnesic" and "atactic" varieties on the basis of where the chain of association from concept to graphic execution was broken or perturbed (Ogle, 1871).

It was Bastian, however, who provided the most thorough-going and wide-ranging analysis. The basic distinction he drew is between Amnesia Verbale and Aphasia/Agraphia (Bastian, 1880). The first category of disorders (sometimes referred to as amnesia *tout court*, a misleading locution from the point of view of current terminology) covers pathology of the afferent input to the auditory and visual word-centres. And it also includes pathology of the centres themselves. Within the general class of Amnesia Verbale, Bastian further distinguished a "paralytic" and an "incoordinate variety". In the first case, the underlying mechanism is "diminished excitability" of the centres; in the second, it is "perverted activity" of the centres. We thus find a firm distinction between 'blocking', which leads to no response, and either 'overexcitability' or 'misplaced' activity, which leads to paraphasic response. The overall framework is not dissimilar from more recent 'threshold' models of lexical access and retrieval (cf. Morton, 1979). In particular, Bastian differentiated between word-finding difficulty consequent upon "lowered activity" in the "word-centres" themselves ('raised thresholds' in modern terminology) and difficulty due to attenuation of the signals that reach the centres *via* sensation or "association channels" (Bastian, 1897a). These formulations are derived from the distinction that the associationists drew between the distinct faculties of *memory* and *recollection*, and Bastian took over the rather precise account of the responsible 'abstract' mechanisms from Sir William Hamilton. In contradistinction to his early writings, Bastian (1880; 1897b) now wholeheartedly embraces the traditional 'central' concepts of association theory, i.e., Ideas. Thus his overall conception of Amnesia Verbale is that it covers "Defects of verbal memory, that is defects in the associations of ideal things or of conceptions with ideal words" (Bastian, 1880, p. 618).

By contrast, aphasia (and agraphia) are characterized as disorders of the "first parts of outgoing tracts" leading from the cerebral word-centres (auditory and verbal) to their respective executive organs. Aphasia and agraphia are thus, for Bastian, 'central' disconnection disorders. The input from the auditory and visual word-centres leads first, however, to the cheiro- and glosso-kinaesthetic centres. These latter centres which are only in part analogous to the speaking and writing centres of the Wernicke-Lichtheim model are specifically conceived of as 'sensory', not 'motor' organs. That is, their internal code is indeed kinaesthetic; they contain representations of the 'positions' that the vocal and graphic tracts take up in linguistic expression, and those representations are in terms of the sensory

feedback of kinaesthetic information from the executive ('motor') organs.
Finally, Bastian distinguished "aphemia" (and its graphic equivalent),
which in their purest forms are consequent upon damage to the "lower"
(i.e. more peripheral) tracts that lead from the kinaesthetic organs to the
motor centres for articulation and graphic expression. The term "aphemia",
for Bastian, also covers the consequences of damage to the actual motor
centres themselves.

The overall structure of Bastian's theory, then, is similar but not identical to the more familiar Wernicke-Lichtheim model. Bastian drew the
demarcation lines of his taxonomy in slightly different positions; and, more
importantly, provided a clearer justification for the classification in terms of
mechanism.

Although Bastian did, frequently, present the theory as a 'punctate'
diagram, he was not insensitive to the notion of a continuous 'associative'
net that links the discrete areas of primary sensory and motor cortex (cf.
Freud, 1891). Thus he expounded as a "working hypothesis" the idea that:

> the tendency to mental impairment with aphasia, and the degree of such
> impairment, will, other things being equal, increase as lesions of the left
> hemisphere recede in site from the 'left frontal convolution' and approach
> the occipital lobe. (Bastian, 1880, p. 687)

> The direction of the gradient seems to contradict the widespread
> nineteenth century claim that the anterior lobes are especially implicated
> in "the carrying on of intellectual and volitional operations. (Bastian,
> 1880, p. 523)

Bastian, by contrast, was struck by "the special frequency with which
lesions of the Occipital Regions of the Hemispheres are apt to be associated
with marked mental degradation" (Bastian, 1880, p. 687).

The first selection (from the Lumleian lectures of 1897a) contains a
particularly clear exposition of Bastian's associationism. The second selection (Chapter XXX from *The Brain as an Organ of Mind*) provides a summary of Bastian's views, and his thoughts on "further problems" that his
approach raises.

References

Bastian, H.C. 1869a. "On the various forms of loss of speech in cerebral disease".
British and Foreign Medical and Chirurgical Review 43: 209-236; 470-492.

———. 1869b. "The physiology of thinking". *Fortnightly Review* 5: 57-71.

———. 1880. *The Brain as an Organ of Mind*. London: Kegan Paul.

———. 1887. "On different kinds of aphasia, with special reference to their classification and ultimate pathology". *British Medical Journal* 2: 931-936; 985-990.

———. 1897a. "On some problems in connexion with aphasia and other speech defects". *The Lancet* 1: 933-942; 1005-1017; 1131-1137; 1187-1194.

———. 1897b. "On a case of amnesia and other speech defects of eighteen years' duration with autopsy". *Medical and Chirurgical Transactions* 80: 61-86.

———. 1898. *Aphasia and Other Speech Defects*. London: H.K. Lewis.

Bouillaud, J.B. 1825. "Recherches cliniques propes à demontrer que la perte de la parole corresponds à la lésion des lobales antérieures en cerveau". *Archives Générales de Médecine* 8:25-45.

Buckingham, H.W. 1984. "Early development of association theory in psychology as a forerunner to connection theory". *Brain and Cognition* 3: 19-34.

Crichton, A. 1798. *An inquiry into the Nature and Origin of Mental Derangement*. London: Cadel and Davies.

Ferrier, D. 1886. *The Functions of the Brain*. London: Smith, Elder & Co.

Freud, S. 1891. *Zur Auffassung der Aphasien*. Wien: Deuticke.

Gall, F.J. 1791. *Philosophisch-medicinische Untersuchungen über Natur und Kunst im Kranken und gesunden Zustand der Menschen*. Wien: Gräffer.

Geschwind, N. 1974. "Le concept de disconnexion: l'histoire d'une idée banale mais importante". *Les syndromes de Disconnexion calleuse chez l'Homme*, ed. by F. Michel and B. Schott, Lyon: SPCM.

Head, H. 1926. *Aphasia and Kindred Disorders of Speech*. Cambridge: Cambridge University Press.

Jackson, J.H. 1870. "A study of convulsions". *Transactions of the St. Andrews Medical Grad. Association* 3: 162-174.

James, W. 1891. *The Principles of Psychology*. London: Macmillan.

Morton, J. 1979. "Word Recognition". *Psycholinguistics Series*, Vol. 2, ed. by J. Morton and J.C. Marshall, London: Elek.

———. 1984. "Brain-based and non-brain-based models of language". *Biological Perspectives on Language*, ed. by D. Caplan, A.R. Lecours and A. Smith, Cambridge, Mass.: MIT Press.

Ogle, W. 1867. "Aphasia and Agraphia". *St. George's Hospital Reports* 2: 83-122.

Riese, W. 1936. "Les discussions des problèmes des localisations cérébrales dans les sociétés savantes du XIXe siècle et leurs rapports avec des vues contemporaines". *L'Hygiène Mentale* 31:137-158.

Zangwill, O.L. 1971. "Diagram makers old and new". *Totus Homo* 3: 53-58.

Selection from the work of Henry Charlton Bastian

THE LUMLEIAN LECTURES
Some Problems in Connection with Aphasia and other Speech Defects*

The various kinds of word memory

According to Sir William Hamilton, "Memory strictly so denominated is the power of retaining knowledge in the mind, but out of consciousness. I say, retaining knowledge in the mind but out of consciousness, for to bring the *retentum* out of memory into consciousness is the function of a totally different faculty (recollection) ... It is not enough that we possess the faculty of acquiring knowledge and of retaining it in the mind but out of consciousness; we must further be endowed with a power of recalling it out of consciousness into consciousness — in short, a reproductive power (recollection). This reproductive power is governed by the laws which govern the succession of our thoughts — the laws, as they are called, of mental association". This definition of memory implies the notion of an organic change taking place in definite nerve elements on the occurrence of each sensory or intellectual process — that is, the notion of a permanent nervous modification of some kind, plus the possibility of its renewal in more complete form from time to time. We may therefore suppose that on fitting occasions, by the intervention of associational activity, there will be revival in more complete form of something like the original molecular activity in

---

* Delivered before the Royal College of Physicians of London, by H. Charlton Bastian, M.A., M.D. Lond., F.R.S., Censor of the College; Physician to University College Hospital and to the National Hospital for the Paralysed and Epileptic. *The Lancet* 1 (1897) 933-942; 1005-1017; 1131-1137; 1187-1194.

the nervous elements concerned with the primary perceptional or intellectual process of this or that kind. It is not essential that the memorial revival of the sensory impression or of the intellectual process should after multitudinous repetition be associated with any distinct conscious phasis. What Sir William Hamilton termed the *retentum* may, indeed be revived as a mere unconscious nerve action — a link in a perceptive process or in a chain of thought represented merely (as John Stuart Mill put it) by "certain organic states of the nerves". This latter consideration is especially worthy of note from the point of view of the importance of revived kinaesthetic impressions for the guidance of movements, seeing that their revival may be unattended by any distinct conscious phasis; and much the same thing may often be said concerning that memorial recall of words in the auditory centre which immediately precedes speech.

From what has already been said it is evident that "loss of recollection" by no means implies nor is it to be taken as synonymous with "loss of memory". For instance, a patient may be unable to recollect words — that is, spontaneously revive them — for ordinary speech when his memory for such words, nevertheless, exists unimpaired, as may be shown by the fact that the patient is able at once to repeat the words in question when he hears them pronounced or sees them written. His defect, therefore, may consist in a mere lowered activity of the auditory word-centre, in which words are primarily revived during thought. "Loss of recollection" may, in fact, depend upon one or other of two causes: either (a) upon some diminished functional activity — that is, diminished readiness to be roused — in the central nerve mechanisms in which the *retentum* is, so to speak, stored or rendered possible of revival; or else (b) upon some defect in this or that set of commissural fibres (associational channels). "Loss of memory", however, in the strict sense of the term implies disease of, or serious damage to, the central nerve units in which the particular *retentum* is stored up or registered.

Although it is important from a scientific point of view to make such a distinction as has been above pointed out, it will be found both convenient and practical to let the term "amnesia" stand for loss of recollection as well as loss of memory of this or that kind.

From what has been said it follows, that all cases of amnesia (in the broad sense of the term) ought, from an anatomical or localising point of view, to be divided into two generic groups: (a) cases in which there is centric defect (either structural or of marked functional type), with which there will often be loss of memory of words as well as loss of recollection; and (b) cases in which there is merely commisural defect (mostly structural), with which there may be loss of recollection of words, but no necessary loss of word-memory. It will be one of my objects in the present lectures to dwell upon the fact (which I pointed out some ten years ago) that it is often in the case of speech defects extremely difficult, if not impossible, from clinical evidence alone to decide whether the underlying lesion or default leading to a particular kind of amnesia be centric or commissural in seat. And yet from the point of view of the localisation of the lesion such a decision may be a matter of much importance, seeing that if the lesion were centric we should look for it in one part of the brain, while if it were commissural it might be found in a region comparatively remote therefrom.

In the case of words there are three distinct kinds or physiological types of memory to be considered — one of them existing in two forms, so as to make four varieties in all. These varieties of verbal memory are as follows: — 1. Auditory memory: the memory of the sounds of words — that is, of the auditory impressions representative of different words. 2. Visual memory: the memory of the visual appearances (printed or written) of words — that is, of the visual impressions corresponding with different words. 3. Kinaesthetic memory.[1] — (a) the memory of the different groups of sensory impressions resulting from the mere movements of the vocal organs during the utterance of words (impressions from muscles, mucous membranes, and skin) — that is, of the kinaesthetic impressions corresponding with the articulation of different words, which for the sake of brevity I have proposed to speak of as "gloss-kinaesthetic" impressions; and (b) the memory of the different groups of sensory impressions emanating from muscles, joints, and skin, during the act of writing individual letters and words that is of the kinaesthetic impressions corresponding with the writing of different letters and words, which I have for similar reasons proposed to speak of as "cheiro-kinaesthetic" impressions.[2]

The organic seat of each of these four different kinds of word-memory is in relation with its own set of afferent fibres; and the several centres must also be closely connected with one another by commissural or associational fibres, so that the memory of a word or the recollection of a word in one or other of these modes doubtless involves some amount of simultaneously revived activity in one or two of the other word-centres.

The relative intensity or importance (in the process of recollection of words for ordinary speech) of the memorial revival in each of these centres

is probably subject to more or less marked variations in different individuals. In the majority of persons, as I pointed out in 1869, the revival of words
in the auditory centre is the most potential process, and that which occurs
first in order of time. This seems to be now very generally admitted.

The localisation of the different word-centres

Although I am not a believer in the complete topographical distinctness of
the several sensory centres in the cerebral hemisphere, I consider it clear
that there must be certain sets of structurally related cell and fibre
mechanisms in the cortex, whose activity is associated with one or with
another of the several kinds of sensory endowment. Such diffuse but functionally unified nervous networks may differ altogether from the common
conception of a neatly defined "centre", and yet for the sake of brevity it is
convenient to retain this word and refer to such networks as so many
"centres".

Looking to the extremely important part that words, either spoken or
written, play in our intellectual life and to the manner in which they are
interwoven with all our thought-processes, it becomes highly probable that
most important sections of the auditory and the visual sensory centress are
devoted to the reception, and consequently to the revival in thought, of
impressions of words: and for convenience of reference it is permissible to
speak of these portions as auditory and visual "word-centres" respectively.
Similarly, there must be what I have termed kinaesthetic word-centres of
two kinds (the one in relation with speech-movements, and the other with
writing movements) holding a like all-important relation to the expression
of our thought by speech and writing. It is possible that the particular parts
of the general auditory and visual centres which are in relation with word-
impressions may be more or less distinctly defined, like the analogous parts
of the general kinaesthetic centre that are in relation with speech or with
writing movements. Certain it is that there are some varieties of amnesia in
which the part of the visual centre in relation with words seems to be specially at fault (as in "word-blindness"), just as there are other cases in which
the part of the auditory centre in relation with words is either wholly or partially inactive (as where we have to do with different degrees of "word-deafness") — in each case without defect in other parts of the general visual or
auditory centres, as evidenced by the fact that the persons so affected can

still quite well see and recognise ordinary objects, or hear and recognise the nature of ordinary sounds.

In regard to the visual centre as a whole, it seems now to be established that it is more or less diffused through the convolutions on the inner aspect of the occipital lobe and probably even more widely throughout this lobe. The particular part of the visual centre that is most concerned with the appreciation and memorial recall of words — or, in other words, the destruction of which most certainly gives rise to word-blindness — is now fairly well settled. There is much evidence to show that this region corresponds with the angular gyrus either alone or in association with part of the supra-marginal lobule — and therefore that it is situated just beyond the confines of the occipital lobe, and in the region originally assigned by Ferrier, upon the basis of his experiments with monkeys, as the centre for vision as a whole.

In regard to the localisation of the general auditory centre considerable doubt now exists, since the researches of Schäfer and Sanger-Brown do not support Ferrier's allotment of this endowment to the upper temporal convolution. Curiously enough, however, it again happens that the localisation of the part of the general auditory centre most concerned with the appreciation of words (as based upon clinico-pathological evidence in man) must be regarded as being in the posterior half or two-thirds of the upper temporal convolution. The above-mentioned results of Schäfer and Sanger-Brown as to the localisation in monkeys of the general sense of hearing were of a negative character, and cannot be said to afford any definite evidence against this presumption as to the site of the auditory word-centre in man.

The situation of one of the two kinaesthetic word-centres can be rather more certainly localised. Having elsewhere stated very fully my reasons for believing that the so-called "motor centres" of Ferrier and others are really sensory centres of kinaesthetic type by means of which movements are guided,[3] I shall not now attempt to set forth the evidence in favour of this opinion, but shall merely state my belief that Broca's region — namely, the posterior part or foot of the third frontal and the inferior part of the ascending frontal convolutions — is in reality the part of the brain to which I have been alluding as the "glosso-kinaesthetic" centre. The situation of the "cheiro-kinaesthetic" centre cannot be localised with nearly as much confidence. The tendency for some years has been to follow Exner, who believes it to be situated in the posterior part of the second frontal gyrus, though, as we shall see later, the ˙evidence in favour of this localisation is at present extremely scanty. All that can be said on this point, therefore, is that we know approximately where to look for the cheiro-kinaesthetic centre.

For the purpose of our discussion, then, it may for the present be assumed that the two kinaesthetic word-centres are situated as above stated: that the auditory word-centre is situated in the posterior half or two-thirds of the upper temporal convolution; and the visual word-centre in the angular and part of the supra-marginal convolutions. It must also be assumed, upon grounds subsequently to be set forth, that these last-named word-centres are connected together by a double set of commissural fibres. We must likewise suppose that two other important sets of commissural fibres exist between the different word-centres — namely, one set through which the auditory word-centre acts upon the glosso-kinaesthetic centre for the production of speech movements, and another by means of which the visual word-centre acts upon the cheiro-kinaesthetic centre for the production of writing movements.

In the study of speech defects it is therefore necessary to consider the effects of lesions in the following situations: (a) in the different kinds of word-centres; (b) in the different commissures by means of which these centres are connected with one another; (c) in the internuncial fibres connecting the two kinaesthetic word-centres with their related motor-centres, in the bulb and in the cervical region of the spinal cord; and (d) in these motor-centres themselves which are concerned with the actual production

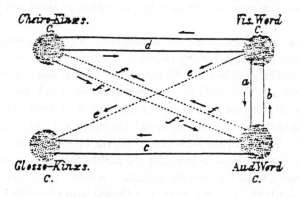

Figure 1. *Diagram showing the approximate sites of the four word-centres and their commissures.*

of speech and writing. But before dealing with any of these problems in detail a few other aspects of the questions relating to word-memory, as well as the modes of activity of the brain in perceptive and speech processes require to be considered.

Further Problems in Regard to the Localization of
Higher Cerebral Functions*

The study of the various defects of Speech, and of Intellectual Expression in general, produced by Cerebral Disease is of great importance in many ways. An accumulation of instances more or less crudely observed must almost necessarily precede the attempt to analyze and classify these various defects. Thereafter observers will work better and with more chance of success in two directions. They will (1) have learned more fully how to observe such cases, that is, what is specially to be looked for in the way of ability or defect in persons so affected; and (2) they may, whenever the precise mental defects manifested during life have been clearly recognized and recorded, as the occasion arises, note with more hope of profitable scientific result the exact region of the Brain which has been damaged.

The error of massing together all the varieties of 'loss of speech' under one name, such as 'Aphasia', and then altogether rejecting doctrines of Cerebral Localization, because the lesions in such dissimilar cases have not always been found in some one part of the Brain, is manifest and absurd, and yet it is one which has been too often repeated in recent years. Even such an accomplished physician as Trousseau spoke of a representative case of Amnesia as a typical instance of Aphasia, and based his explanation of the Aphasic condition a good deal upon the phenomena by which it was characterized. This massing together, under one name, of wholly dissimilar defects, and the confusion thus created, would, of course, so long as it lasted, effectually defeat all attempts at Cerebral Localization.

It is, therefore, absolutely necessary if further advance is to be made in regard to the 'localization' of higher Cerebral Functions, first, that we should learn carefully to discriminate the different Speech-defects from one another during life; and, secondly, that where opportunities occur, the locality of lesions should be principally observed and recorded in typical and uncomplicated cases.

---

* From: H.C. Bastian. *The Brain as an organ of mind*. London: Kegan Paul. 1880. Chapter 3, p. 673-690.

A few brief additional details (beyond those which it has been found convenient to mention in the last chapter) will now be given as to the extent of knowledge already garnered within this second sphere of observation and inference — which, though not at present co-extensive with the other, nevertheless includes some facts of a rather startling description.

In 1825, Bouillaud affirmed that the Frontal Lobes of the Brain were the parts principally concerned with Speech, because, as he said, these were the organs "for the formation and recollection of words, or the principal signs which represent our ideas". He had collected 114 observations of disease of the Frontal Lobes accompanied by loss or defect of Speech, and upon these he based his views.

Andral, however, in 1833, recorded fourteen cases where Speech was abolished without any alteration in the Frontal Lobes, but in which a lesion existed in the Parietal or in the Occipital Lobes.

In 1836 Dr. Marc Dax called attention to the great frequency of loss of Speech in association with right rather than with left-sided Paralysis. The title of his essay was this: — "Lesions of the left half of the Brain coinciding with the loss of memory of the Signs of Thought".[4] In support of this view that loss of Speech depended especially upon lesions of the left half of the Brain, Dr. Dax brought forward 140 observations.

But in 1861, Broca went still further. Whilst affirming, with Dr. Marc Dax, that the left Hemisphere was the one principally concerned with articulate Speech, he precisely defined the seat of lesion in that condition which we now call Aphasia as *"the posterior part of the third frontal convolution of the left hemisphere"*.

This view, originally based upon a very small number of cases, was received at first with the greatest surprise and scepticism. It was thought by many to be most improbable that such a faculty as Speech should depend upon the integrity of one small portion of only one of the two Cerebral Hemispheres. Yet by reason of the observations which have accumulated during the last eighteen years, it is now admitted by most of those who are best entitled to judge, that Broca's localization is in a certain sense correct, and that in the instances of real typical Aphasia the lesion is, in a large majority of cases, found to involve the posterior part of the third frontal gyrus on the left side, or else the immediately subjacent white substance intervening between this convolution and the Corpus Striatum. The reason why lesions in other parts may, according to their situation, either occasionally or invariably lead to a more or less similar Speechless condition, is a question upon which we shall hope to throw additional light in this chapter.

Many cases are on record in which a lesion of the posterior part of the third frontal gyrus of the right Hemisphere has existed, without producing any loss of Speech. So that we have both positive and negative evidence in favour of Broca's association of the power of Articulate Speech with the integrity of the third left *frontal* convolution, especially if we extend the depth of the region cited by him so as to make it include the outgoing fibres from this part of the third frontal gyrus.

It is, however, also true that in a certain small proportion of cases a similar condition of speechlessness has been induced where a lesion has been found in the corresponding parts of the right Hemisphere. In some of these exceptional cases the persons have been left-handed, though in others even this reason for the change of sides has been absent. The writer has himself met with a most typical instance of this. But it is of importance to note that even in these very exceptional cases, though the side affected has been different, Speech has equally been lost by a unilateral damage of the same definite and extremely limited region of the Hemisphere.

Thus it would follow, that the motor incitations sufficing to call the articulatory centres into activity during Speech, are accustomed, in the large majority of cases, to emerge from the third frontal gyrus of the left side: though in a small minority of persons it may happen that the effective motor stimuli are wont to pass off instead from the right third frontal gyrus. The halves of the bilateral Articulatory Centres in the Pons, Medulla, and upper part of the Spinal Cord are so welded together by commissures that each of them practically constitutes one double Centre. And these may (after the manner of such bilateral Centres) be incited to action by stimuli coming through the Corpus Striatum either from the left or from the right Cerebral Hemisphere — though, as a matter of fact, as above stated, such stimuli seem to reach it, in the large majority of persons, from the left side of the Brain.

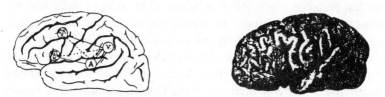

Figure 2. *Brain of a Woman who suffered from Aphasia, showing the traces of a lesion in the posterior part of the third frontal Convolution. (Prevost.) — See Nature*, March 16, 1876, p. 400.

But if bilaterally-acting muscles are always in association with closely welded bilateral Motor Centres, and if such Centres may generally be called into activity by stimuli reaching them from either side or from both sides simultaneously, then the habitual excitation of the Speech Centres and their related muscles from the left side, must be regarded as a remarkable peculiarity.

There is, however, some reason for believing that if the habitual outgoing channels of the left side are damaged (so that Speech has been lost), the route for stimuli from the *right* third frontal gyrus to the corresponding Corpus Striatum may, under certain circumstances, be more effectively opened up, so that the power of Speaking is after a time regained. In such a case the stimuli would, of course, impinge upon the right rather than upon the left side of the lower bilateral Articulatory Centres.

Broadbent indeed maintains that, as a rule, loss of Speech is only temporary with lesions of the left Corpus Striatum, or of those parts of the outgoing fibres from the third frontal gyrus which are contiguous to this body. And he ingeniously attempts to explain its supposed speedy restoration in these cases. If the left third frontal gyrus be itself undamaged, and if the fibres of the Corpus Callosum which extend from it to the right third frontal gyrus be intact, then the outgoing stimuli not being able to take their usual course may, he thinks, find their 'way round' from the left to the right third frontal and thence downwards to the Corpus Striatum of the right side.[5] In these cases loss of Speech would possibly only exist for a few weeks, till the new route and new mode of action could be thoroughly opened up and established. It is difficult, however, to understand how the previous education and organization of this right Corpus Striatum can have been brought up to the stage necessary to enable it speedily to assume such functions, if, to take the most favourable supposition, only feeble and ineffective stimuli have previously been reaching it.

There are difficulties also in the way of the acceptance of some of the reasoning upon which this theory is based.

Broadbent says: — "In its first attempts to talk the child is influenced by imitation and guided by the ear; that is, as the grouping of the motor cells of the cord is effected through the sensory cells, by cell processes passing from the posterior to the anterior nerve nuclei, so the grouping of the cells in the corpus striatum will be effected through the cells of the auditory perceptive centre by means of the fibres connecting together the two ... And, as the motor nuclei of the cord can still be employed in reflex action through the sensory nuclei, as well as in voluntary motion by means of descending fibres from the corpus striatum, *so may the word groups in the corpus striatum be reached imitatively through the auditory perceptive centre, as well as through the third frontal gyrus"*. Consequently he assumes that there is a double action of a consensual character from both Auditory Centres, and that in the early 'imitative' Speech-processes these parts would both react upon their respective Corpora Striata. There is also, as he thinks, a higher or volitional unilateral action through the left third frontal gyrus — an action which is unilateral because, as he puts it, "The left hemisphere alone is educated for intellectual expression".

But, Sensori-motor and Ideo-motor acts of Speech are dependent upon processes occurring (in a slightly different manner) in identically the same cerebral regions — and these would correspond with Broadbent's 'imitative' modes of Speech. Yet, as the writer has previously endeavoured to show (pp. 550-557), no valid demarcation can be established between Ideo-motor and Voluntary acts of Speech, and the distinction conferred upon the latter by the addition of an 'emotion of desire' does not make it the less necessary for the outgoing stimulus primarily to pass off from the Auditory Centre; nor, on the other hand, is there any distinct evidence to show that the incitations in 'imitative' Speech do not, like those in Voluntary Speech, also find their 'way out' through the third frontal gyrus. In fact, we have every reason to believe that the route from the Auditory Perceptive Centre to the Corpus Striatum is one and the same for every kind of Speech, whether its mode of incitation may be strictly 'imitative', Ideo-motor, or distinctly Volitional.

This latter conclusion is found to be in accordance with the evidence derived from disease. No fact has been more certainly established in regard to Aphasic patients, than that there is in them a loss not only of Voluntary, but of Ideo-motor, and, to just as marked an extent, a loss of 'imitative' Speech. A really Aphasic patient cannot copy the simplest word or vowel sound, which he has just heard, nor does he even do it unbidden and echolike, in the most purely imitative reflex style.

Others again have assumed that a separate route exists by which Emotional stimuli may be transmitted to the lower centres for Articulation in the Pons and Medulla, without passing through the Corpus Striatum, simply because aphasic patients occasionally utter new words of an interjectional order — as oaths, or such phrases as 'Oh dear!', 'Thanks!' and other simple exclamations, under the influence of a strong emotional stimulus.

Even for this kind of connection, however, no independent evidence exists (see p. 580); and perhaps the facts can be equally well explained by the supposition that Emotional stimuli of greater energy, or which emanate from a wider area, may occasionally force their way through damaged tracks, the resistance in which could not be overcome by mere Volitional stimuli.

As to the causes which have determined the greater or almost exclusive influence of the left Hemisphere in inciting Speech-movements, only conjectures can be offered. It has been thought that a certain more forward condition of development of the left hemisphere — as a result of hereditary right-handedness recurring through generation after generation — might gradually become sufficient to cause the left Hemisphere to 'take the lead' in the production of Speech-movements. Some little evidence exists — though at present it is very small — to show that it is left-handed people more especially who may become Aphasic by a lesion of the *right* third frontal gyrus. It is practically certain, indeed, that the great preponderance of right-hand movements in ordinary individuals must tend to produce a more complex organization of the left than of the right Hemisphere, and this both in its sensory and its motor regions. We may confidently look for the existence in it of the organic basis of a vastly greater and more complex Tactile experience; and as movements of the right arm and hand are more frequent, both as associated factors of this experience and in other ways, we have also a right to expect that the Kinaesthetic Centres will be similarly developed to a notably greater degree in the left Hemisphere. And as a matter of course also the nervous mechanisms for the movements with which these sensory impressions are associated would be much more complex in the Motor Ganglion of the left than in that of the right Hemisphere.

Many years ago, moreover, the writer ascertained a fact which at the time seemed very difficult to understand — viz., that the specific gravity of the cortical Grey Matter of the Brain in left frontal, parietal, and occipital regions is often distinctly, though slightly, higher than that from corresponding regions of the right Hemisphere.[6] But such an increase in specific gravity might be produced by the existence of the greater number of cells and commissural fibres which the extra sensory and derivative functions above referred to would probably entail.

Having considered some of the questions of 'cerebral localization' relating to the production of Aphemia, Agraphia, and Aphasia, something must now be said in regard to the seat of lesions productive of the very varied conditions comprised under the term Amnesia.

Our knowledge on this point is at present rather vague and indefinite, since it is only quite recently that the necessity of not confounding such cases with Aphasia has been at all generally recognized. Moreover, no distinct attempt has hitherto been made to analyze and classify the various conditions comprised under this one term 'Amnesia'. Much more will doubtless soon be ascertained, in reference to this subject, by future workers, especially when the examination of cases is more thoroughly and systematically undertaken.[7]

Still the knowledge we possess of Amnesic conditions, as well as of the distribution of 'ingoing' fibres in their passage from the base of the Brain to the Convolutions, already enables us to point roughly to the neighbourhood in which lesions or injuries would be likely to produce defects of Speech and Writing of this type.

Lesions of the convolutions *about the posterior extremity of the Sylvian Fissure of the left Hemisphere* will probably prove almost as instrumental in producing one or other variety of Amnesia, as lesions of or about the third left frontal are of inducing Aphasia. In Broadbent's case (p. 645) the lesion was found in this region, and in a fairly typical unpublished example of Amnesia the writer has also recently found a lesion in the same situation.

The reason for looking to this region will, moreover, be obvious if the reader will recollect that the posterior third of the peduncular fibres (that is of the co-called 'internal capsule') spread out from beneath the posterior part of the Thalamus; and that, stretching backward and outwards across the floor of the lateral ventricle from near the beginning of the descending cornu, they distribute themselves in the main to the Occipital and the Temporal Convolutions. And if the conclusions of Ferrier in regard to the important relations of the 'supra-marginal lobule' and the 'angular gyrus' with the Visual Centre, and of the posterior part of the 'upper temporal convolution' with the Auditory Centre should prove to be correct, there would be these still more precise reasons for expecting to find the lesions productive of Amnesia, with some frequency, in or about the situation indicated. Such a 'localization' may, therefore, be provisionally entertained, and no more promising means of ultimately ascertaining with tolerable certainty the situation of the most important parts of the Visual and Auditory Perceptive Centres in man would seem to present themselves, than the careful clinico-pathological study of typical Amnesic cases whenever the opportunities may occur.

Another question of great interest now arises, and that is, whether it will be found that lesions productive of Amnesia are also in the main limited to the left Hemisphere. Some eminent observers, such as Brown-Séquard and Hughlings Jackson, believe that a limitation of this kind does obtain. But whilst the writer freely admits that lesions of the left are more likely to be potential than those of the right Hemisphere in the production of such states, it seems to him that both facts and theory tend to negative the idea that similar defects would not be induced by lesions in certain parts of the right Hemisphere.

It will be found that many such cases are already on record — one of the most typical being that of Marcou, as given by Trousseau (see p. 621). And if we bear in mind that corresponding Perceptive Centres in the two Hemispheres are almost habitually called into simultaneous activity, and are in structural continuity with one another through the Corpus Callosum, it might be expected that irritative or destructive lesions of the Auditory or the Visual Word-Centres of the right side could scarcely occur without producing distinct derangement, at all events for a time, in the functional activity of the similar centres in the left Hemisphere — which, as one is bound to admit, seem to take the lead in the expression of Thought by Speech and Writing. On this very interesting subject much further information is needed, and we have previously (p. 493) had to refer to the doubt that exists as to the extent to which one Hemisphere alone may suffice for ordinary mental activity. It may fairly be expected, perhaps, that Amnesia produced by a lesion of the right side would have a tendency to be more temporary than such a condition when occasioned by similar lesions of the left Hemisphere.

Finally, another consideration of some importance in connection with 'cerebral localizations' now suggests itself. The condition of Amnesia may merge by insensible gradations into one of Aphasia — so that the latter state, with certain extra peculiarities, may at times result from a lesion altogether away from the third left frontal gyrus, if, as we at present suppose, the regions in which lesions have the greatest tendency to produce one or other of the forms of Amnesia should be situated around the posterior extremity of the left Sylvian Fissure.

This may be easily understood. Suppose a person to be suffering from a defective activity of the Auditory Word-Centre, so that Names cannot be recalled 'voluntarily' or by 'association'. There would already be great hesitations and difficulties in the expression of Thoughts, both in Speech and in Writing. But suppose this mere defective activity to be replaced by actual destruction of the left Auditory Word-Centre, so that its functional activity became entirely lost: words could then, of course, neither be recalled 'voluntarily' nor by 'association'; and still further, they could not be perceived and consequently could not be imitated. An individual thus affected would neither be able to Speak nor to Write, that is, he would be completely Aphasic with the superadded peculiarity that he would not readily comprehend spoken and perhaps written Language. The latter ability might persist to some extent, because the molecular equilibrium of the Auditory Word-Centre and of the related Visual-Centre of the opposite Hemisphere might not be sufficiently disturbed to prevent all apprehension of spoken or of written symbols. We might, in fact, have in such a case, the production of a complex Aphasic condition almost precisely similar to that met with in the girl whose case was recorded by Bazire, (p. 653) or even one like that recorded by the writer at p. 655, and yet such an Aphasic condition might have been caused by a lesion far away from the left third frontal convolution. And if this were so, such cases might have been quoted with much apparent effect against existing doctrines in regard to 'cerebral localization'.

Similarly, it is possible that Agraphia, accompanied by 'word-blindness', might result from a lesion of the left Visual Word-Centre, and that the site of such lesion might be contiguous to the posterior extremity of the left Sylvian Fissure.

Aphemia (that is, mere loss of Speech) could not be produced by a lesion of this region of the Brain, because destruction of the Auditory Word-Centre would destroy the revival of words for spontaneous Writing, as well as for Speech — so that the double condition Aphasia (or an approximate state in which 'imitative' Writing only is possible), would necessarily result, instead of the more special Aphemic state.

It is clear, also, that if important tracts of the Auditory and Visual Word-Centres are in reality situated somewhere about the end of the Sylvian Fissures, and if the Kinaesthetic Word-Centres, both for Speech and Writing, are situated in or somewhere in the neighbourhood of the third frontal convolutions, Aphasia might in addition be caused by lesions cutting across the commissural fibres in any part of their course between these pairs of centres.

Clearly, if stimuli caused by the mental revival of words do not (a) issue from the Auditory and Visual Word-Centres; if they (b) are stopped on their way therefrom to the corresponding Kinaesthetic Word-Centres;

or (c) if they are stopped in or on the other side of these latter Centres, that is on their way to the left Corpus Striatum, the result would, in each case, be the production of Aphasia, although the situations of the lesions in these cases would be altogether different. In the first case, too, we should have Aphasia with much mental impairment; in the second case we should have Aphasia with trifling mental impairment; whilst in the third case we should have the typical Aphasia, in which little or no mental degradation is to be detected.

This being true, a general law may provisionally be formulated, as a future working hypothesis: that *the tendency to mental impairment with Aphasia, and the degree of such impairment, will, other things being equal, increase as lesions of the left Hemisphere recede in site from the 'third frontal convolution' and approach the Occipital Lobe.* The general doctrine of Marc Dax seems to be justified, whilst Broca's more special localization must be held to hold good only for one particular though very common form of Loss of Speech — or, to use the broader and more accurate phraseology, loss of the power of Intellectual Expression.

The conclusions above arrived at are found to afford a new and quite unlooked for confirmation of the view already announced as to the special frequency with which lesions of the Occipital Regions of the Hemisphere are apt to be associated with marked mental degradation; they will also tend to make us appreciate more fully the real validity of the objections raised by some against the doctrine that the posterior part of the left 'third frontal gyrus' is the region always damaged in cases of Aphasia; and they may pave the way for new and more exact differential observations, by means of which alone we can expect to make real progress in a task of extreme difficulty, in which we are now only breaking ground in a tentative manner — that is, in the endeavour to determine what kind of functions are principally carried on in different regions of the Cerebral Cortex.

If we have said nothing in regard to the 'localization' of certain higher Intellectual and Moral Powers, the reason for this will be obvious to all thoughtful readers. No step can be taken with any chance of success in this direction till the preliminary enquiries to which we have been devoting our attention have been reduced to a more settled condition. The foundations of the subject must clearly be laid before we can begin to rear a superstructure.

Yet that every higher Intellectual and Moral Process — just as much as every lower Sensorial or Perceptive Process — involves the activity of cer-

tain related cell-and-fibre networks in the Cerebral Cortex, and is absolutely dependent upon the functional activity of such networks, the writer
firmly believes. He, however, as decidedly rejects the notion which some
would associate with such a doctrine, viz., the supposition that Human
beings are mere 'Conscious Automata'.

It must be conceded that if Conscious States or Feelings have in reality
no bond of kinship with the molecular movements taking place in certain
Nerve Centres; if they are mysteriously appearing phenomena, differing
absolutely from, and lying altogether outside, the closed 'circuit of motions'
with which they coexist, no way seems open by which such Conscious States
could be conceived to affect or alter the course of such Motions. The logic
of this seems irresistible. The conclusion can, indeed, only be avoided by a
repudiation of the premises: and this the writer does. He altogether rejects
the doctrine that there is no kinship between States of Consciousness and
Nerve Actions, and consequently would deny the view that the 'causes' of
Conscious States lie altogether outside the circuits of Nerve Motions.

Consciousness or Feeling must be a phenomenon having a natural origin, or else it must be a non-natural, non-material entity. For reasons which
have been set forth in various parts of the present volume the writer adopts
the former of these views.

It is commonly believed that 'living matter' has now, or has had in past
times, a natural origin; Nerve Tissues also have a natural origin in or from
elemental forms of 'living matter'; and if Conscious States or Feelings are
admitted to be an appanage only of Nerve Actions, so also (as far as we can
ascertain) does their mode of appearance, their increase in intensity, their
modifiability by agents modifying the nerve tissues, and the limitation by
which they occur only in association with certain nerve actions taking place
in the higher and most complex of an animal's Nerve Centres, harmonize
with the notion that they are in some way an actual outcome of such Nerve
Actions — no more capable of being dissevered from the physical conditions on which they depend, than is Heat to be dissevered from its physical
conditions (see p. 142). To say that Heat is a 'mode of motion', takes for
granted the underlying fact that we cannot have motion except through a
something which moves. Heat has no abstract and isolated existence as an
entity. Consciousness also is a result of a something which moves. But just
as it is the very material motions on which Heat depends which do the work
ascribed to Heat, so do the very material motions on which Consciousness
or Feeling depends, do the work which we ascribe to Feeling. These par-

ticular motions, be it remarked, enter as components into the 'circuit of motions' constituting Nerve Actions, and may, therefore, easily co-operate as real motors. Hence it is that States of Feeling may, in very truth, and in accordance with popular belief, react upon Nerve Tissues so as to alter the molecular motions taking place therein. Feelings, whether purely personal or of the moral order, thus have, as they seem to have, an indubitable effect in modifying our Intellectual Operations, our Volitions, or our Movements.

To show how these particular motions in Nerve Tissue arise which underlie Conscious States, and how they again subside into more ordinary nerve actions, must, from the very nature of the problem, ever remain impossible. But we certainly should not on this account allow ourselves to be mentally paralysed by a belief in the existence of a metaphysical gulf between what is termed the Subjective and the Objective — the 'Ego' and the 'Non-Ego'. Yet, even some believers in the philosophy of evolution have thus been led to deny the natural origin of Conscious States, and have as a consequence found themselves forced to hold a doctrine of thorough-going 'Automatism' — one in which all notions of Free Will, Duty, and Moral Obligation would seem from this theoretical basis to be alike consigned to a common grave, together with the underlying powers of self-education and self-control.

Notes

1. These forms of word-memory were first definitely stated by me to be purely sensory in papers on the Physiology of Thinking and on the Muscular Sense; and the name "kinaesthetic" was subsequently (*The Brain as an Organ of Mind*) applied to the complex groups of impressions resulting from movements of this or that part of the body.

2. Other French writers, as well as Ballet, attribute to Charcot the doctrine that ["le mot n'est pas une unité, mais un complexus" (*Le Langage Intérieur*, 1886, p.13) because he also dwelt upon these four different kinds of word-memory. Charcot's lectures on Aphasia were delivered in 1883, but M. Ballet will find a full description of these four different kinds of word-memory in my book *The Brain as an Organ of Mind* (1880), p. 696, or in the French translation (*Le Cerveau et la Pensée*, tome li., p. 222), published in 1882.

3. "*The Muscular Sense: its Nature and Cortical Localisation*" (1887), and "*On the Neutral Processes Underlying Attention and Volition*" (1892).

4. Republished in Dax, 1865.

5. Inability on the part of an Aphasic person to learn to Speak from the right side of the Brain would thus be found to depend upon conditions precisely analogous to those producing in a right-sided Hemiplegic an inability to learn to Write with the left hand (i.e., from the right side of the Brain). Speech would be impossible if the Auditory Centre, and

Writing would be impossible if the Visual Centre, in the left Hemisphere were destroyed; or, similar disabilities would exist if the fibres of the Corpus Callosum respectively connecting either of these left Centres with its corresponding Centre of the opposite Hemisphere were cut across by disease.

6. See a paper "On the Specific Gravity of the Human Brain" [Bastian] 1886.

7. In all cases of Amnesia, or of mixed Aphasia and Amnesia, details should among other things always be given in reference to the following points: — (1) The patient's ability to understand spoken words (not being deaf); (2) to repeat sounds or words when requested; (3) to write from dictation; (4) to understand and therefore to point out printed letters and words (not being blind); (5) to copy written words,, or printed words into written words; and (6) to name printed letters or objects, or read aloud.

References

Bastian, H.C. 1869a. "On the various forms of loss of speech in cerebral disease". *British and Foreign Medical and Chirurgical Review* 43: 209-236; 470-492.

———. 1869b. "The physiology of thinking". *Fortnightly review* 5: 57-71.

———. 1869c. "On the muscular sense". *British Medical Journal* 1:394.

———. 1880. *The Brain as an Organ of Mind*. London: Kegan Paul.

———. 1886. "On the specific gravity of the human brain". *Journal of Mental Science* : 28-32.

———. 1887. "On the muscular sense: its nature and cortical localisation". *Brain* 10: 1-89.

———. 1892. "On the neural processes underlying attention and volition". *Brain* 13.

Bouillaud, J.B. 1825. *Traité clinique et physiologique de l'eucephalité et de ses suites*. Paris: J.B. Baillière.

Broca, P. 1861b. "Remarques sur le siège de la faculté de langage articulé, suivie d'une observation d'aphémie (perte de la parole)". *Bulletins de la Société Anatomique* 6:330-357.

Charcot, J.M. 1886. "Le langage interieur". *Revue de Médecine* 6: 97-138.

Dax, M. 1865. "Lesions de la moitié gauche de l'encephale coincidant avec l'oubli des signes de la pensée (lu à Montpellier en 1836)". *Gazette Hebdomadaires de Médicine et de Chirurgie* 2: 259-260.

John Hughlings Jackson

Introduced by

BENTO P. M. SCHULTE†
*Institute of Neurology, University of Nijmegen
Nijmegen, The Netherlands*

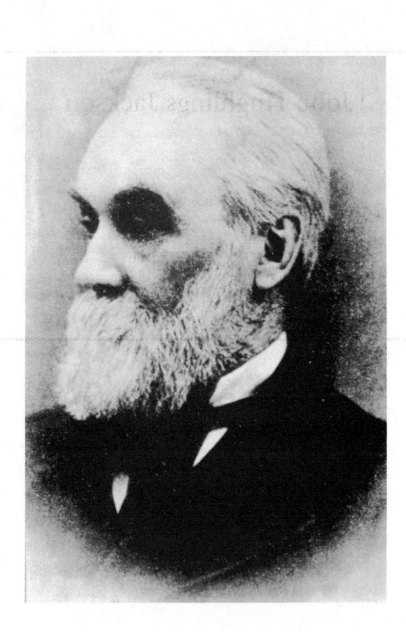

John Hughlings Jackson
1835-1911

Biography

John Jackson was born a farmer's son at Providence Green, Hammerton,
Yorkshire, England on 4 April 1835. The matronymic Hughlings, from his
mother Sara Hughlings, became attached to the Jackson family name. His
elementary education was poor. In 1856 he qualified for medicine at York,
where he came under the influence of the neurologist Thomas Laycock, who
considered the brain as subject to the laws of reflex action. Highly impressed
by the writings of the philosopher and early evolutionist Herbert Spencer
(1820-1903), Jackson gave serious consideration to the thought of abandon-
ing medicine in favor of philosophy. When Jackson had come to London in
1859, Jonathan Hutchinson (1828-1913) persuaded him to pursue his medical career. With the help of Hutchinson, Jackson started in London as a medical journalist and thus became acquainted with the chief London hospitals.
In 1862 he became assistant physician to the National Hospital, Queen
Square, where Jackson's interest in neurology was encouraged above all by
Edouard Brown-Séquard (1817-1894). In 1864 he was appointed to the staff
of the London Hospital. In 1867 he joined the staff of the National Hospital,
at that time named Hospital for the Epileptic and Paralysed, where he
worked as a staff member up to 1896, and as a consultant from 1896 to 1906.
More than 300 papers from his hand, written in a meticulous but difficultly
readable style with many footnotes, were mainly published in medical journals of limited circulation at first. In 1878 he joined J.C. Bucknill, J.
Crichton-Brown, and D. Ferrier as founder and editor of the famous journal
Brain. About 1865 he married his cousin Elisabeth Jackson, who suffered
from what we now call Jacksonian epilepsy and who died childless eleven
years later. Jackson was a modest, even shy man of big stature, restless, who
abhorred sports or even walking, suffered from migraine, vertigo, and progressive hearing deficiency. The reading of novels and even of penny thrillers
was his only hobby. The "father of British neurology" died of pneumonia on
October 7, 1911. (see McHenry, 1969; Holmes, 1956 and Lennox, 1970 for
appraisals of his life and work.)

Selected Bibliography

Hughlings Jackson, John. 1866. "Notes on the physiology and pathology of language".
    Medical Times and Gazette 1: 659.

――――. 1874. "On the nature of the duality of the brain". *Medical Press and Circular* 1: 19; 41; 63.

――――. 1879. "On affections of speech from disease of the brain". *Brain* 1: 304-330; *Brain* (1880) 2: 203-222; *Brain* (1880) 2: 323-356.

――――. 1884. "Evolution and dissolution of the nervous system". *Popular Science Monthly* 25: 171-180.

――――. 1893. "Words and other symbols in mentation". *Medical Press and Circular* 2: 205-208.

Introduction

Jackson's Neurology

Jackson's clinical observations of epilepsy are the key to his neurology. As he was convinced that "idiopathic epilepsy" was far too difficult a subject for precise investigation, the simpler cases of partial convulsion had his particular interest (Taylor, 1931). These partial seizures were named by Jackson for Bravais, who described them in 1827, or he called some of them, after their anatomic origin, uncinate seizures. Charcot suggested the now generally accepted name Jacksonian seizures. Jackson considered an epileptic seizure as a symptom of disease of the brain and as *an experiment made on the brain by disease*. In the study of these fits, or of any kind of disease of the nervous system, there are three lines of investigation: to find the organ damaged (anatomical localization), to find the functional affection of nervous tissue (physiology), and to find the alteration in nutrition (pathology). Jackson stresses the opinion that the mode of onset is the most important matter in the anatomical investigation in any case of epilepsy. This fundamental methodological statement opened the door for understanding the experiments made by disease on the nervous system. It resulted for instance in Jackson's description and analyses of observations on the localization of movements in the cerebral hemisphere, as revealed in cases of convulsion, chorea, and aphasia. These and many other observations lead to Jackson's conclusion that in cases of disease of the nervous system the condition is duplex: negative and positive. He was strongly convinced that destructive lesions never cause positive effects, but induce a negative condition which permits positive symptoms to appear. The function of "nervous arrangements" (a typical Jacksonian term) may be lost temporarily (as in aftereffects of epileptic fits) or permanently (as in hemiplegia after a stroke): this is the patient's negative condition. The function of the same nervous elements may be exalted temporarily (as in epileptic seizures) or permanently (as in increased reflexes that are released from higher control after a stroke): this is the patient's positive condition. The negative and the positive condition of nervous disease are opposites. There are no degrees from one to the other, they depart from normal function, the one upwards, the other downwards. Upwards and downwards must be understood in Jackson's concept of the three levels of evolution of the central nervous system. The lowest level comprises spinal cord, medulla oblongata, and pons Varolii; the middle level consists of the basal ganglia and the cerebral cortex before and behind the central sulcus (fissure of Rolando); the highest level comprises the prefrontal and the occipital lobes of the brain. In the nervous system evolution developed from the most automatic movements in the lowest level to the most voluntary movements in the highest level. On the contrary, disease of the highest or of the middle level causes dissolution of those parts of the nervous system and loss of control of these parts over the next lower level. It is notable how in this concept of Jackson the motor aspects in the nervous system prevail.

The concept of evolution and dissolution of the nervous system is fundamental in Jackson's neurology. In his first Croonian Lecture of 1884, Jackson stated:

> The doctrine of evolution daily gains new adherents. It is not simply synonymous with Darwinism. Herbert Spencer applies it to all orders of phenomena. His application of it to the nervous system is most important for medical men. I have long thought that we shall be very much helped in our investigations of diseases of the nervous system by considering them as reversals of evolution, that is, as dissolutions. Dissolution is a term I take from Spencer as a name for the reverse of the process of evolution. The subject has been worked at for many years. About half a century ago, Laycock applied the doctrine of reflex action to the brain. Sir Charles Bell, in speaking of degrees of drunkeness, and Baillarger, in speaking of aphasia, have pointed out that there is a reduction from the voluntary towards the most automatic. (Taylor, 1931)

Jackson refers in his papers on many occasions to Spencer's Principles of Psychology of 1855 (Spencer, 1855). Autodidact Herbert Spencer was one of the most discussed English philosophers of the Victorian era. In his theory of evolution he argues that a continuing development from lower to higher stages is present in every aspect of reality. But evolution would be followed by dissolution. His idea of the evolution of species was published before Charles Darwin's *On the Origin of Species* (1859). Jackson derived, as Henry Head remarked, all his psychological knowledge from Herbert Spencer, and adopted his phraseology almost completely. Without knowledge of Spencer's ideas, Jackson's interpretation of his masterly clinical observations remains unintelligible.

Jackson's Aphasiology

In 1864 Jackson published his first papers on loss of speech and on defects of expression, in 1894 his last, with a total number of 28. The theme of loss of speech is seldom discussed separately, but almost always in connection with other neurological phenomena as hemiplegia and epileptic seizures.

In these papers it is clear from the beginning that Jackson, unlike his contemporaries, is critical about *localization* of the "faculty of speech" in a circumscribed part of the brain. In 1866 he expressed his disagreement with Broca with a gentle introduction: "I must here say that I believe less in some of the views propounded by Broca than I did, although I think the scientific world is under vast obligation to him for giving precision to an important inquiry", but then he states: "I think, then, that the so-called 'faculty' of language has no existence". The medieval doctrine of the faculties and its transformation by Franz-Joseph Gall into the doctrine of speech centers in the brain were not accepted by Jackson. In Jackson's interpretation the nervous system is an organ of movements, even for the most voluntary and complex movements serving in speech. In his paper "On the nature of the duality of the brain" (1874) he states: "To locate the damage which destroys speech and to locate speech are two different things". In 1868 Broca presented his views in a meeting of the British Association at Norwich. Jackson contributed to the discussion and from the abstract "Observations on the physiology of language" (1868) it is clear that Jackson opposed Broca. On that occasion Jackson stressed his opinion that destructive lesions never cause positive effects, but only negative ones, and that any positive symptoms are the consequences of the released activity of lower centers. In every case of affection of speech there exists, according to Jackson, a negative and a positive condition. The patient may be not able to speak, to write, or to read, and expression by signs may be impaired: this is the negative condition. At the same time the patient may be able to write his signature, to swear or utter other emotional expressions: this is the positive condition (Head, 1926). In other words, Jackson applied his ideas on evolution and dissolution of the nervous system also on affections of speech.

Jackson makes a distinction between *voluntary* and *involuntary* language. He acknowledges his indebtedness to the ideas of Jules Baillarger (1809-1890), physician to the Salpêtrière at Paris. In his "Notes on the physiology and pathology of language" (1866) Jackson states:

> M. Baillarger has already, I find, considered this question in an admirable manner. He says: "L'analyse des phénomènes conduit à reconnaître, dans certains cas de ce genre, que l'incitation verbale involontaire persiste, mais que l'incitation verbale volontaire est abolie. Quant à la perversion de la faculté du langage caractérisée par la prononciation de mots incohérents, la lésion consiste encore dans la substitution de la parole automatique à l'incitation verbale volontaire.

In his book *De l'aphasie au point de vue psychologique* (1865) Baillarger distinguished between "aphasie simple" and "aphasie avec perversion de la faculté du langage", an automatic–voluntary dissociation being possible in the former and usually present in the latter. Baillarger considered the automatic–voluntary dissociation essential for the classification of aphasia (Baillarger, 1865). Jackson called this the "Baillarger principle". The aphasia classification Jackson presented as his own at the forementioned Norwich meeting in 1868 was very similar to that of Baillarger. Recently Alajouanine (1968) called the distinction between voluntary and automatic language "le principe de Baillarger-Jackson dans l'aphasie".

From 1874 Jackson expressed his views based on the Baillarger principle. The right half of the brain, he says, is the half for the automatic use of words, the left is the half for both the automatic and the voluntary use. The left is the leading half. Thus, both halves serve in verbalizing, but the left half of the brain is that by which we speak. In cases with disease of the left half, near to or involving the corpus striatum, the patient is speechless. But he can still utter words. Speechlessness does not imply wordlessness. But speaking is not simply the utterance of words. Speech consists of words referring to one another in a particular manner: *speaking is propositionizing*. Words are in themselves meaningless, Jackson says; they are only *symbols* of things or of "images" of things. A proposition symbolizes a particular relation of some images. The unit of speech is a proposition. A proposition is defined as such a relation of words that it makes one new meaning, not by mere addition of what we call the separate meanings of the several words; the terms in a proposition are modified by each other. But a proposition is not a string of symbols, each word referring independently to that perception of which it is a symbol. The meaning of a proposition is one, not two meanings in juxtaposition. In his paper "Words and other symbols in mentation" (1893) Jackson summarized the forementioned ideas in the statement: "Speaking is symbolising, a mental operation". It is thus understandable why Jackson preferred as name for loss of speech Hamilton's term *asemasia* to Trousseau's term *aphasia*.

As the term *proposition* is so fundamental in Jackson's ideas on aphasia it is interesting to note that the term and concept of proposition are significant constituents of Aristotelian logic, as Walther Riese pointed out (Riese, 1977). A second Aristotelian source of Jackson's view on aphasia may be seen, according to Riese, in Jackson's definition of written language. Jackson defined written words as *symbols of symbols*. In Aristotle's "De interpretatione" one finds Jackson's definitions of spoken and of written words: "Spoken words are the symbols of mental experience and written words are the symbols of spoken words". Jackson was, after all, a clinician and a philosopher.

On the expressive side of language Jackson interprets loss of speech as loss of symbols. On the receptive side of language loss of perception (imperception) means loss of images. Speech and perception cooperate intimately in mentation. In the process leading to speech there is, in Jackson's views, a double revival of words. Nervous arrangements for words used in speech lie chiefly in the left half of the brain, and nervous arrangements for words used in understanding speech lie in the right half also. Automatic (unconscious or subconscious) revival occurs first in the right half of the brain and voluntary (conscious) revival, being speech, occurs afterwards in the left half of the brain. Similarly there is first involuntary (unconscious or subconscious) revival of images ("image symbols"), followed by a voluntary (conscious) revival of images, being perception. In the case of perception there is a vivid image; in the case of thinking of an object in its absence (ideation) the image is faint. In a similar way, in internal speech there is faint excitation of the same sensorimotor processes which for external speech need to be strongly excited.

After his famous lecture on "Loss of speech" at the London Hospital in 1864, Jackson was at first cited by all the writers on aphasia in the same way as Broca. But soon his views on affections of speech no longer held the interest of his collegues. Henry Head offered four reasons for this neglect of Jackson's works: he published in journals that were not easily accessible, his papers were and are difficult to read, his Spencerian phraseology tended to alienate psychologists, and the nature of his ideas was foreign to the current views of the day (Head, 1926). Sigmund Freud was one of the few on the continent who paid attention to him. But Freud did not understand Jackson fully and conceived Jackson's concept of evolution in Darwinian terms (Freud, 1891). The only seemingly Darwinian term in Jackson's writings, however, is "survival of the fittest". And even this term was not coined by Charles Darwin but by Herbert Spencer. In our century things changed. In 1913 Arnold Pick dedicated *Die agrammatischen Sprachstörungen* to "Hughlings Jackson, the deepest thinker in neuropathology of the past century" (Pick, 1913). In 1915 Henry Head, who followed Jackson's footsteps in his monumental work *Aphasia and kindred disorders of speech* (1925), reprinted some of Jackson's more important papers on aphasia in *Brain* (Head, 1915). In 1931, Jackson's pupil James Taylor edited, with the advice and assistance of Gordon Holmes and Frances Walshe, Jackson's selected writings in two volumes (reprinted in 1958). The second volume of this work contains a list of Jackson's writings.

In *"The Founders of Neurology"* William Lennox ended his biography of Jackson as follows: 'Father of British neurology', he appears to us as having been foremost on the brilliant staff that made 'Queen Square' a centre of world neurology. Yet partially eclipsed during life by some more mundane contemporaries Jackson's light acquired even greater brilliance in the afterglow" (Lennox, 1970, p. 459).

References

Alajouanine, Th. 1968. "Le principe de Baillarger-Jackson dans l'aphasie". *L'Aphasie et le langage pathologique*. Paris: Baillière.
Baillarger, J.G.F. 1865. *De l'aphasie au point de vie psychologique*. Paris: Masson.
Freud, S. 1891. *Zur Auffassung der Aphasien*. Wien: Deuticke.
Head, H. 1915. "Hughlings Jackson on aphasia and kindred affections of speech". *Brain* 38: 1-190.
———. 1926. *Aphasia and Kindred Disorders of Speech*. Cambridge: Cambridge University Press.
Holmes, G. 1956. "John Huglings-Jackson". *Grosse Nervenärzte*, Band 1, p. 135-144. Stuttgart: Georg Thieme.
Lennox, W.G. 1970. "John Huglings-Jackson". *The Founders of Neurology*, ed. by W. Haymaker and F. Schiller, pp. 456-459. Springfield: C. Thomas.
McHenry, L.C. 1969. "John Huglings-Jackson". *Garrison's history of neurology*, pp. 307-312. Springfield: C. Thomas.

Pick, A. 1913. *Die agrammatischen Sprachstörungen*. Berlin: Springer.

Riese, W. 1977. "The sources of Hughlings Jackson's view on aphasia". *Selected Papers on the History of Aphasia*, ed. by R. Hoops. Lisse: Swets and Zeitlinger.

Spencer, H. 1855. *The Principles of Psychology*. London: Williams and Norgate.

———. 1864. *The Principles of Biology*. London: Williams and Norgate.

Taylor, J. 1931. *Selected Writings of John Hughlings Jackson*, Vol. I. London: Hodder and Stoughton. (Reprint: New York, Basic Books, 1958).

Selection from the work of John Hughlings Jackson

On Affections of Speech from Disease of the Brain*

It is very difficult for many reasons to write on Affections of Speech. So much, since the memorable researches of Dax and Broca, has been done in the investigation of these cases of disease of the brain, that there is an *embarras de richesse* in material. To refer only to what has been done in this country, we have the names of Gairdner, Moxon, Broadbent, William Ogle, Bastian, John W. Ogle, Thomas Watson, Alexander Robertson, Ireland, Wilks, Bristowe, Ferrier, Bateman, and others. To Wilks, Gairdner, Moxon, Broadbent, and Ferrier, I feel under great obligations. Besides recognising the value of Broadbent's work on this subject, I have to acknowledge a particular indebtedness to him. Broadbent's hypothesis — a verified hypothesis — is, I think, essential to the methodical investigation of affections of speech. Let me give at once an illustration of its value. It disposes of the difficulty there otherwise would be in holding (1) that loss of speech is, on the physical side, loss of nervous arrangements for highly special and complex articulatory *movements*, and (2) that in cases of loss of speech the articulatory *muscles* are not paralysed, or but slightly paralysed. I shall assume that the reader is well acquainted with Broadbent's researches on the representation of certain movements of the two sides of the body in each side of the brain; the reader must not assume that Broadbent endorses the applications I make of his hypothesis. The recent encyclopaedic article on Affections of Speech, by Kussmaul, in Ziemssen's 'Practice of

*By J. Hughlings Jackson, M.D., F.R.C.P., F.R.S., Physician to the London Hospital, and to the Hospital for the Epileptic and Paralysed. Originally published in *Brain*, 1., 304-330 (1879).

Medicine', is very complete and highly original. It is worthy of most careful study.

The subject has so many sides — psychological, anatomical, physiological, and pathological — that it is very difficult to fix on an order of exposition. It will not do to consider affections of speech on but one of these sides. To show how they mutually bear, we must see each distinctly. For example; we must not confound the physiology of a case with its pathology, by using for either the vague term "disease". Again, we must not ignore anatomy when speaking of the physical basis of words, being content with morphology, as in saying that words "reside" in this or that part of the brain. Supposing we could be certain that this or that grouping of cells and nerve-fibres was concerned in speech, from its being always destroyed when speech is lost, we should still have to find out the anatomy of the centre. Even supposing we were sure that the psychical states called words, and the nervous states in the "centre for words", were the same things, we should still have the anatomy of that centre to consider. The morphology of a centre deals with its shape, with its "geographical" position, with the sizes and shapes of its constituent elements. A knowledge of the anatomy of a centre is a knowledge of the parts of the body represented in it, and of the ways in which these parts are therein represented. Whilst so much has been learned as to the morphology of the cerebrum — cerebral topography — it is chiefly to the recent researches of Hitzig and Ferrier that we are indebted for our knowledge of the anatomy of many of the convolutions, that is, a knowledge of the parts of the body these convolutions represent. It is supposed that the anatomy of the parts of the brain concerned with words is that they are cerebral nervous arrangements representing the articulatory muscles in very special and complex movements. Similarly, a knowledge of the anatomy of the centres concerned during visual ideation is a knowledge of those regions of the brain where certain parts of the organism (retina and ocular muscles) are represented in particular and complex combinations. A merely materialistic or morphological explanation of speech or mind, supposing one could be given, is not an anatomical explanation. Morphologically, the substratum of a word or of a syllable is made up of nerve-cells and fibres: anatomically speaking, we say it is made up of nerve-cells and fibres representing some particular articulatory movement.

Unless we most carefully distinguish betwixt psychology and the anatomy and physiology of the nervous system in this inquiry, we shall not see the fundamental similarity there is betwixt the defect often described in psychological phraseology as "loss of memory for words", and the defect called ataxy of articulation. A method which is founded on classifications which are partly anatomical and physiological, and partly psychological, confuses the real issues. These mixed classifications lead to the use of such expressions as that an *idea* of a word produces an articulatory *movement*; whereas a psychical state, an "idea of a word" (or simply "a word") cannot produce an articulatory movement, a physical state. On any view whatever as to the relation of mental states and nervous states such expressions are not warrantable in a *medical* inquiry. We could only say that discharge of the cells and fibres of the anatomical substratum of a word produces the articulatory movement. In all our studies of diseases of the nervous system we must be on our guard against the fallacy that what are physical states in lower centres fine away *into* psychical states in higher centres; that, for example, vibrations of sensory nerves *become* sensations, or that somehow or another an idea produces a movement.

Keeping them distinct, we must consider now one and now another of the several sides of our subject: sometimes, for example, we consider the psychical side — speech — and at other times the anatomical basis of speech. We cannot go right on with the psychology, nor with the anatomy, nor with the pathology of our subject. We must consider now one and now the other, endeavouring to trace a correspondence betwixt them.

I do not believe it to be possible for any one to write methodically on these cases of disease of the nervous system without considering them in relation to other kinds of nervous disease; nor to be desirable in a medical writer if it were possible. Broadbent's hypothesis is exemplified in cases of epilepsy and hemiplegia, as well as in cases of affections of speech, and can only be vividly realised when these several diseases have been carefully studied. Speech and Perception ("words" and "images") co-operate so intimately in Mentation (to use Metcalfe-Johnson's term) that the latter process must be considered. We must speak briefly of Imperception — loss of images — as well as of loss of Speech — loss of symbols. The same general principle is, I think, displayed in each. Both in delirium (partial imperception) and in affections of speech the patient is reduced to a more automatic condition; respectively reduced to the more organised relations of images and words. Again, we have temporary loss or defect of speech after certain epileptiform seizures: temporary affections of speech after these seizures are of great value in elucidating some difficult parts of our subject, and cannot be understood without a good knowledge of various other kinds of epileptic and epileptiform paroxysms, and post-paroxysmal states. After a convulsion beginning in the (right) side of the face or tongue, or in both these parts, there often remains temporary speechlessness, although the articulatory muscles move well. Surely we ought to consider cases of discharge of the centres for words as well as cases in which these centres are destroyed, just as we consider not only hemiplegia but hemispasm. Before trying to analyse that very difficult symptom called ataxy of articulation, we should try to understand the more easily studied disorder of co-ordination, locomotor ataxy; and before that, the least difficult disorder of co-ordination of movements resulting from ocular paralysis. Unless we do, we shall not successfully combat the notion that there are centres for co-ordination of words which are something over and above centres for special and complex movements of the articulatory muscles, and that a patient can, from lesion of such a centre, have a loss of co-ordination, without veritable loss of some of the movements represented in it.

It might seem that we could consider cases of aphasia, as a set of symptoms at least, without regard to the pathology of different cases of nervous disease. We really could not. It so happens that different morbid processes have what, for brevity, we may metaphorically call different seats of election; thus, that defect of speech with which there are frequent mistakes in words is nearly always produced by local cerebral softening; that defect which is called ataxy of articulation, is, I think, most often produced by haemorrhage. Hence we must consider hemiplegia in relation to affections of speech; for it so happens that the first kind of defect mostly occurs, as Hammond has pointed out, without hemiplegia, or without persistent hemiplegia, a state of things producible by embolism and thrombosis, and the latter mostly with hemiplegia and persistent hemiplegia, a state of things usually produced by haemorrhage. From ignoring such considerations, the two kinds of defects are by some considered to be absolutely different, whereas on the anatomico-physiological side they are but very different degrees of one kind of defect.

There are certain most general principles which apply, not only to affections of speech, but also to the commonest variety of paralysis, to the simplest of convulsive seizures, and to cases of insanity.

The facts that the speechless patient is frequently reduced to the use only of the most general propositions "yes" or "no", or both; that he may be unable to say "no" when told, although he says it readily in reply to questions requiring dissent; that he may be able ordinarily to put out his tongue well, as for example to catch a stray crumb, and yet unable to put it out when he tries, after being asked to do so; that he loses intellectual language and not emotional language; that although he does not speak, he understands what we say to him; and many other facts of the same order, illustrate exactly the same principle as do such facts from other cases of disease of the nervous system as — that in hemiplegia the arm suffers more than the leg; that most convulsions beginning unilaterally begin in the index finger and thumb; that in cases of post-epileptic insanity there are degrees of temporary reduction from the least towards the most "organised actions", degrees proportional to the severity of the discharge in the paroxysm, or rather to the amount of exhaustion of the highest centres produced by the discharge causing the paroxysm. In all these cases — except in the instance of convulsion, which, however, illustrates the principle in another way — there are, negatively, degrees of loss of the most voluntary processes with, positively, conservation of the next most voluntary or next more automatic; otherwise put, there are degrees of loss of the latest acquirements with conservation of the earlier, especially of the inherited, acquirements; speaking of the physical side, there are degrees of loss of function of the least organised nervous arrangements with conservation of function of the more organised. There is in each reduction to a more automatic condition: in each there is Dissolution, using this term as Spencer does, as the opposite of Evolution.[1]

In *defects* of speech we may find that the patient utters instead of the word intended a word of the same class in meaning, as "worm-powder" for "cough-medicine"; or, in sound, as "parasol" for "castor oil". The presumption is that the patient uses what is to him a more "organised" or "earlier" word, and if so, Dissolution is again seen. But often there is no obvious relation of any sort betwixt the word said and the one appropriate, and thus the mistake does not appear to come under Dissolution. If, however, we apply the broad principles which we can, I think, establish from other cases of Dissolution, viz. from degrees of insanity — especially the slight degrees of the post-epileptic insanity just spoken of — we shall be able to show that many of the apparently random mistakes in words are not real exceptions to the principle of Dissolution.

For the above reasons I shall make frequent references to other classes of nervous disease. The subject is already complex without these excursions, but we must face the complexity. Dr. Curnow has well said (*Medical Times and Gazette*, Nov. 29, p. 616), "The tendency to appear exact by disregarding the complexity of the factors is the old failing in our medical history".

Certain provisional divisions of our subject must be made. The reader is asked to bear in mind that these are admittedly arbitrary; they are not put forward as scientific distinctions. Divisions[2] and Arrangements are easy, Distinctions and Classifications are difficult. But in the study of a very complex matter, we must first divide, and then distinguish. This is not contradictory to what was said before on the necessity of encountering the full complexity of our subject. Harm comes, not from dividing and arranging, but from stopping in this stage, from taking provisional divisions to be real distinctions, and putting forward elaborate arrangements, with divisions and subdivisions, as being classifications. In other words, we shall, to start with, consider our subject empirically, and afterwards scientifically; we first arbitrarily divide and arrange for convenience of obtaining the main facts which particular cases supply, and try to classify the facts, in order to show their true relations one to another, and consider them on the psychical side as defects of mind, and on the physical side as defects of the nervous system. Empirically, we consider the cases of affection of speech we meet with, as they *approach* certain nosological types (most frequently occurring cases), scientifically we classify the facts thus obtained, to show how affections of speech are *departures from* what we know of healthy states of mind and body. The latter study is of the cases as they show different degrees of nervous Dissolution.

Let us first of all make a very rough popular division. When a person "Talks" there are three things going on — Speech, Articulation, and Voice. Disease can separate them. Thus from disease of the larynx, or from paralysis of its nerves, we have loss of voice, but articulation and speech remain good. Again, in complete paralysis of the tongue, lips, and palate, articulation is lost, but speech is not even impaired; the patient remains able to express himself in writing, which shows that he retains speech — internal speech — that he propositionises well. Lastly, in extensive disease in a certain region in one half of the brain (left half usually) there is loss of speech, internal and external, but the articulatory muscles move well.

Let us make a wider division. Using the term Language, we make two divisions of it, Intellectual and Emotional. The patient, whom we call speechless (he is also defective in pantomime), has lost intellectual language and has not lost emotional language.

The kind of case we shall consider first is that of a man who has lost speech, and whose pantomime is impaired, but whose articulatory muscles move well, whose vocal organs are sound, and whose emotional manifestations are unaffected. This is the kind of case to be spoken of as No. 2 (p. 314).

The term Aphasia has been given to affections of speech by Trousseau; it is used for defects as well as for loss of speech. I think the expression Affections of Speech (including defects and loss) is preferable. Neither term is very good, for there is, at least in many cases, more than loss of *speech*; pantomime is impaired; there is often a loss or defect in symbolising relations of things in any way. Dr. Hamilton proposes the term Asemasia, which seems a good one. He derives it "from α and σημαινω, an inability to indicate by signs or language". It is too late, I fear, to displace the word aphasia. Aphasia will be sometimes used as synonymous with Affections of Speech in this article.

We must at once say briefly what we mean by speech, in addition to what has been said by implication when excluding articulation, as this is popularly understood, and voice. To speak is not simply to utter words, it is to propositionise. A proposition is such a relation of words that it makes one new meaning; not by a mere addition of what we call the separate meanings of the several words; the terms in a proposition are modified[3] by each other. Single words are meaningless, and so is any unrelated succession of words. The unit of speech is a proposition. A single word is, or is in effect, a proposition, if other words in relation are implied. The English tourist at a French *table d'hôte* was understood by the waiter to be asking for water when his neighbours thought he was crying "oh!" from distress. It is from the use of a word that we judge of its propositional value. The words "yes" and "no" are propositions, but only when used for assent and dissent; they are used by healthy people interjectionally as well as propositionally. A speechless patient may retain the word "no", and yet have only the interjectional or emotional, not the propositional, use of it; he utters it in various tones as signs of feeling only. He may have a propositional use of it, but yet a use of it short of that healthy people have, being able to reply "no", but not to say "no" when told; a speechless patient may have the full use of it. On the other hand, elaborate oaths, in spite of their propositional structure, are not propositions, for they have not, either in the mind of the utterer or in that of the person to whom they are uttered, any meaning at all; they may be called "dead propositions". The speechless patient may occasionally swear. Indeed he may have a recurring utterance, e.g. "Come on to me", which is propositional in structure but not, to him, propositional in use; he utters it on any occasion, or rather on no *occasion*, but every time he tries to speak.

Loss of speech is therefore the loss of power to propositionise. It is not only loss of power to propositionise aloud (to talk), but to propositionise either internally or externally, and it may exist when the patient remains able to utter some few words. We do not mean, by using the popular term power, that the speechless man has lost any "faculty" of speech or prop-ositionising; he has lost those words which serve in speech, the nervous arrangements for them being destroyed. There is no "faculty" or "power" of speech apart from words revived or revivable in propositions, any more than there is a "faculty" of co-ordination of movements apart from move-ments represented in particular ways. We must here say too that besides the use of words in speech there is a service of words which is not speech; hence we do not use the expression that the speechless man has lost words, but that he has lost those words which serve in speech. In brief, Speechlessness does not mean entire Wordlessness.

It is well to insist again that speech and words are psychical terms; words have of course anatomical substrata or bases as all other psychical states have. We must as carefully distinguish betwixt words and their phys-ical bases, as we do betwixt colour and its physical basis; a psychical state is always accompanied by a physical state, but nevertheless the two things have distinct natures. Hence we must not say that the "memory of words" is a *function* of any part of the nervous system, for function is a physiologi-cal term (*vide infra*). Memory or any other psychical state arises *during* not *from* — if "from" implies continuity of a psychical state with a physical state functioning of nervous arrangements, which functioning is a purely physical thing — a discharge of nervous elements representing some impressions and movements. Hence it is not to be inferred from the rough division we just made of the elements of "talking", and from what was said of their "separation" by disease, that there is anything in common even for reason-able contrast, much less for comparison, betwixt loss of speech (a psychical loss) and immobility of the articulatory muscles from, say disease of the medulla oblongata, as in "bulbar paralysis" (a physical loss). As before said, we must not classify on a mixed method of anatomy, physiology, and psychology, any more than we should classify plants on a mixed natural and empirical method, as exogens, kitchen-herbs, graminaceae, and shrubs. The things comparable and contrastable in the rough division are (1) the two physical losses: (a) loss of function of certain nervous arrangements in the cerebrum, which are not speech (words used in speech), but the anatomical substrata of speech; and (b) loss of function of nervous arrangements in the medulla oblongata. (2) The comparison, on the psychical side, fails. There is no psychical loss in disease of the medulla oblongata to compare with loss of words, as this part of the nervous system, at least as most suppose,[4] has no psychical side; there is nothing psychical to be lost when nervous arrangements in the medulla oblongata are destroyed.

The affections of speech met with are very different in degree and kind, for the simple reason that the exact position of disease in the brain and its gravity differ in different cases; different amounts of nervous arrangements in different positions are destroyed with different rapidity in different persons. There is, then, no single well-defined "entity" — loss of speech or aphasia — and thus, to state the matter for a particular practical purpose, such a question as, "Can an aphasic make a will?" cannot be answered any more than the question, "Will a piece of string reach across this room?" can be answered. The question should be, "Can this or that aphasic person make a will?" Indeed, we have to consider degrees of affection of Language, of which speech is but a part. Admitting the occurrence of numerous degrees of affection of Language, we must make arbitrary divisions for the first part of our inquiry, which is an empirical one.

Let us divide roughly into three degrees: (1) *Defect of Speech*. — The patient has a full vocabulary, but makes mistakes in words, as saying "orange" for "onion", "chair" for "table"; or he uses approximative or quasi-metaphorical expressions, as "Light the fire up there", for "Light the gas". "When the warm water comes the weather will go away", for "When the sun comes out the fog will go away". (2) *Loss of Speech*. — The patient is practically speechless and his pantomime is impaired. (3) *Loss of Language*. — Besides being speechless, he has altogether lost pantomime, and emotional language is deeply involved.

To start with, we take the simplest case, one of loss of speech, No.2 ("complete aphasia"). Cases of defect of speech (1) are far too difficult to begin with, and so, too, are those cases (3) in which there is not only loss of speech, but also deep involvement of that least special part of language which we call emotional language. Moreover, we shall deal with a case of permanent speechlessness. I admit that making but three degrees of affection of language, and taking for consideration one kind of frequently occurring case, is an entirely arbitrary proceeding, since there actually occur very numerous degrees of affection of language, many slighter than, and some severer than, that degree (No.2) we here call one of loss of speech. But, as aforesaid, we must study subjects so complex as this empirically before we study them scientifically; and for the former kind of study we must have what are called "definitions" by type, and state exceptions. This is the plan adopted in every work on the practice of medicine with regard to all diseases. Let us give an example of the twofold study. Empirically or clinically, that is for the art of medicine, we should consider particular cases of epilepsy as each *approaches this or that nosological type* ("le petit mal, le grand mal", &c.). For the science of medicine we should, so far as is possible, consider cases of epilepsy as each is dependent on a "discharging lesion" of this or that part of the cortex cerebri, and thus as it is a *departure from healthy states* of this or that part of the organism. We cannot do the latter fully yet, but the anatomico-physiological researches of Hitzig and Ferrier have marvellously helped us in this way of studying epilepsies, as also have the clinical researches of Broadbent, Charcot, Duret, Carville, and others.[5]

The following are brief and dogmatic statements about a condition which is a common one — the kind of one we call loss of speech, our second degree (No.2) of Affection of Language. The statements are about two equally important things: (1) of what the patient has lost in Language — his negative condition, and (2) of what he retains of Language — his positive condition. Here, again, is an illustration of a general principle which is exemplified in many if not in all cases of nervous disease, and one of extreme importance when they are scientifically considered as instances of nervous Dissolution. We have already stated the duality of many symptomatic conditions in the remarks on p. 308. Without recognising the two elements in all cases of affections of speech, we shall not be able to classify affections of speech methodically. If we do not recognise the duplex (negative and positive) condition, we cannot possibly trace a relation betwixt Nos.1, 2 and 3 (p. 314). There can be no basis for comparison betwixt the wrong utterances in No.1 and the non-utterances in Nos. 2 and 3 — betwixt a positive and a negative condition — betwixt speech, however bad, and no speech. There is a negative and a positive condition in each degree; the comparison is of the three degrees of the negative element and the three degrees of the positive element; the negative and positive elements vary inversely. The condition of the patient No. 1, who made such mistakes as saying "chair" for "table" was duplex; (a) negatively in not saying "table", and (b) positively, in saying "chair" instead; there is in such a case *loss* of some speech, with *retention* of the rest of speech. Hence the term defect of speech applied to such a case is equivocal; it is often used as if the actual utterance was the *direct* result of the disease. The utterance is wrong in that the words of it do not fit the things intended to be indicated; but it is the best speech under the circumstances, and is owing to activity of healthy (except perhaps slightly unstable) nervous elements. The real, the primary, fault is in the nervous elements which do not act, which are destroyed, or are for the time *hors de combat*. If then we compare No. 1 with No. 2, we compare the two negative conditions, the inability to say "table", &c. (the loss of some speech) in No. 1, with the loss of nearly all speech in No. 2, saying the latter is a greater degree of the former, and we compare the two positive conditions, the retention of inferior speech (the wrong utterances) in No. 1, with in No. 2 the retention of certain recurring utterances and with the retention of emotional language, saying the latter is a minor or lower degree of language than the former. Unless we take note of the duplex condition in imperception (delirium and ordinary insanity), we shall not be able to trace a correspondence betwixt it and other nervous diseases. There are necessarily the two opposite conditions in all degrees of mental affections, from the slightest "confusion of thought" to dementia, unless the dementia be total.

The Patient's Negative Condition

(1) He does not speak. — He can, the rule is, utter some jargon, or some word, or some phrase. With rare exceptions, the utterance continues the same in the same patient: we call these Recurring Utterances. The exceptions to the statement that he is speechless are two. (a) The recurring utterance may be "yes" or "no", or both. These words are propositions when used for assent or dissent, and they are so used by some patients who are for the rest entirely speechless. (b) There are Occasional Utterances. Under excitement the patient may swear: this is not speech, and is not exceptional; the oath means nothing; the patient cannot repeat it, he cannot "say" what he has just "uttered". Sometimes, however, a patient, ordinarily speechless, may get out a phrase appropriate to some simple circumstance, such as "good-bye" when a friend is leaving. This is an exception, but yet only a partial exception; the utterance is not of high speech

value;[6] he cannot "say" it again, cannot repeat it when entreated; it is inferior speech, little higher in value than swearing. However, sometimes a patient, ordinarily speechless, may get out an utterance of high speech value; this is very rare indeed.

(2) *He cannot write*; that is to say, he cannot express himself in writing. This is called Agraphia (William Ogle). It is, I think, only evidence of the loss of speech, and might have been mentioned in the last paragraph. Written words are symbols of symbols. Since he cannot write, we see that the patient is speechless, not only in the popular sense of being unable to talk, but altogether so; he cannot speak internally. There is no fundamental difference betwixt external and internal speech; each is propositionising. If I say "gold is yellow" to myself, or think it, the proposition is the same; the same symbols referring to the same images in the same relation as when I say it aloud. There is a difference, but it is one of degree; psychically "faint" and "vivid", physically "slight" and "strong" nervous discharges. The speechless patient does not write because he has no propositions to write. The speechless man may write in the sense of penmanship; in most cases he can copy writing, and can usually copy print into writing, and very frequently he can sign his name without copy. Moreover he may write in a fashion without copy, making, or we may say drawing, a meaningless succession of letters, very often significantly the simplest letters, pothooks. His handwriting may be a very bad scrawl, for he may have to write with his left hand. His inability to write, in the sense of expressing himself, *is* loss of speech; his ability to make ("to draw") letters, as in copying, &c., shows that his "image series" (the materials of his perception) is not damaged.

Theoretically there is no reason why he should not write music without copy, supposing of course that he could have done that when well; the marks (artificial images) used in noting music, have no relation to words any way used. On this matter I have no observations. Trousseau writes in his Lecture on Aphasia (*Syd. Soc. Trans.*, vol.i, p. 270), "Dr. Laseque knew a musician who was completely aphasic, and who could neither read nor write, and yet could note down a musical phrase sung in his presence".

(3) In most cases the speechless patient *cannot read at all*, obviously not aloud, but not to himself either, including what he has himself copied. We suppose our patient cannot read. This is not from lack of sight, nor is it from want of perception; his perception is not itself in fault, as we shall see shortly.

(4) His power of making signs is impaired (pantomimic propositionis-

ing). We must most carefully distinguish pantomime from gesticulation. Throwing up the arms to signify "higher up", pantomime, differs from throwing up the arms when surprised, gesticulation, as a proposition does from an oath.

So far we have, I think, only got two things, loss of speech (by simple direct evidence, and by the indirect evidence of non-writing and non-reading) and defect of pantomime. There are in some cases of loss of speech other inabilities; the most significant are that a patient cannot put out his tongue when he tries, or execute other movements he is told, when he can move the parts concerned in other ways quite well.

The Patient's Positive Condition

(1) He can understand what we say or read to him; he remembers tales read to him. This is important, for it proves that, although Speechless, the patient is not Wordless. The hypothesis is that words are in duplicate; and that the nervous arrangements for words used in speech lie chiefly in the left half of the brain; that the nervous arrangements for words used in understanding speech (and in other ways) lie in the right also. Hence our reason for having used such expressions as "words serving in speech"; for there is, we now see, another way in which they serve. When from disease in the left half of the brain speech is lost altogether, the patient understands all we say to him, at least on matters simple to him. Further it is supposed that another use of the words which remain is the chief part of that service of words which in health precedes speech; there being an unconscious or subsconscious revival of words in relation before that second revival which is speech. Coining a word, we may say that the process of Verbalising is dual; the second "half" of it being speech. It is supposed also that there is an unconscious or subsconscious revival of relations of images, before that revival of images in relation which is Perception.

(2) His articulatory organs move apparently well in eating, drinking, swallowing, and also in such utterances as remain always possible to him (recurring utterances), or in those which come out occasionally. Hence his speechlessness is not owing to disease of those centres in the medulla oblongata for immediately moving the articulatory muscles; for in other cases of nervous disease, when these centres are so damaged that the articulatory muscles are so much paralysed that *talking* is impossible, the patient

remains able to *speak* (to propositionise) as well as ever; he has internal speech, and can write what he speaks.

The following dicta may be of use to beginners. Using the popular expression "talk", we may say that if a patient does not talk because his brain is diseased, he cannot write (express himself in writing), and can swallow well; if he cannot talk because his tongue, lips, and palate are immovable, he can write well and cannot swallow well.

(3) His vocal organs act apparently well; he may be able to sing.

(4) His emotional language, is apparently unaffected. He smiles, laughs, frowns, and varies his voice properly. His recurring utterance comes out now in one tone and now in another, according as he is vexed, glad, &c.; strictly we should say he sings his recurring utterance; variations of voice being rudimentary song (*Spencer*); he may be able to sing in the ordinary meaning of that term. As stated already, he may swear when excited, or get out more innocent interjections, simple or compound (acquired parts of emotional language). Although he may be unable to make any but the simplest signs, he gesticulates apparently as well as ever, and probably he does so more frequently and more copiously than he used to do. His gesticulation draws attention to his needing something, and his friends guess what it is. His friends often erroneously report their guessing what he wants when his emotional manifestations show that he is needing something, as his expressing what thing it is that he wants.

So far for the negative and positive conditions of Language in our type case of Loss of Speech — No. 2 in Defect of Language.

Words are in themselves meaningless, they are only symbols of things or of "images" of things; they may be said to have meaning "behind them". A proposition symbolises a particular relation of some images.[7]

We must then briefly consider the patient's condition in regard to the images symbolised by words. For although we artificially separate speech and perception, words and images co-operate intimately in most mentation. Moreover, there is a morbid condition in the image series (Imperception), which corresponds to aphasia in the word series. The two should be studied in relation.

The speechless patient's perception (or "recognition", or "thinking" of things) (propositions of images) is unaffected, at any rate as regards simple matters. To give examples: he will point to any object he knew before his illness which we name; he recognises drawings of all objects which he knew before his illness. He continues able to play at cards or dominoes; he recognises handwriting, although he cannot read the words written; he knows poetry from prose, by the different endings of the lines on the right side of the page. One of my patients found out the continuation of a series of papers in a magazine volume, and had the right page ready for her husband when he returned from his work; yet she, since her illness, could not read a word herself, nor point to a letter, nor could she point to a figure on the clock. There is better and simpler evidence than that just adduced that the image series is unaffected; the foregoing is intended to show that the inability to read is not due to loss of perception nor to nonrecognition of letters, &c., as particular marks or drawings, but to loss of speech. Written or printed words cease to be symbols of words used in speech for the simple reason that those words no longer exist to be symbolised; the written or printed words are left as symbols of nothing, as mere odd drawings. The simplest example showing the image series to be undamaged is that the patient finds his way about; this requires preconception, that is "propositions of images" of streets, &c. Moreover, the patient can, if he retains the propositional use of "yes" and "no", or if he has the equivalent pantomimic symbols, intelligently assent or dissent to simple statements, as that "Racehorses are the swiftest horses", showing that he retains organised nervous arrangements for the images of the things "swiftness" and "horse"; this has already been implied when it was asserted that he understands what we say to him, a process requiring not some of his words only, but also some of his "images" of things, of which the words are but symbols.

Such facts as the above are sometimes adduced as showing that the patient's "memory" is unaffected. That expression is misleading, if it implies that there is a general faculty of memory. There is no faculty of memory apart from things being remembered; apart from having, that is, now and again, these or those words, or images, or actions (faintly or vividly). We may say he has not lost the memory of images, or, better, that he has the images actually or potentially; the nervous arrangements being intact and capable of excitation did stimuli come to them; we may say that he has lost the memory of those words which serve in speech. It is better, however, to use the simple expression that he has not lost images, and that he has lost the words used in speech.

These facts as to retention of images are important as regards the writing of speechless patients. The printed or written letters and words are images, but they differ from the images of objects, in being artificial and arbitrary, in being acquired later; they are acquired after speech and have their meaning only through speech; written words are symbols of symbols of images. The aphasic patient cannot express himself in writing because he cannot speak; but the nervous arrangements for those arbitrary images which are named letters are intact, and thus he can reproduce them as mere drawings, as he can other images, although with more difficulty, they, besides lacking their accustomed stimulus, being less organised. He can copy writing, and he can copy print into writing. When he copies print into writing, obviously he derives the images of letters from his own mind (physically his own organisation). He does not write in the sense of expressing himself, because there are no words reproduced in speech to express. That series of artificial images which makes up the signature of one's name has become almost as fully organised as many ordinary images; hence in many cases the speechless man who can write nothing else without copy can sign his name.

For the perception (or recognition or thinking) of things, at least in simple relations, speech is not necessary, for such thought remains to the speechless man. Words are required for thinking, for most of our thinking at least, but the speechless man is not wordless; there is an automatic and unconscious[8] or subconscious service of words.

It is not of course said that speech is not required for thinking on novel and complex subjects, for ordering images in new and complex relations (i.e. to the person concerned), and thus the process of perception in the speechless, but not wordless, man may be defective in the sense of being inferior from lack of co-operation of speech: it is not itself in fault, it is left unaided.

To understand anything novel and complex said to him, the healthy man speaks it to himself, e.g. repeats, often aloud, complex directions of route given to him.

The word "thing" has not been used as merely synonymous with "substance"; nor is it meant that anybody has nervous arrangements for the images of "swiftness" and "horse", but only for images of some swiftly-moving thing or things, and for images of some particular horse or horses.

It may be well here to give a brief recapitulation of some parts of our subject and, also very briefly, an anticipation of what is to come; the latter is given partly as an excuse for having dwelt in the foregoing on some points not commonly considered in such an inquiry as this, and partly to render clearer some matters which were only incidentally referred to.

The division into internal and external speech is not that just made into the dual service of words. Internal and external speech differ in degree only: such a difference is insignificant in comparison with that betwixt the prior unconscious, or subconscious, and automatic reproduction of words and the sequent conscious and voluntary reproduction of words; the latter alone is speech, either internal or external. Whether I can show that there is this kind of duality or not, it remains certain that our patient retains a service of words, and yet ordinarily uses none in speech. The retention of that service of words which is not a speech use of words, is sometimes spoken of as a retention of "memory of" words, or of "ideas of" words. But as there is no memory or idea of words apart from having words, actually or potentially, it is better to say that the patient retains words serving in other ways than in speech; we should say of his speechlessness, not that he has lost the memory of words, but simply that he has lost those words which serve in speech.

When we consider more fully the duality of the Verbalising process, of which the second "half" is speech, we shall try to show that there is a duality also in the revival of the images symbolised; that perception is the termination of a stage beginning by the unconscious or subconscious revival of images which are in effect "image symbols"; that we think not only by aid of those symbols, ordinarily so-called (words), but by aid of symbol-images. It is, I think, because speech and perception are preceded by an unconscious or subconscious reproduction of words and images, that we seem to have "faculties" of speech and of perception, as it were, above and independent of the rest of ourselves. We seem to have a memory or ideas[9] of words *and* words; having really the two kinds of service of words. The evidence of disease shows, it is supposed, that the highest mentation arises out of our whole organised states, out of ourselves — that Will, Memory, &c., "come from below", and do not stand automatically "above", governing the mind; they are simply the now highest, or latest, state of our whole selves. In simple cases of delirium (partial imperception with inferior perception) as when a patient takes his nurse to be his wife, we find, I think, a going down to and a revelation of what would have been when he was sane, the lower and earlier step towards his true recognition or perception of the nurse.

The first step towards his recognition of her when he was sane, would be the unconscious, or subconscious, and automatic reproduction of his, or of one of his, well-organised symbol-images of woman; the one most or much organised in him would be his wife. To say what a thing is is to say what it is like; he would not have known the nurse even as a woman, unless he had already an organised image of at least one woman. The popular notion is, that by a sort of faculty of perception, he would recognise her without a prior stage in which, he being passive, an organised image was roused in him by the mere presence of the nurse; the popular notion almost seems to imply the contradiction that he first sees her, in the sense of recognising her, and then sees her as like his already acquired or organised image of some woman. We seem to ourselves to Perceive, as also to Will and to Remember, without prior stages, because these prior stages are unconscious or subconscious. It seems to me that in delirium the patient is reduced to conditions which are revelations of, or of parts of, the lower earlier and prior stages; the lower or earlier stages are then conscious. They are the *then* highest or latest conscious states. When the patient becomes delirious, he takes the nurse to be his wife. More or fewer of the highest nervous arrangements being then exhausted, the final stage is not possible; there is only the first stage; the reproduction of his well organised symbol-image is all there is, and that is all the nurse can be to him; she is, to him, his wife. The symbol-image is then vividly reproduced because the centres next lower than those exhausted are in abnormally great activity (note, that there are two conditions, one negative and the other positive). There is a deepening of consciousness in the sense of going down to lower earlier and more organised states, which in health are mostly unconscious or subconscious, and precede higher conscious states; in other words with loss or defect of object consciousness, even in sleep with dreaming, there is increasing subject consciousness; on the physical side, increasing energising of those lower centres which are in the day time more slightly energising during that unbroken subconscious "dreaming", from which the serial states, constituting our latest or highest object consciousness, are the continual "awakenings".

It is supposed that the well organised images spoken of — in effect arbitrary images, symbol-images, those which *become* vivid and are "uppermost" in delirium, and then cease to be mere symbols — constitute what seems to be a "general notion" or "abstract idea" of such things as "horse", "swiftness", &c.; their particularity (that they are only images of some horse or horses, of some swift moving thing or things) not appearing, because they are unconscious or subconscious; they served once as images of particular things, and at length as symbol-images of a class of images of things, as well as images of the particular things.

At page 319 we spoke of the right half of the brain as being the part during the activity of which the most nearly unconscious and most automatic service of words begins, and of the left as the half during activity of which there is that sequent verbal action which is Speech. The division is too abrupt; some speech — voluntary use of words — is, as we have seen, when alluding to Occasional Utterances, possible to the man who is rendered practically speechless by disease in the left half. Again, from disease of the right half, there is not loss of that most automatic service of words which enables us to understand speech. The thing which it is important to show is, that mentation is dual, and that physically the unit of function of the nervous system is double the unit of composition; not that one half of the brain is "automatic" and the other "voluntary".

Having now spoken of the kind of case we shall consider, and having added remarks, with the endeavour to show how the several symptoms — negative and positive are related one to another, we shall be able to give reasons for excluding other kinds of cases of speechlessness.

We are not concerned with cases of all persons who do not speak. We shall not, for example, deal with those untrained deaf-mutes who never had speech, but with the cases of those persons only who have had it, and lost it by disease. The condition of an untrained deaf-mute is in very little comparable with that of our arbitrarily-taken case of loss of speech. The deaf-mute's brain is not diseased, but, because he is deaf, it is uneducated (or in anatomical and physiological phraseology undeveloped) so as to serve in speech. Our speechless patient is not deaf. Part of our speechless patient's brain is destroyed; he has *lost* nervous arrangements which had been trained in speech. Moreover, our speechless man retains a service of words which is not speech; untrained deaf-mutes have no words at all. Further, the untrained deaf-mute has his natural system of signs, which to him is of speech value so far as it goes. He will think by aid of these symbols as we do by aid of words.[10] Our speechless patient is defective even in such slight pantomime as we may reasonably suppose to have been easy to him before his illness. The deaf-mute may have acquired for talking and thinking the common arbitrary system of deaf-mute signs (finger-talk), or he may have been taught by the new method to speak as we do, and thus have ceased to be mute. But when not taught to speak, he is not in a condition even roughly comparable with that of a man who has *lost* speech. No doubt by disease of some part of his brain the deaf-mute might lose his natural system of signs, which are of some speech value to him, but he could not lose speech, having never had it. Much more like our speechless patient's condition is that of the little child which has been taught to understand speech, and has not yet spoken.

There is another set of cases of so-called loss of speech, which we shall not consider as real loss of speech. I prefer to say that these patients *do* not speak: cases of some persons are meant, who do not talk and yet write perfectly. This may seem to be an arbitrary exclusion. There is in most of these cases an association of symptoms, which never arises from any local disease of any part of the nervous system; the so-called association is a mere jumble of symptoms. Let us state the facts. The patients are nearly always boys or unmarried women. The bearing of this is obvious. The so-called loss of speech is a total non-utterance, whereas it is an excessively rare thing for a patient who does not speak, because his brain is locally diseased, to have no utterance whatever; I do not remember seeing one such case in which there was not some utterance (recurring utterance) a few days or a few weeks after the onset of the illness; the absolute pseudo-speechlessness may remain for months. They cannot be mute from paralysis of the articulatory muscle, because they swallow well. Frequently there is loss of voice also — they get out no sounds except, perhaps, grunts, &c. — and yet they cough ringingly and breathe without hoarseness or stridor; there is no evidence of laryngeal disease. Now loss of voice never occurs with loss of speech from local disease of one side of the brain. No disease of the larynx would cause loss of speech or loss of articulation. The patients often "lose" their speech after calamity or worry. In these cases there is no hemiplegia and no other one-sided condition from first to last. They often, after months of not-speaking, recover absolutely and immediately after some treatment which can have no therapeutical effect, e.g. a liniment rubbed on the back, a single faradaie stimulation of the vocal cords or of the neck. Dr. Wilks has reported a case of "cure" of a girl who had not spoken for months; she had also "lost" the use of her legs. Knowing well what was the general nature of the case, Dr. Wilks, by speaking kindly to her, and giving her an excuse for recovery in the application of faradisation, got her well in a fortnight. Sometimes the so-called speechless patient speaks inadvertently when suddenly asked a question, and then goes on talking; is well again. Sometimes speech is surprised out of her. Thus a woman, whose case is recorded by Durham, when told to cry "ah!" when the spatula was holding down her tongue, pushed his hand away, saying, "How can I, with that thing in my mouth?" She then said, "Oh! I have spoken". She was "cured". I believe that patients, "speechless" as described, might be "cured" by faradisation of the vocal cords, or by a thunderstorm, or by quack medicines or appliances, or by mesmerism, or by wearing a charm, or not speaking flippantly — by being "prayed over".

Sometimes these cases are spoken of as cases of "emotional aphasia" — the speechlessness is said to be "caused by" emotional excitement, because it often comes on *after* emotional disturbance.

I submit that the facts that the patients do not talk and *do* write and *do* swallow are enough to show that there is no disease at all, in any sense except that the patients are hysterical (which is saying nothing explanatory), or that they are pretending. There can be no *local* disease, at any rate.

These cases are spoken of at length, although they are excluded, because they are sometimes adduced as instances of aphasia, or loss of speech proper, with ability to write remaining. I confess that were I brought face to face with a man whom I believed to *have* local disease of his brain, who did not *talk*, and yet wrote well, I should conclude that he did *speak* internally although he could not talk. To say that *he* cannot speak and yet can express himself in writing is equivalent, I think, to saying *he* cannot speak and yet *he* can speak.

Notes

1. Here I must acknowledge my great indebtedness to Spencer. The facts stated in the text seem to me to be illustrations from actual cases of disease, of conclusions he has arrived at deductively in his Psychology. It is not affirmed that we have the exact opposite of Evolution from the apparently brutal doings of disease; the proper opposite is seen in healthy senescense, as Spencer has shown. But from disease there is, in general, the corresponding opposite of Evolution.

2. "How often would controversies be sweetened were people to remember that 'Distinctions and Divisions are very different things', and that 'one of them is the most necessary and conducive to true knowledge that can be: the other, *when made too much of*, serves only to puzzle and confuse the understanding.' Locke's words are the germ of that wise aphorism of Coleridge: 'It is a dull or obtuse mind that must divide in order to distinguish; but it is a still worse that distinguishes in order to divide'. And if we cast our eyes back over time, it is the same spirit as that which led Anaxagoras to say, 'Things in this one connected world are not cut off from one another as if with a hatchet'". — Westminster Review (art. Locke), January 1877 (no italics in original).

3. On this matter see an able article in the Cornhill Magazine, May 1866. See also Waitz, *Anthropology* (Collingwood's Translation), p. 241 et seq.

4.   I, however, believe as Lewes does, that in so far as we are physically alive, we are psychically alive; that some psychical state attends every condition of activity of every part of the organism. This is, at any rate, a convenient hypothesis in the study of diseases of the nervous system.

5.   See Moxon (1869). In this paper Moxon shows conclusively the necessity of keeping the clinical, or what is above called empirical — not using that term in its popular bad signification — and scientific studies of disease distinct. After reading this paper, my eyes were opened to the confusion which results from mixing the two kinds of study. It is particularly important to have both an empirical arrangement and a scientific classification of cases of Insanity. An example of the former is the much-criticised arrangement of Skae; the scientific classification of cases of insanity, like that of affections of speech, would be regarding them as instances of Dissolution; the Dissolution in insanity begins in the highest and most complex of all cerebral nervous arrangements, the Dissolution causing affections of speech in a lower series. The one kind of classification is for diagnosis (for direct "practical purposes"), the other is for increase of knowledge, and is worthless for immediate practical purposes. The fault of some classifications of insanity is that they are mixed, partly empirical and partly scientific.

6.   What is meant by an utterance of high speech value and by inferior speech will later on be stated more fully than has been just now stated by implication. When we cease dealing with our subject empirically and treat it scientifically, we hope to show that these so-called exceptions come in place under the principle of Dissolution. We may now say that speech of high value, or superior speech, is new speech, not necessarily new words and possibly not new combinations of words; propositions symbolising relations of images new to the speaker, as in carefully describing something novel; by inferior speech is meant utterances like, "Very well", "I don't think so", ready fitted to very simple and common circumstances, the nervous arrangements for them being well organised.

7.   The term "image" is used in a psychical sense, as the term "word" is. It does not mean "visual" images only, but covers all mental states which represent things. Thus we speak of auditory images. I believe this is the way in which Taine uses the term image. What is here called "an image" is sometimes spoken of as "a perception". In this article the term perception is used for a *process*, for a "proposition of images", as speech is used for propositions, i.e. particular inter-relations of words. The expression "organised image" is used briefly for "image, the *nervous arrangements for which* are organised", correspondingly for "organised word", &c.

8.   The expression "*unconscious* reproduction of words", involves the same contradiction as does the expression, "unconscious sensation". Such expressions may be taken to mean that energising of lower, more organised, nervous arrangements, although unattended by any sort of conscious state, is essential for, and leads to, particular energisings of the highest and least organised — the now-organising — nervous arrangements, which last mentioned energising is attended by consciousness. I, however, think (as Lewes does) that some consciousness or "sensibility" attends energising of all nervous arrangements (I use the term subconscious for slight consciousness). In cases where from disease the highest nervous arrangements are suddenly placed *hors de combat*, as in sudden delirium, the next lower spring into greater activity; and then, what in health was a subordinate subconsciousness, becomes a vivid consciousness, and is also the highest consciousness there then can be.

9.   The so-called *idea* of a word, in contradistinction to *the* word, is itself a word subconsciously revived, or revivable, before the conscious revival or revivability of the same word, which latter, in contradistinction to the so-called *idea of* a word, is the so-called *word itself — the* word.

10.   We must not confound the finger-talk with the "natural" system of signs. They are essentially different. No one supposes that words are essential for thought, but only that some symbols are essential for conceptual thought, although it may be that people with "natural" symbols do not reach that higher degree of abstract thinking which people do who have words.

References

Moxon, W. 1869. "On the necessity for a Clinical Nomenclature of Disease". *Guy's Hospital Reports*, 15:479-500.
Spencer, H. 1855. *The Principles of Psychology*. London: Williams and Norgate.

Sigmund Freud

Introduced by

Otto R. HOMMES
Institute of Neurology, University of Nijmegen
Nijmegen, The Netherlands

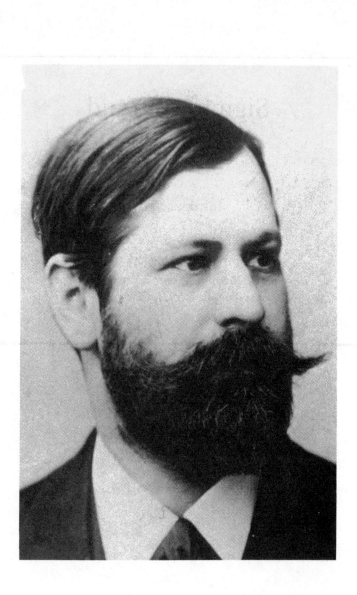

Sigmund Freud
1856-1939

Biography

Sigmund Freud is perhaps the best known physician of modern times. His work has had a major impact, not only on medicine, but also on anthropology, psychology, and sociology. Recently strong influences on linguistics and philosophy have developed. Freud's work and thought have had and still have lasting significance for all students of man's behavior and drives.

Sigmund Freud was born of Jewish parents on 6 May 1856 in Freiberg, Moravia, then part of the Austrian Empire and presently the city of Pribor in the Czech Republic. He studied medicine in Vienna, specializing in neuroanatomy, physiology, and neuropathology. In 1885 a three month stay with the famous Paris neurologist Jean Martin Charcot was the turning point in his career. Freud developed the first parts of psychoanalytic theory and practice in cooperation with Joseph Breuer. Initially his new theories were totally ignored by the academic world. Recognition came slowly.

Strong opposition to Freud's leadership and scientific views in the small group of collaborators resulted in definite breaks with Carl Jung and Alfred Adler. Freud's daughter Anna became a famous child-analyst in her own right. She was a great help to him in his later years, as he suffered from a maxillary malignancy. A year before his death Freud had to leave Vienna under pressure of the Nazis. He emigrated to London, where he died on 23 September, 1939.

Introduction

Historical setting of Freud's work on aphasia

Freud was trained as a neurologist and at the time of writing *Zur Auffassung der Aphasien* had held a position as "Privatdozent für Neuropathologie an der Universität Wien" since 1885. This position was approximately at the level of an assistant professorship. It was and is in German-speaking countries the first rung on the academic ladder.

The study on aphasia was written at the request of A. Villaret as part of the *Handwörterbuch der gesamten Medizin* and appeared in 1888 in the first volume of this medical dictionary. It was edited as a separate booklet in 1891. Freud was in his mid-thirties when he wrote this study. He dedicated the work to Dr. Joseph Breuer, with whom he did his first studies on hypnosis. It was Breuer who showed Freud that drives and wishes, hidden from clear consciousness, can produce abnormal behavior and that these abnormalities will disappear when the original emotions can be expressed freely. This insight was strengthened by Freud's visit to Paris in 1885-1886. On his return to Vienna he found absolute rejection and open hostility towards these new ideas. This caused Freud to give up his university position and start a private practice, where he treated hysterical patients very successfully.

In these years before publishing the famous studies on hysteria in 1895, Freud had to work practically in complete isolation, even losing his long-time friend Breuer. He kept a meticulous record of all his findings and discoveries. "The multiplicity and novelty of those problems must have had a completely bewildering effect on him, especially as it became clearer and clearer that he had touched upon facts which contradicted all established ways of thinking and traditional concepts" (Eissler 1978, p. 18). His thinking and vocabulary on sexuality and the open treatment of the "unspeakable", and his discoveries about the sexual activities of small children were, in particular, clearly contrary to the prudish social attitudes of those times.

The ethical paradigm was that the "unspeakable" should be unthinkable.

It is in this period of scientific and social isolation that Freud's *Zur Auffassung der Aphasien* was published as a "critical study". In the introduction he stated that he had not done any new clinico-pathological studies on that problem, but that he aimed at a new theoretical treatment of various clinical aspects of aphasia. In essence the study discusses the question of the relation between brain lesions on the one hand and disturbances of higher human behavior on the other hand. He reviewed critically the theory on brain function of Wernicke which was then dominant. Two assumptions of this theory had to be changed, according to Freud:

1.   brain functions are related to brain centers.
2.   brain functions are related to relations between centers and conduction between centers.

At that time it was accepted that every "function" would have its "brain center", or could be explained by cooperation between various centers. This was stimulated by the very productive clinical activity of finding brain lesions accompanied by specific functional defects. Pathology was the main reference of thinking for physiology. Freud brought to the reader's attention new theoretical concepts that appeared at that time in England and were formulated mainly by Bastian and Hughlings-Jackson. These theories favor the central concept that brain functions are dependent on and have to be defined by *levels of organization*. As such, Freud's concepts of brain function are "structuralisme avant la lettre". It is stated that every part of the brain has its place in organizational levels, but that these parts are largely interchangeable on one level. Dependent on the type, the localization, and the extent of the brain lesion, cerebral organization will be changed or reduced in level. The brain's work is not dependent on "centers" and "wiring", but the brain as a whole organizes itself, structures itself. The way it reacts to lesions is also an organizational response, defined as higher and lower in complexity and as more or less effective in response to the demands of body and environment.

In the period in which Freud was busy formulating these concepts, he also found overwhelming evidence that organizational principles (drives) were behind behavioral abnormalities (symptoms and signs). As such his study *Zur Auffassung der Aphasien* can be seen as the major step away from the clinical neurologist that he was, thinking in terms of centers and tracts, toward what he became: the founder of psychoanalysis, understanding human behavior as levels of organization, governed by basic principles. From this point of view Freud's work on aphasia surpasses by far the "telephone" or the more refined "computer" thinking that is still prominent today in clinical neurology. Freud's views are, at least and at last, adequate to the unheard and unthought complexities of brain activity and human behavior in relation to the brain.

The theme

Wernicke's interpretattion of aphasia can be described by what, at that time, was called a cerebral reflex. In Figure 1 the positions of sensory (receptive) aphasia, conduction aphasia, and motor (productive) aphasia in this reflex system are given.

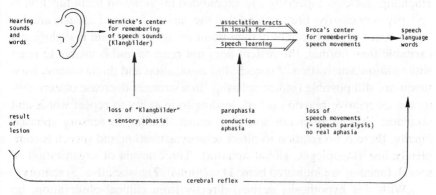

Figure 1. Wernicke's theory on aphasias as disturbances of a cerebral reflex

Freud indicates that a lesion of association tracts should block words and sentence repetition, but should leave spontaneous speech intact. As this is never found clinically, Freud claims that conduction aphasia as such does not exist.

The hypothesis that speech learning is done with association tracts is refuted by Freud, as never having been proven clinically. Then the evidence is reviewed that clinical signs and symptoms make the assumption of speech centers necessary. He concludes that such evidence does not exist and that the logical necessity of the assumption of speech centers is absent.

Freud then goes on to discuss "inner speech". Freud indicates that it is an important aspect of all knowledge of speech and should be included in considerations on aphasia.

In the discussion of clinical aspects of paraphasia, Freud showed that in this condition the right word is replaced by another because of similar significance or similar sound; condensation and generalization of words also occurs. It is as if Freud presaged here his later studies in hysteria and dreams, where he described the same dynamics for contents of the unconsciousness. In the whole discussion of the prevailing theory of aphasia, it is remarkable how carefully Freud investigated all the relevant clinical signs and symptoms, without jumping to conclusions. Finally, he demonstrated so many lapses in the existing theory on aphasia that the way was free for a more adequate and encompassing hypothesis.

For the functional hypothesis that Freud then proposed, he referred to Charlton Bastian and John Hughlings Jackson, two British neurologists. Hughlings Jackson especially had expounded his views on brain function in epilepsy very clearly. Freud stated that the various forms of aphasia are different states of excitation of certain brain areas. If the brain is slightly less excitable than normal, the patient does not react to and is unable to react with volitional activation of speech, but association and direct sensory excitation are still possible (motor aphasia). In a stronger decrease of excitability the associative reaction is lost, leading to inability to repeat words and sentences, but spontaneous speech is intact, leading to sensory aphasia. Finally, there is no relation to direct sensory activation and speech is completely lost (logoplegia, global aphasia). Three levels of organization of speech function are indicated here: 1) volitional, 2) associative, 3) sensory.

With this hypothesis, derived directly from clinical observation, no centers are needed to explain the various forms of aphasia. Only one large cortical area is assigned to speech functions. The various clinical forms are described as different levels of disorganization in this area. This hypothesis is also able to explain other functional activities and functional states of parts or of the whole of the central nervous system. However, it has some other implications that may be even more important. The hypothesis also explains the reverse, from complete logoplegia to normal speech. And it can be easily adapted to explain the development of speech in children. This lucidly explained hypothesis was completely new at that time and has, even now, not lost any of its splendor.

Levels of organization and aphasia

In short, Freud stated that global aphasia (logoplegia) indicates a total loss of functional organization of the speech area of the brain. The lowest level of organization is observed in sensory aphasia. The next higher level makes associative speech possible (conduction aphasia), but with anomia (amnestic aphasia). The amnestic aphasia or anomia Freud explained, following Grashey, with what we now would call extinction. This form of aphasia occurs when the functional activation of the brain is not of sufficient duration or of sufficient intensity. Special situations such as tiredness and drowsiness may increase the threshold and so produce insufficient activation and amnestic aphasia. Amnestic aphasia can thus be described as extinction of speech that can be corrected by intensification or longer duration of activation. The levels of organization of speech described above can also be found in individual speech development of the child. The hypothesis encompasses normal development and abnormal clinical symptomatology.

It is clear that Freud rejected localization of words, images of sounds (*Klangbilder*), and images of movement (*Bewegungsbilder*) in "centers". He proposed that larger areas of the brain are functionally related to the interpretation of information from our body and our world. What happens in the brain Freud called a *"Vorgang"*, a process, a happening. Implicitly he refused to classify these processes as physical or psychic. The functional organization of these interpretive processes from our body and our world are localized in cortical areas, which in modern neuro-anatomy are called projection areas: motor, somatosensory, acoustic, and visual. These areas surround the area that organizes speech. Clinical interpretation of functional loss after a lesion has to take that into account.

In the functional organization of the cortical areas various levels are found, as discussed earlier for the speech area. Freud assumed that the organizational level of speech is higher than those of the surrounding cortical regions of somatosensory projection areas. In these regions parts of bodily and environmentally perceived significance are organized. In the speech area this all has to be integrated into a higher level of organization of symbolic structures. Starting from this point Freud discussed what the study of clinical speech disturbances can teach us about the function of the brain. Disturbances of speech can now be divided in three levels of organization.

1. Aphasia of the first order — verbal aphasia — shows disturbances of highest integrative and associative use of words. It is a disturbance of organization of the speech area itself, and not of the surrounding areas.

2. Aphasia of the second order — asymbolic aphasia — shows disturbances of the speech area in its relations to the surrounding functional organization of motor activities, somatosensory, optic, and acoustic representations.

3. Aphasia of the third order — agnostic aphasia — shows disturbances of the surrounding motor acoustic, somatosensory, and visual functional representations between them.

Conclusions

Freud's hypotheses on the clinical significance of aphasia may be represented as in Figure 2.

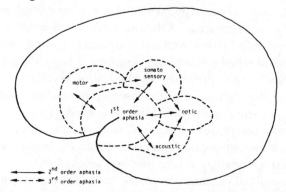

Figure 2. *Freud's hypothesis on functional and regional organization of speech in human cortical areas. Lesions of areas are indicated as 1st, 2nd, and 3rd order aphasia.*

In each of the functional organizations several levels of activation may be found. The forms of aphasia known from clinical observation can each find their place very easily in this schema, without losing their localizational aspect too much, but also not giving too much weight to the topographical aspects. It is a functional theory relating domains to functional organizations. It can be applied to all higher integrative organismal activities. The problem is that these activities have to be defined first, before defects in clinical neurology can be detected. From Freud's later work we might suppose that he would call such higher integrative organizational activities sexual drive, unconsciousness, ego, self, id, or even complex formations. It would be highly rewarding to study some aspects of Freud's theory combined with data of modern neurophysiology and neurology of human behavior and also in the light of Lacan's psychiatry.

References

Eissler, K.R. 1978 "Biographical Sketch". *Sigmund Freud: his life in Pictures and Words*, ed. by E. Freud, L. Freud and J. Grubich-Simites. New York: Harcourt, Brace and Jovanovich.
Freud, S. 1891. *Zur Auffassung der Aphasien*. Wien: Deuticke.
Lacan, J. 1958. *Les Psychoses*. Paris: P.U.F.
Wernicke, C. 1874. *Der aphasische Symptomencomplex*. Breslau: Cohn & Weigert.

Selection from the work of Sigmund Freud

On Aphasia*

We have rejected the assumptions that the speech apparatus consists of distinct centres separated by functionless areas, and that ideas (memories) serving speech are stored in certain parts of the cortex called centres while their association is provided exclusively by subcortical fibre tracts. It only remains for us to state the view that the speech area is a continuous cortical region within which the associations and transmissions underlying the speech functions are taking place; they are of a complexity beyond comprehension.

How can such a theory explain the existence of the speech centres, especially of the areas of Broca and Wernicke established by morbid anatomy? A glance at the convexity of a left hemisphere will enlighten us; the situation of the so-called speech centres suggests an explanation which fits well into our theory. These centres lie far apart; according to Naunyn, they are situated in the posterior part of the first temporal convolution, the posterior part of the third frontal gyrus and in the inferior part of the parietal lobe where the angular gyrus merges into the occipital lobe; the site of a fourth centre, for writing, does not seem to be definitely established (?posterior part of the middle frontal gyrus). These areas are situated in such a way that there lies between them a large cortical region, i.e., the

---

* Reprinted from "On Aphasia", London: Imago Publishing Co., pp. 62-83 (1953)

insula with the convolutions covering it; the lesion of any part of this area is probably always associated with speech disorder. Although the extent of this area cannot be exactly delineated from a survey of lesions found in cases of aphasia, one can nevertheless say that the so-called speech centres form the outlying parts of the speech area assumed by us, and that speech disorders occur when lesions are situated within the external boundaries of these centres; i.e., towards the centre of the hemisphere, while lesions in cortical areas lying outside them are of a different significance. Thus the "centres" appear as the corner stones of the speech territory. Next we have to consider the areas adjoining these centres from outside. Broca's area is immediately adjacent to the centres of the bulbar motor nerves. Wernicke's area is situated in a region which also contains the acoustic termination, the exact location of which is unknown; the visual speech centre borders on those parts of the occipital lobe in which we know the optic nerve to terminate. An arrangement such as this, though meaningless from the point of view of the centre theory, has for us the following significance:

The association area of speech, into which visual, auditory, and motor (or kinaesthetic) elements enter, extends for that very reason between the cortical areas of those sensory nerves and the motor regions concerned with speech. If we now imagine a movable lesion of constant size within this association area, its effect will be the greater the more it approaches one of these cortical fields, i.e., the more peripherally it is situated within the speech area. If it borders immediately on one of these cortical fields it will cut off the association area from one of its tributaries, i.e., the mechanisms of speech will be deprived of the visual, or auditory, or some other element, as every association of that nature used to come from that particular corti-cal field. If the lesion is moved towards the interior of the association area its effect will be more indefinite; in no event will it be able to destroy all possibilities of one particular category of associations. Thus the parts of the speech region bordering on the cortical fields of the optic, auditory and motor cranial nerves have gained the significance demonstrated by morbid anatomy which has established them as centres of speech. This significance, however, holds only for the pathology, and not for the physiology of the speech apparatus, because it cannot be maintained that in these parts other, or more important, processes take place than in those parts of the speech area the damage of which is better tolerated. This view follows directly from our refusal to separate the process of the idea (concept) from that of association, and to localize the two in separate parts.

Wernicke came near to these views only in his last observations on this subject when he expressed doubt as to whether we were justified in assuming separate centres for reading within the visual receptive area of the cortex, and for writing within the so-called motor arm-region [Wernicke 1881, p. 477]. But his doubt was not of a fundamental nature; it amounted to no more than an anatomical amendment implying that the visual and cheiromotor impressions so important for speech, were situated among other impressions contributing to speech. Heubner, on the contrary, in discussing his case felt compelled to ask a question similar to the one raised here for speech in general: "Are there perhaps no cortical areas for mind blindness, mind deafness and mind muteness? Are these symptoms not rather simply due to the separation of the cortical areas subserving these functions from the rest of the cortex by lesions localized in their vicinity?"

There are two possible objections against the validity of our views about the centres:

(1) If destruction of the parts of the speech area bordering directly on a cortical receptive or motor field has the described effect on the speech function only because it has severed the connections with the respective sources of association, the destruction of these receptive and cortical areas themselves ought to have the same result. This, however, is contrary to clinical experience which has established that all such lesions cause localized symptoms without speech disorder. This first objection can easily be disposed of if one considers that all these cortical areas are bilateral, while that of the association area of speech is organized in one hemisphere only. Destruction of one visual cortical area, for example, will not interfere with the utilization of visual stimuli for speech, i.e., with reading, because the speech area retains its connections with the contralateral visual cortex, which, in this particular case, is provided by crossed white fibres. If, however, the lesion moves to the boundary of the visual receptive area, alexia ensues, probably because the connection not only with the homolateral, but also with the contralateral visual area has been severed. We therefore have to add to our theory: the appearance of centres is also created by the fact that the fibres from the cortical receptive fields of the other hemisphere enter at the same place, i.e., on the periphery of the speech area where, in case of lesion, the connection with the homolateral receptive areas is also effected. This is plausible, because for the function of speech association the presence of a bilateral origin of visual, auditory and other stimuli is physiologically irrelevant.

The assumption, by the way, that the speech region is connected with cortical areas of both hemispheres is not new, but has been taken over from the theory of the centres. The precise anatomy of these crossed connections has not yet been established, but when it is known it might explain some peculiarities in the localization and extent of the so-called centres, as well as some of the individual features of the speech disorders.

(2) The question may be raised what advantage there be in denying the existence of special centres for speech while we have to assume cortical fields, i.e., centres, for the visual and auditory nerves, and for the motor organs of speech. The answer is that there is no reason why these areas should not be subjected to similar considerations. However, their existence cannot be disputed; their extent is defined by the anatomical fact of the termination of the sensory nerves and the origin of the pyramidal tract in circumscribed areas of the cortex. The region of speech associations, however, lacks these direct relations to the periphery of the body. It certainly has no sensory and most probably no special motor "projection fibres".[1]

VI

Our concept of the organization of the central apparatus of speech is that of a continuous cortical region occupying the space between the terminations of the optic and acoustic nerves and of the areas of the cranial and certain peripheral motor nerves in the left hemisphere. It probably covers, therefore, the same area which Wernicke was inclined to allocate to speech in his first paper, i.e., all the convolutions forming the Sylvian fissure. We have refused to localize the psychic elements of the speech process in specified areas within this region; we have rejected the supposition that there were areas within this region which were excluded from the speech function in general and kept in reserve for the acquisition of new knowledge of speech. Finally, we have attributed the fact that pathology has demonstrated centres of speech, though of indefinite delimitation, to the situation of the adjoining receptive and motor cortical areas and of the crossed fibre tracts. Thus the speech centres are, in our view, parts of the cortex which may claim a pathological but no special physiological significance. We feel justified in rejecting the differentiation between the so-called centre or cortical aphasias and the conduction (association) aphasias, and we maintain that all aphasias originate in interruption of associations, i.e., of conduction.

Aphasia through destruction or lesion of a centre is to us no more and no less than aphasia through lesion of those association fibres which meet in that nodal point called a centre.

We have also asserted that every aphasia is directly, or through some remote effect, caused by disturbance within the cortex itself. This implies that the speech area has no afferent or efferent pathways of its own extending to the periphery of the body. This statement is proved by the fact that subcortical lesions of any location are incapable of producing aphasia, provided anarthria is excluded by definition. Nobody has even been known to become word deaf as the result of a lesion in the auditory nerve, in the medulla oblongata, in the posterior corpora quadrigemina or in the internal capsule unless he had been deaf already; nor has anybody ever been made word blind by a partial lesion of the optic nerve, or of the diencephalon, etc. However, Lichtheim differentiates a subcortical word deafness and a subcortical motor aphasia, and Wernicke postulates subcortical alexia and agraphia. They do not attribute these types of speech disorder to lesions of subcortical fascicles of association fibres, which in our view cannot be differentiated from association fibres within the cortex itself, but to lesions of radial, i.e., afferent or efferent speech tracts. It is therefore necessary to analyse these subcortical aphasias more precisely.

The characteristic features of a subcortical sensory aphasia can easily be deduced from Lichtheim's schema which postulates a special auditory tract α A (Fig. 1) for speech. The patient is supposed to be unable to perceive word sounds, yet capable of availing himself of previously acquired sound impressions and of carrying out all other speech functions faultlessly. Lichtheim actually found such a case; although the early stages of this patient's illness had not been fully elucidated, his final state entirely conformed to the picture supposed to be caused by interruption of α A. I confess that in view of the importance of the sound images for the speech function I have found it exceedingly difficult to find another explanation for this subcortical sensory aphasia which would make the assumption of an afferent auditory tract A unnecessary. I was already inclined to explain Lichtheim's case by assuming that individual speech might be independent of the sound images; the patient was a highly educated journalist. But such an explanation would quite rightly have been regarded as a mere subterfuge.

I therefore searched the literature for similar cases. Wernicke, in reviewing Lichtheim's paper, stated that he had made a similar observation which he was going to publish in the regular reports from his clinic. Unfortunately I have not been able to find this report in the literature.[2] However, I found a case described by Giraudeau[3] which closely resembled Lichtheim's patient. Giraudeau's patient (Bouquinet) was able to speak perfectly well but she showed a severe word deafness without being deaf. However, the data concerning her hearing ability were incomplete. She could understand questions addressed to her but only after they had been repeated several times, and even then she failed frequently. Once a question had been understood and answered, all following replies would continue in the same train of thought, the patient not taking any notice of later questions. The two patients appear even more alike if we consider that the behaviour of Lichtheim's patient differed from that commonly observed in cases of word deafness. He did not make any effort to understand questions addressed to him; he gave no reply nor did he appear to pay any attention to what he heard. Perhaps the patient, by this apparently purposive behaviour, gave the wrong impression of being completely word deaf, while possibly repeated and urgent requests might have made him, like Bouquinet, understand. Word deaf patients, as a rule, perceive language which they are unable to understand; they believe, however, that they have understood something and, as a result, tend to give inappropriate answers.

The post-mortem examination of Giraudeau's patient revealed a lesion of the first and second temporal convolution, such as has so frequently been found to underlie ordinary sensory aphasia. Nobody, looking at the drawing attached to Giraudeau's communication, would have thought that this lesion had caused anything but the common form of sensory aphasia. But there is another aspect to be considered. The lesion in Giraudeau's case was again an unusual one, i.e., a tumour (gliosarcoma). In discussing transcortical motor aphasia, I ventured the opinion that probably a lesion of the speech apparatus did not only cause localizing signs, but that the special nature of the disease process might be revealed by a functional modification of its symptoms. Giraudeau's case, therefore, does not prove the existence of the subcortical fibre tract A. The tumour found at the post-mortem examination had not proliferated from the white matter outwardly, having perhaps in an earlier state caused a subcortical lesion only. On the contrary, it was attached to the meninges and could easily be lifted from the softened white matter. I therefore feel justified in assuming that the subcortical sensory aphasia is not due to a lesion of a subcortical pathway A, but to damage of the same localization as found in cases with cortical sensory aphasia.

However, I am unable to throw light on the specific functional state of the area thus affected.[4]

Subcortical motor aphasia can be dealt with more briefly. According to Lichtheim it is characterized by intact writing ability in the presence of symptoms of cortical motor aphasia. Wernicke, who made a careful analysis of the disorders of written language, refused to accept this criterion. To him the one characteristic feature of the subcortical motor aphasia is the patient's ability to state the number of syllables. The controversies over Lichtheim's test have been mentioned earlier in this book. Some observations made by Dejerine (1891) have in the meantime confirmed the significance of Lichtheim's syllable test for the diagnosis of subcortical motor aphasia. However, this particular speech disorder could with equal justification be classified as anarthria rather than aphasia.

Several well observed cases, the most recent one by Eisenlohr (1889), suggest that damage underneath Broca's area causes a speech disorder which can be described as literal paraphasia and which represents a transition to dysarthria. For the motor part of the speech apparatus alone, therefore, a special pathway to the periphery may have to be conceded. However, in attributing a special efferent tract to the motor speech area, we want to point out that the deeper the lesion is situated the more closely the disability resembles anarthria. Aphasia still remains a cortical phenomenon.

Therefore, the speech apparatus as conceived by us, has no afferent or efferent pathways of its own, except for a fibre tract the lesion of which causes dysarthria. We shall refer to the so-called subcortical reading and writing disorders later on.

We now propose to inquire what kind of hypotheses have to be made about the causation of aphasias following lesions of a speech apparatus thus organized; or, in other words, what does the study of the aphasias teach us about the function of this apparatus? In doing this we shall endeavour to separate the psychological from the anatomical aspect of the problem as much as possible.

From the psychological point of view the "word" is the functional unit of speech; it is a complex concept constituted of auditory, visual and kinaesthetic elements. We owe the knowledge of this structure to pathology which demonstrates that organic lesions affecting the speech apparatus result in a disintegration of speech corresponding to such a constitution. We have learned to regard the loss of any one of these elements as the most important pointer to the localization of the damage. Four constituents of the word concept are usually listed: the "sound image" or "sound impression", the "visual letter image", the "glosso-kinaesthetic and the cheiro-kinaesthetic images or impressions". However, this constitution appears even more complicated if one considers the probable process of association involved in the various speech activities.

(1) We learn to speak by associating a "word sound image" with an "impression of word innervation". When we have spoken we are in possession of a "kinaesthetic word image", i.e., of the sensory impressions from the organs of speech. The motor aspect of the "word" therefore is doubly determined. Of its two elements the former, i.e., the impression of word innervation, seems to be the least important psychologically. Its existence as a psychological element may even be disputed. We also perceive, after having spoken, a "sound image" or "sound impression" of the spoken word. As long as we have not perfected our speech, the second sound image, though associated with the first, need not be identical with it. At this stage, which is the phase of speech development in childhood, we use a language built up by ourselves; in associating various other word sounds with the one produced by ourselves we behave like the motor aphasics.

(2) We learn the language of others by endeavouring to equate the sound image produced by ourselves as much as possible to the one which had served as the stimulus for the act of innervation of our speech muscles, i.e., we learn to "repeat". In "continuous speech" we produce a series of words by waiting with the innervation of the speech muscles until the word sound, or the kinaesthetic word impression of the preceding word, or both, have been perceived. The safeguards of our speech against breakdown thus appear over-determined, and it can easily stand the loss of one or the other element. However, the loss of the correcting function of the second sound image and of the kinaesthetic word image explains some peculiarities of paraphasia, both physiological and pathological.

(3) We learn to spell by associating the visual images of the letters with new sound images which inevitably recall word sounds already known. We immediately repeat the word sound characteristic of the letter. Thus, in spelling aloud, the letter, too, appears determined by two sound impressions which tend to be identical, and two motor impressions which closely correspond to each other.

We learn to read by linking up with each other, according to certain rules, a succession of word innervation impressions and kinaesthetic word impressions perceived in enunciating individual letters. As a result, new kinaesthetic word images originate, but as soon as they have been enunciated we detect from their sound images that both kinaesthetic and sound images so perceived have long been familiar to us, being identical with those used in speaking. Next, we associate with those word images acquired by spelling the significance attached to the original word sounds. Now we read with understanding. If we have originally spoken a dialect instead of a literary language, we have to super-associate the kinaesthetic and sound impressions perceived in spelling aloud over the original ones, and we have to acquire a new language in this way; this process is facilitated by the resemblance between dialect and literary language.

This presentation shows that the process of learning to read is very complicated indeed and entails a frequent shift of the direction of the associations. It also suggests that the defects of reading in aphasia originate in various ways. Impairment of reading letters is characteristic of a defect of the visual element. The assembling of letters to a word takes place in the process of transmission to the speech tract; it will therefore be abolished in motor aphasia. The understanding of what has been read is effected only with the aid of the sound images produced by the words uttered, or through the kinaesthetic impressions produced in speaking. Reading with understanding thus proves to be a function which disintegreates as the result not only of motor but also of auditory defects, furthermore a function which is independent of the act of reading itself. Everybody knows from self observation that there are several kinds of reading some of which proceed without understanding. When I read proofs with the intention of paying special attention to the letters and other symbols, the meaning of what I am reading escapes me to such a degree that I require a second perusal for the purpose of correcting the style. If, on the other hand, I read a novel, which holds my interest, I overlook all misprints and it may happen that I retain nothing of the names of the persons figuring in the book except for some meaningless feature, or perhaps the recollection that they were long or short, and that they contained an unusual letter such as x or z. Again, when I have to recite, whereby I have to pay special attention to the sound impressions of my words and to the intervals between them, I am in danger of caring too little about the meaning, and as soon as fatigue sets in I am reading in such a way that the listener can still understand, but I myself no longer know what I have been reading. These are phenomena of divided attention which are of particular importance here, because the understanding of what is read takes place over circuitous routes. It is clear from the analogy with our own behaviour that understanding becomes impossible once reading itself has become difficult, and we must beware of regarding this as an indication of a lesion in a fibre tract. Reading aloud is not to be regarded as a different function form reading to oneself, except that it tends to distract attention from the sensory part of the reading process.

(5) We learn to write by reproducing the visual images of the letters with the help of kinaesthetic impressions received from the hand (cheiro-kinaesthetic impressions) until we have obtained identical or similar pictures. As a rule, the pictures produced in writing are only similar to, and super-associated over those perceived in reading, as we learn to read print but have to use different characters in handwriting. Writing is comparatively simpler and less vulnerable than reading.

(6) It can be assumed that the various speech activities continue to be performed by way of the same associations by which we learned them. Abbreviations and substitutions may be employed, but their nature is not always easy to recognize. Their significance is still further reduced by the consideration that in cases of organic lesion the speech apparatus as a whole probably suffers some damage and is forced into a return towards the primary and secure, though more cumbersome modes of associations. In the case of the experienced reader the influence of the "visual word image" makes itself felt, with the result that single words, especially proper names, can be read even without recourse to spelling.

The word, then, is a complicated concept built up from various impressions, i.e., it corresponds to an intricate process of associations entered into by elements of visual, acoustic and kinaesthetic origins.

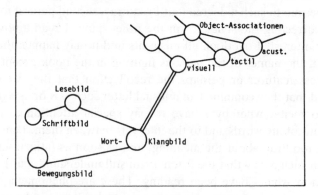

Figure 1. *Psychological schema of the word concept*

The word concept appears as a closed complex of images, the object concept as an open one. The word concept is linked to the concept of the object via the sound image only. Among the object associations, the visual ones play a part similar to that played by the sound image among the word associations. The connections of the word sound image with object associations other than the visual are not presented in this schema.

However, the word acquires its significance through its association with the "idea (concept) of the object", at least if we restrict our considerations to nouns. The idea, or concept, of the object is itself another complex of associations composed of the most varied visual, auditory, tactile, kinaesthetic and other impressions. According to philosophical teaching, the idea of the object contains nothing else; the appearance of a "thing", the "properties" of which are conveyed to us by our senses, originates only from the fact that in enumerating the sensory impressions perceived from an object, we allow for the possibility of a large series of new impressions being added to the chain of associations (J.S. Mill). This is why the idea of the object does not appear to us as closed, and indeed hardly as closable, while the word concept appears to us as something that is closed though capable of extension.

In the light of observations in speech disorders we have formed the view that the word concept (the idea of the word) is linked with its sensory part, in particular through its sound impressions, to the object concept. In consequence, we have arrived at a division of speech disorders into two classes: (1) verbal aphasia, in which only the associations between the single elements of the word concept are disturbed; and (2) asymbolic aphasia, in which the association between word concept and object concepts are disturbed.

I am using the term asymbolia in a different sense from that given to it by Finkelnburg[5] because "asymbolic" seems more appropriate a designation for the relationship between the word and the idea of the object than for that between the object and its idea. For disturbances in the recognition of objects, which Finkelnburg called asymbolia, I should like to propose the term "agnosia". It is quite possible that agnostic disturbances which occur only in cases of bilateral and extensive cortical lesions, may also entail a disturbance of speech as all stimuli to spontaneous speech arise from object associations. Such speech disorders I should call the third group of aphasias, or "agnostic aphasias". Clinical experience has in fact acquainted us with several cases which call for such a concept.

The first case of agnostic aphasia is that of Farges (1885) which was inadequately observed and most inappropriately interpreted as *"aphasie chez une tactile"*; but I hope the clinical facts will speak for themselves. The patient was a case of cerebral blindness, probably due to bilateral cortical lesions. She did not reply when addressed, and when one tried hard to contact her she kept on repeating, *"Je ne veux pas, je ne peux pas!"* in a tone of extreme impatience. She was unable to recognize her doctor by his voice. However, as soon as he felt her pulse, i.e., as soon as he provided her with the opportunity of a tactile association, she at once recognized him, called him by his name and chatted with him without any sign of aphasia, until he let her hand go and thus again became inacessible to her. The same happened in relationship to objects when she was given the opportunity of producing associations of touch, smell or taste by being offered the respective sensory stimuli. As long as they lasted she had the necessary words at her command and behaved in a purposeful manner; however, as soon as she was deprived of them she resumed her monotonous expressions of impatience or uttered incoherent syllables and proved unable to understand what was said to her. This patient therefore had a completely intact speech apparatus which she was unable to utilize unless it was stimulated by those object associations which had remained intact.

A second observation of this type caused C.S. Freund (1889) to postulate the category of "optic aphasia". His patient showed difficulties in spontaneous speech and in naming objects very similar to those observed in sensory aphasia. The following is a sample of his reactions: he called a candlestick "spectacles", and on looking again he said, "It is for putting on, a top hat" and immediately afterwards: "It is a stearin light". If, however, he was allowed to take the object into his hands with his eyes closed he quickly found the correct name. His speech apparatus, therefore, was intact, but it failed when stimulated by way of visual object associations only, while it worked correctly when stimulated through tactile object associations. However, in Freund's case the effect of the disturbance of the object associations had a less severe effect than in Farges' case. Freund's patient deteriorated and later became completely word deaf. The post-mortem examination revealed lesions involving not only the visual but also the speech area.

The disabling effect which disturbances of the visual object associations may have on the speech function can be explained by the special importance that they assume in certain cases. In an individual whose thought processes depend largely on visual images, a peculiarity which according to Charcot is determined by individual predisposition, bilateral lesions in the visual cortext are bound to cause in addition disorders of the speech function which go far beyond what can be accounted for by the localization of the lesions. *"Aphasie chez une visuelle"* would have been a far more appropriate description for Farges' observation than *"aphasie chez und tactile"*.

While agnostic aphasia was in these cases caused by a remote functional effect in the absence of an organic lesion of the speech apparatus itself, the verbal and asymbolic aphasias are manifestations of such a lesion. We shall endeavour as far as possible to differentiate the functional from the topographical factors in the analysis of these speech disorders.

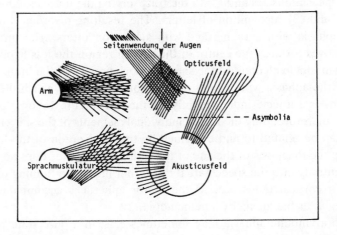

Figure 2. Anatomical schema of the area of the speech associations demonstrating how the appearance of speech centres is created. The auditory and visual receptive fields and the motor areas for the muscles serving articulation and writing are represented by circles. The association tracts connecting them with the interior of the speech area are represented by radiating fascicles. The area in which the latter are crossed by the corresponding fascicles from the other hemisphere becomes a centre for the respective associative element when the tracts are cut off from the fields represented by circles. The crossed connections of the auditory receptive field have been omitted from the schema to avoid confusion, and also because of the uncertainty of the connections between the auditory receptive field and the sensory speech centre. The separation of the connections with the visual receptive field into two fascicles is based on the consideration that the eye movements play an important part in the associations contributing to the act of reading.

We have designed a schema (Fig. 2) which is meant to illustrate the relations between the various elements of speech associations without taking into account anatomical details. In this schema the circles do not represent the so-called speech centres but show the receptive and motor cortical fields between which the speech associations take place. The parts of the speech area bordering on these cortical fields acquire the significance of centres by virtue of their crossed connections with the other hemisphere: those connected with the cortical fields for the hand, the speech muscles and the optic nerve can be seen in the schema. It follows that in the case of a verbal aphasia, three symptoms can be accounted for by the localization of the lesion: if the latter is situated within the "speech centres", the following functions will be impaired: (1) transmission of stimuli to the tracts serving the speech muscles and (2) to the tract serving the muscles employed in writing, and (3) recognition of letters. The resulting disorder is a typical motor aphasia with agraphia and with alexia for letters. The further the lesion moves towards the centre of the speech region the less likely it is to cut off any single element of the speech associations, and the more the features of the aphasia will depend on functional factors to which the speech apparatus is subject, independently of the site of the lesion. In verbal aphasia, therefore, only the loss of individual elements of the speech associations can be related to and explained by the localization of the lesion. It will help the diagnosis of the site of the lesion if the latter does not extend more centrally into the speech area, but rather into the adjoining receptive or motor cortical fields, i.e., if the motor aphasia is accompanied by a hemiplegia, or the alexia by a hemianopia.

The asymbolic aphasia may sometimes exist in a pure state resulting from a cicumscribed lesion lying across the path of the association tracts. This had happened in Heubner's patient who presented an almost ideal example of the separation of the speech region from its associations by a vascular lesion encircling the auditory area which is a nodal point of the speech region. Asymbolic speech disorder without complications, i.e., without disturbance of the word associations, may also result from a merely functional state of the speech apparatus as a whole; there are some indications that the link between word associations and object associations is the most easily exhaustible component of the speech function, its weakest point as it were. This was illustrated in an interesting paper by Pick (1889) who had noted transient word deafness following epileptic fits. The patient observed by him showed an asymbolic speech disorder in the course of her recovery from the fit. Even before the understanding returned she was able to repeat words spoken to her.

The phenomenon of echolalia, i.e., the repetition of questions asked, appears to belong to the asymbolic disorders. In some of these cases, e.g., in those observed by Skwortzoff (1881) (case X) and Fränkel (quoted by Ballet 1886), echolalia proved to be a means of overcoming the difficulties in relating the words perceived to the object associations by reinforcement of the word sounds. These patients failed to understand questions at first, but were able to understand and answer them after they had repeated them. This phenomenon also calls to mind Bastian's thesis that a speech centre, the function of which is impaired, loses first the ability to respond to "volitional" stimuli, while still able to react efficiently to sensory stimulation and in association with other speech centres. Every "volitional" excitation of the speech centres, however, involves the area of the auditory images and results in its stimulation by object associations.

Notes

1. I reported the main contents of this study in a paper read to the "Wiener physiologischer Club" (Vienna Physiological Club) as early as 1886. However, the statutes of this club do not allow for a claim to priority to be based on its proceedings. In 1887 Nothnagel and Naunyn presented their well-known review on the localization of brain diseases to the Congress of Internal Medicine at Wiesbaden. Their views agree with those presented here in several important points. Nothnagel's observations on the concept of cerebral centres as well as Naunyn's remarks on the topography of the speech areas are likely to make readers suspect that my study was influenced by their highly significant review. This was not the case; the stimulus to this study came, in fact, from papers published by Exner jointly with my late friend Josef Paneth in Pflüger's Archiv.

2. A private enquiry at the Breslau Clinic revealed that the cases mentioned in this context by Wernicke have not yet been published.

3. Giraudeau: *Revue de Médecine, 1882*; also quoted by Bernard, *De l'aphasie et de ses diverses formes*, Paris, 1885.

4. Notwithstanding these considerations, I still find it very difficult to explain the subcortical sensory aphasia, i.e., word deafness without impairment of spontaneous speech, while Lichtheim's schema disposes of the problem by simply assuming interruption of a tract A. It was therefore of great value to me to come across a paper by Adler (1891) in which a similar case was described as "a combination of subcortical and transcortical sensory aphasia".

    A comparison of Adler's case with those of Lichtheim and Wernicke contributes to the understanding of the so-called subcortical sensory aphasia. Two points in particular are illuminating. (1) Lichtheim mentioned the possibility that his patient may have been slightly deaf as the data about his hearing ability were incomplete. Wernicke's patient had a defect for higher tones. Adler's patient had definitely diminished hearing, which according to the author was most probably due to a disturbance in the apparatus of sound conduction. It is, therefore, possible that ordinary deafness, peripheral or central in origin, may play a part in this disorder, such as was the case in Arnaud's patients to be referred to later. (2) More decisive still is the following conformity which can hardly be incidental. Both cases (Lichtheim and Adler; Wernicke's brief note is silent on this point) developed the picture of subcortical sensory aphasia only after repeated cerebral accidents of which at least one had involved the minor hemisphere; Lichtheim's patient had a left-sided facial palsy, Adler's case a left-sided hemiplegia. Adler mentioned this coincidence without recognizing its significance for the explanation of pure word deafness. I feel justified in assuming that subcortical sensory aphasia is caused not, as postulated in Lichtheim's schema, by a simple tract interruption, but through incomplete bilateral lesions in the receptive field of hearing, perhaps combined with peripheral deafness, as was the case in Arnaud's patients. Such complicated conditions for an apparently simple speech disorder fit better into my conception of the sensory aphasias than into that of Lichtheim.

5.   Quoted from Spamer (1876).

References

Adler, A. 1891. "Beitrag zur Kenntnis der selteneren Formen der sensorischen Aphasie". _Neurologischer Controlblatt_ 15:296.

Ballet, G. 1886. Le langage interieur et les diverses formes de l'aphasie. Paris: Félix Alcan.

Dejerine, J. 1891. "Contribution à l'etude de l'aphasie motrice sous-corticale et de la localisation cérébrale des centres larynges (muscles phonateurs)". _Mémoires de la Société de Biologie_ 3: 155-162.

Eisenlohr, C. 1889. "Beitrage zur Lehre von der Aphasie". _Deutsche Medische Wochenschrfit_ 36:737-742.

Farges, L. 1885. "Aphasie chez une tactile". _L'Encephale_ No. 5.

Freund, C.S. 1889. "Ueber optische Aphasie und Seelenblindheit". _Archiv für Psychiatrie und Nervenkrankheiten_, 20:276-297; 375-416.

Heubner, E. 1889. "Ueber Aphasie." _Schmidt's Jahrbücher_, Bd. 224, p. 220.

Lichtheim, L. 1885. "Ueber Aphasie." _Deutsches Archiv für Klinische Medizin_ 36:204-268.

Pick, A. 1889. "Zur Lokalisation einseitiger Gehörshallicinationen, nebst Bemerkungen über transitorische Worttaubheit". _Jahrbuch für Psychiatrie_ 8:1-2.

Pick, A. 1891. "Neue Beiträge zur Pathologie der Sprache." _Archiv für Psychiatrie und Nervenkrankheiten_ 28:1-52.

Pick, A. 1891. "Ueber die sogenannte Re-evolution (Hughlings Jackson) nach epileptischen Anfällen, nebst Bemerkungen über transitorische Worttaubheit". _Archiv für Psychiatrie und Nervenkrankheiten_ 22:3.

Skwortzoff, A. 1881. _De la Cécité et de la Surdité des Mots dans l'Aphasie._ Paris: Masson & Cie.

Spamer, F. 1876. "Ueber Aphasie und Asymbolie, nebst Versuch einer Theorie der Sprachbildung". _Archiv fuer Psychiatrie und Nervenkrankheiten_ 6:496-542.

Wernicke, C. 1881. _Lehrbuch der Gehirnkrankheiten._ Vol. 1. Berlin: Fischer.

Jules Dejerine

Introduced by

Willy O. RENIER
Institute of Neurology, University of Nijmegen
Nijmegen, The Netherlands

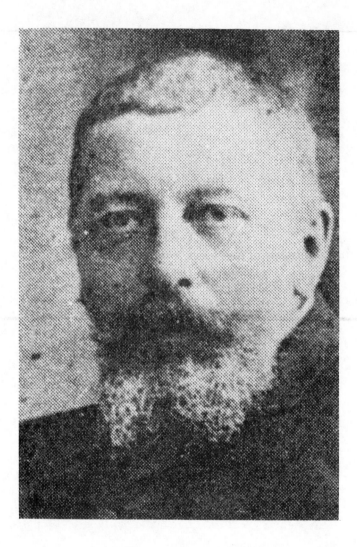

Jules Dejerine
1849-1917

Biography

Dejerine was born near Geneva, Switzerland, in 1849. At school he was not regarded as an outstanding student. He became interested in biology and comparative anatomy. At the age of twenty-two he went to pursue his clinical studies in Paris, where he was a pupil of Vulpian and was connected to the Salpêtrière as well as the Bicêtre. In 1910 he was elected 'Professeur de clinique des maladies du système nerveux à la Faculté de Médicine' in Paris. Dejerine owed much to his wife, Augusta Marie Klumpke, whom he married in 1888. She had studied medicine in Paris and became the first woman to receive the title of 'interne des hôpitaux' in 1887. When Dejerine died in 1917, having spent himself in the exhausting service of an army hospital, it was his wife who carried on the bulk of his work, both in practice and in research. Dejerine published studies on topics such as progressive muscular dystrophy, olivopontocerebellar atrophy, and the thalamic syndrome, but among aphasiologists he is best known for his studies on alexia.

Selected Bibliography

Dejerine, J. 1885. "Etude sur l'aphasie dans les lésions de l'insula de Reil". *Revue de Médecine* 5: 174-191.

———. 1891. "Sur un cas de cécité verbale avec agraphie suivi d'autopsie". *Mémoires de la Société de Biologie* 3: 197-201.

———. 1892. "Contribution à l'étude anatomique et clinique des différentes variétés de cécité verbale". *Mémoires de la Société de Biologie* 4: 61-90.

——— and André-Thomas, J. 1904. "Un cas de cécité verbale avec agraphie suivi d'autopsie". *Revue Neurologique* 12: 655-664.

———. 1906. "L'Aphasie Sensorielle". *La Presse Médicale* 14: 437-439.

———. 1906. "L'Aphasie Motrice". *La Presse Médicale* 14: 453-457.

———. 1914. *Sémiologie des affections de système nerveux*. Paris: Masson et Cie.

——— and P. Sérieux. 1897. "Un cas du surdité verbale pure, terminé par aphasie sensorielle, suivi d'autopsie." *Mémoires de la Société de Biologie* 10: 1074-1077.

Introduction

Dejerine's terminology

In the second chapter of his book *Sémiologie des affections du système nerveux*, entitled 'Troubles du langage', written in 1914, Dejerine argued that there are four types of language disturbance: aphasia, dysarthria or anarthria, mutism, and stuttering. Only the first two are caused by brain damage. When disturbances of verbal communication, that is, the exchange of ideas between persons, exists, there are three possible causes:

- disturbance of intelligence: in this condition the patient cannot understand speech or written text; he can no longer reason in a concrete or abstract manner;
- lesion of language centers or connections with the sensoric or motoric apparatus, which he calls 'les aphasies proprement dites': intelligence is not affected in these cases;
- lesions of the bucco-pharyngo-laryngeal system, resulting in dysarthria or anarthria.

The concept of intelligence clearly plays an important role in this classification scheme. Later in his book he argues that in cases of total aphasia "le déficit intellectuel est souvent plus marqué que dans l'aphasie sensorielle ou motrice". In fact the concept of intelligence as used by Dejerine is closely related to consciousness or alertness and to the possibility of inner speech. Intelligence is said to be affected if a patient cannot cooperate when he is tested.

Dejerine's views on aphasia are perhaps best expressed in his definition: "l'aphasie est la perte de la mémoire des signes aux moyens desquels l'homme civilisé échange ses idées avec ses semblables." Aphasia, therefore, is not restricted to spontaneously spoken language but to all the different ways in which verbal concepts can be expressed. Dejerine distinguished two major groups of disturbances on clinical and pathological grounds: sensory aphasia (les aphasies de compréhension) and motor aphasia (les aphasies d'expression).

Although Dejerine was well respected by his colleagues, his contribution to the area of aphasia lies more in his teaching of the 'classical' theories on language centers than in research. He attempted to fit all the different varieties of aphasia into a single scheme. From his somewhat polemic style of writing one gets the impression that an important purpose of his papers was to defend the views of authors such as Broca, Wernicke, and Kussmaul against the attacks of authors such as Pierre Marie, rather than to present a new model of language disorders.

Dejerine is well known for his study of specific reading and writing disorders after brain damage. After the introduction of the concept of sensory aphasia by Wernicke (1874) and the subsequent subdivision by Kussmaul (1876) into word-deafness and word-blindness, Dejerine was able, in 1887, to state that there are four 'centers' in the left hemisphere that are involved in language disorders (see Figure 1, p. 212):

a.   the third frontal gyrus (Broca's area): affected in motor aphasia;
b.   the posterior part of the first temporal gyrus (Wernicke's area): affected in word deafness;
c.   the gyrus angularis ('pli courbe'): involved in word blindness (discovered by Dejerine);
d.   the foot of the second frontal gyrus (area of Exner): affected in agraphia.

The existence of the writing center (area of Exner) was later refuted by Lichtheim and Wernicke. Dejerine subscribed to their view: if a patient cannot write anymore, this is to be ascribed to a disturbance of the 'inner speech' and not to damage of the center for writing words. In 1891 Dejerine described two cases which support his position. The first case was a 63-year-old sailor who suddenly became word blind and agraphic. He could not read letters nor words except for his own name. There was no naming problem. For a month the patient made paraphasic errors. After 8 months the patient died and autopsy was performed. A yellow cone-shaped softening in the area of the gyrus angularis of the left hemisphere was found. The base was located in the cortex of the angular gyrus and the top was situated in the ependym of the occipital part of the lateral ventricle.

One year later Dejerine published a second case. The patient was a 61-year-old intellectual and educated businessman. After several attacks lasting several minutes that gave rise to a numb feeling in his right extremities, he also perceived some difficulty in speaking. He then suddenly became word blind. He was seen by an ophtalmologist, who could not find any disturbance except for a slight right homonymous hemianopia and hemiachromatopia. The patient could not read words or letters. Moreover, he could not recognize music notes, but had no difficulties with digits. Inner speech, color naming, singing, and calculation were intact. He could write spontaneously or to dictation. However, he was not able to copy from text. He could not produce the normal handwritten version of a letter shown to him in print. Tactile inspection of letters improved letter recognition. The patient reported that he could see in his mind the word he wanted to write but he could not read the same word after it was written down by him. Intelligence seemed intact as well as his ability to play cards. This condition remained stable for four years. After a period of agitation and depression his writing became irregular. He then became paretic on his right side and had articulation problems. The following day the paresis had disappeared but now he was clearly aphasic. The patient died ten days later.

At autopsy the right hemisphere was completely intact. In the left hemisphere two types of lesions were observed. Firstly, there were two older lesions, one in the occipital cortex and one in the splenium. Secondly, a relatively fresh softening of the gray and white matter of the parietal lobe and the angular gyrus was found.

On the basis of these two cases Dejerine discriminated two forms of word blindness, resulting from lesions at two different sites.

a) word blindness with agraphia: produced by a lesion of the angular gyrus, where visual images of letters and words are stored. This lesion gives rise to agraphia and possibly to paraphasia, due to the fact that the kinesthetic information is lost.

b) word blindness without agraphia, or pure word blindness: the lesion is located in the visual cortex. The patient cannot copy letters and words at will; however, auditory and muscle information can activate visual images, and therefore spontaneous writing and writing to dictation remain possible.

These two types of word blindness correspond with the cortical and subcortical forms of alexia described by Wernicke. By means of the same two studies, Dejerine came to the conclusion that the area of Exner could not be maintained as a center for writing. Another important argument against the notion of a writing center in Exner's area was that patients with left frontal lesions can write if they use their left hand or foot.

After this period of synthesis and classification of the clinical types on the basis of aphasia and cerebral localization of the lesion responsible, discussions arose on the functional relations between these centers. As a sign of the times a mechanistic relation was elaborated. While Magnan believed that a primary role is played by the motor center in the mechanism of language pathology, Wernicke ascribed a regulating role to the sensory center. Charcot and his followers, including Dejerine, on the other hand argued in favor of autonomy of the centers. Charcot explained the variation in which the aphasia is expressed according to the 'psychic type' of the individual person. This type is determined by education: education and study may make someone more motorically, visually, auditorily, or graphically oriented. According to Dejerine there are two mechanisms involved in the affection of language, namely lesions of cortical language areas and subcortical lesions that isolate the language centers from other parts of the brain. In the former case inner speech is usually lost. Pure word blindness is an example of the latter mechanism: association fibers between the visual center (occipital lobe) and the center for visual images of words are disconnected.

References

Wernicke, C. 1874. *Der aphasische Symptomencomplex: Eine psychologische Studie auf anatomischer Basis*. Breslau: Cohn & Weigert.
Kussmaul, A. 1876. *Die Störungen der Sprache*. Leipzig: Vogel.

Selection from the work of Jules Dejerine

Contribution to the Anatomical-Pathological and Clinical Study of the different Varieties of Word Blindness*

At present two different varieties of *word blindness* are known in the clinic. The symptom of word blindness, which is characterized by more or less completely lost comprehension of the signs represented by script, is the same in both varieties, but the state of writing distinguishes one from the other. In the one, the patient who cannot read printing or handwriting, is also incapable of writing spontaneously or from dictation, or can only write very defectively. In the other, in contrast, the patient who is unable to read or to read back his own handwriting writes easily and correctly, either spontaneously or from dictation; only the action of copying is more or less defective. In other words, the first variety is attended with more or less total agraphia, while this is not the case in the second variety.

First variety: — *Word blindness with agraphia.* This variety is often accompanied by other forms of aphasia: motor aphasia, particularly with paraphasia, or even with word deafness. But it can also be observed in isolation.

Associated to word deafness, it corresponds to the clinical syndrome described by Wernicke as *sensory aphasia*, and in general it results from an extensive lesion of the posterior part of the gyrus surrounding the Sylvian fissure. *In isolation*, it results from a lesion of the angular gyrus; this locali-

---

* Translated from "Contribution à l'étude anatomique et clinique des différentes variétés de cécité verbale" *Mémoires de la Société de Biologie* 4: 61-65 (1892)

zation has only recently been determined. In earlier observations (Broadbent, Dejerine, d'Heilly and Chentemesse, Rosenthal), however, either word blindness did not exist in isolation, but was combined with other forms of aphasia, in particular with word deafness, or the lesion found at autopsy, whether more or less extensive, was not exclusively limited to the angular gyrus.

Last year, I reported to the Society an example of isolated word blindness with total agraphia due to a lesion precisely to the angular gyrus (Dejerine, 1891). Since then Berkhan[1] and Sérieux (1892) both reported similar cases. Today, the location of the first variety of word blindness (*word blindness with agraphia or with strongly marked disturbance of writing*) is therefore well established. It depends upon a destruction of the angular gyrus of the left hemisphere, as these three observations have shown, having exhibited extremely clear symptomatology and a clearly localized lesion.

Thus, the agraphia which in this variety accompanies word blindness depends, as in the latter variety, on a single lesion only, localized in the angular gyrus, and not on two different lesions, one (destruction of the visual verbal center) to explain word blindness and the other (destruction of the so-called writing center, second frontal) the symptom of agraphia.

The determination of that localization was important to establish, because we possess a detailed case of word blindness with agraphia published by Henschen (1890)[2] in which the autopsy brought to view two very limited lesions, one in the angular gyrus and the other at the foot of the second frontal gyrus. The author raises the question, without resolving it, whether the agraphia was, in this case, the necessary consequence of word blindness or a secondary symptom depending on the lesion of the second frontal gyrus. I consider that question as solved now on account of the three observations just mentioned and in which a lesion which was strictly limited to the angular gyrus had brought about word blindness with total agraphia in two cases, and strongly marked difficulties in writing in the third one.

Second variety: — word blindness with intact spontaneous writing and writing from dictation. Pure word blindness. We possess several nice clinical observations of the second variety of word blindness (for example those that are reported by Bernard (1885)). Writing, either spontaneously or from dictation, is completely preserved; only the act of copying is more or less disturbed. Sometimes the copy is produced only with great difficulty, with some sort of technical drawing or line drawing and on the condition that the model remains continuously before the eye. Sometimes the patient cannot translate print into handwriting.

However, the patient who cannot read or read back his own script can manage via a trick using his muscle sense. By following the contours of the characters with his finger, or by tracing them in the palm of his hand, he succeeds in spelling letters and words.

The anatomical location of the second variety of word blindness, *word blindness without disturbance of writing, pure word blindness*, has not yet been determined.

Wernicke (1885), speaking theoretically, accepted for the first variety a lesion of the center of visual images of letters and he called it *cortical alexia*. He restricted the name *subcortical alexia* to the second variety, thus indicating that in the latter, the center of visual images of words is intact and the lesion on which it depends consists of a separation of that center from the central terminations of the optic nerve.

In that variety, however, the whole symptomatology favors preservation of the center of optical images, as was indicated correctly by Wernicke, because spontaneous writing and writing from dictation can only be possible if that center is preserved. The following observation, from autopsy, will show the correctness of that hypothesis.

The clinical history of this patient forms the finest example of pure word blindness without agraphia that has ever been published, and the autopsy adds a document of the utmost importance to the doctrine of sensory aphasia, because it shows that two locations that are anatomically absolutely distinct correspond to the two clinical forms of word blindness hitherto known.

In November 1887 my friend Dr. Landolt sent a patient to me at Bicêtre in whom he had diagnosed word blindness with hemianopsia and hemiachromatopsia of the right side; he published the clinical observation in 1888. I observed that patient many times in the course of the winter of 1887-1888 in my institution, where he regularly came twice a week for a long time. I saw him again during the years 1889-1890 and 1891. He died a few days after the beginning of this year (1892), and the family authorized me to perform the autopsy at their home.

Observation. Total word blindness — for letters and words — lasting four years in a man of 68 years, very intelligent and well educated. — Total loss of comprehension of musical notation — music blindness. Complete preservation of the reading of numbers as well as of the ability to calculate.

— No trace of word deafness. — No trace of trouble with articulated speech. — Inner speech intact. — No psychic blindness or optical aphasia. — Perfect, very expressive mimicry. — Perfect preservation of spontaneous writing or writing from dictation; the Patient can correctly write whole pages either spontaneously or from dictation. — Copying from text: difficult and defective. — Lateral right homonymous hemianopsia with hemiachromatopsia of the same side. — Intactness of motricity, of sensation in general as well as of the muscle sense. — Persistence of the same symptoms for four years. Sudden death, after exhibiting paraphasia with total agraphia for six days, without a trace of word deafness. — Perfect preservation of intelligence and mimicry.

Autopsy: Left hemisphere. Recent lesions due to red softening in the inferior parietal lobe and the angular gyrus. Old lesions — atrophical yellow spots — localized in the lingual lobe, the fusiform lobe, the cuneus and the tip of the occipital lobe as well as a strongly marked atrophia of the optical radiations in the fold of the corpus callosum.

Right hemisphere intact.

C..., 68 years old, always enjoyed excellent health. He never had any serious illness, was not an alcoholic and never had syphilis. His intelligence was higher than average. Having been a dry goods wholesaler for a long time he earned a little fortune, allowing him, for several years, to live on his private means. He was married and never had any children. His marriage was very harmonious; his wife, a few years younger than her husband, is also well educated; she has a fine ear for music and she pressed this interest on her husband for a long time. C. played a lot of music with his wife, sight-read difficult scores very easily and sang, either alone or with his wife. C. kept abreast of literature and read a great deal. On the whole it was easy, while talking to him, to form a clear idea of his intelligence and his knowledge.

His father died at eighty-two, his mother at sixty-three of cerebral softening; she was half paralyzed during the last ten years of her life and was senile.

C. was never taken ill, except for some indigestion which was accompanied by dizziness and loss of consciousness and especially after always eating the same foods. His sight was always excellent. While he was occupied with selling material, he was forced to do work which was very tiring to the eyes. He designed the patterns for the textiles and transferred them to millimeter graph paper, counted the threads of the textiles, and so on. He had no migraine and no cerebral problems before the end of October 1887.

Mrs. C. reports that on October 19th 1887 her husband suddenly and without loss of consciousness felt recurrent stiffness of the right leg for just a few minutes. These minor attacks recurred frequently over the following days and were accompanied by a feeling of stiffness and a certain degree of weakness in the right arm and leg, as well as very slight trouble with speech. All these problems, however, did not prevent the patient from walking or even from going on long errands. On October 23rd, in particular, in spite of about ten attacks of stiffness, the patient took walks and remembered being perfectly able to read the signboards of the shops and the posters in the street. According to Mrs. C. (for the patient had no memory of the problems mentioned above), the weakness of the right leg and arm was worse the next day and the day after that, the patient suddenly noticed that he could not read a word anymore, *while being perfectly able to write and talk and to distinguish the objects and persons surrounding him as well as ever.* Convinced of the fact that he was only struck by problems of vision which would yield to the use of proper glasses, he consulted Dr. Landolt a fortnight after the appearance of these symptoms.

[Same text, p. 83-90]

In sum, the clinical history of this patient consists of two stages. During the first stage, which lasted four years, the patient showed the purest clinical picture to be imagined of the second variety of word blindness, *pure word blindness without disturbance of spontaneous writing or writing from dictation.* During the second stage, which only lasted about ten days, total agraphia with paraphasia complicated the word blindness. In that second stage, the clinical pictures corresponds to that of the first variety of word blindness, *word blindness with marked disturbance of writing.*

As the autopsy showed, two anatomically different lesions of the left hemisphere corresponded to these two clinical stages: the older one took up the occipital lobe and more particularly the convolutions of the tip of the occipital lobe, on the base of the cuneus, as well as those of the lingual lobe and the fusiform lobe. The convolutions of that region were small, shrivelled, atrophied, and yellow. The lesion continued in the underlying white matter and penetrated in a wedge into the depth, reaching the ventricular ependyma of the occipital horn and the optical radiations, which were gray, atrophied, and degenerate. At the cortical side this focus had destroyed the gray matter of the convolutions that border on the posterior part of the internal temporal occipital fissure. Therefore, that lesion was situated in the middle of the visual zone of the cortex.

The other lesion, which was of recent date, took up the angular gyrus and the inferior parietal lobe, the region which we are accustomed to see as lesioned in cases of word blindness with writing problems. It explains perfectly the symptoms observed during the last days of the life of this patient. Does the older lesion in the same way explain the symptoms of the first stage of the affection, namely: pure word blindness without writing problems, hemianopsia, and hemiachromatopsia? Before discussing this question, I shall briefly summarize our current knowledge of the intracerebral stretch of the optic nerves and of the cortical regions that function during reading.

We know that the optic nerves, after arriving at the level of the chiasm, cross incompletely and in such a way that the external part of each optic nerve, which comes from the temporal part of the retina, passes directly into the optic tract on the same side, while the internal part, which comes from the nasal side of the retina, crosses and passes into the tracts of the opposite side. Each tract emerges into the homonymous half of the two retinas or, in other words, the right optic tract emerges into the right half of the two retinas, the left tract into the left half of the two retinas.

Each optic tract passes round the cerebral pedunculi and splits up at the level of the posterio-inferior part of the optical layer into two roots: one, small, internal, emerges into the internal geniculate body and from there on to the posterior quadrigeminal tubercle. The other, more voluminous, external, emerges into the external geniculate body, the anterior quadrigeminal tubercle, and the posterior part of the optical layer. That external root only seems to be part of the optic nerve; it degenerates, however, only with the external geniculate body, the anterior quadrigeminal tubercle, and the posterior part of the optical layer as a result of any lesion which invokes an atrophy of the eyeball or as a result of the excision of the eye, whether applied to man or to young animals shortly after birth.

The degeneration of the two optic nerves also involves the degeneration of the largest part of the optic tracts, those of the external geniculate bodies, of the anterior quadrigeminal tubercles, and of the posterior part of the two optical layers. But the internal geniculate bodies, the posterior quadrigeminal tubercles are not degenerated and at the internal side of each of the optic tracts healthy fibres are found, which cross at the level of the chiasm where they take up the posterior part, and they form a fissure between the two internal geniculate bodies, known as the *inferior commissure* or the *Gudden commissure*. These fibres are not part of the optic nerve, but seem to communicate with the temporal lobe, through the posterior quadrigeminal tubercle (Monakow).

Thus, the optic nerves and optic tracts show an ascending degeneration, but they can also show a descending degeneration as a result of cortical lesions. The external geniculate bodies, the anterior quadrigeminal tubercles, and the posterior extremity of the optical layer, which form the *first optic centers*, indeed show a thick bundle of cortical fibres, already described by Gratiolet as *optic radiations*; those fibres, lying in the most posterior part of the internal capsule, go horizontally backwards, pass around the external wall of the occipital continuation of the lateral ventricle, where they are separated from the ventricular ependyma by vertical fibres of the tapetum which cross their direction; they end in the cuneus and convolutions of the occipital tip, regions that form the *visual centers* or *cortical optics*. One lesion of these cortical centers involves, as a result, a degeneration of the optic radiations and of the posterior part of the optical layer. In newborn animals and sometimes in man, that degeneration ranges up to the external geniculate body, the anterior quadrigeminal body, and the tract and optic nerve of the same side as well as the optic nerve of the opposite side (Monakow).

In summary, then, a lesion of the cortical visual center, of the optic radiations or of the optic tract involves for both eyes loss of the retinal sensitivity of the corresponding part and, as the visual rays cross each other at the level of the lens, it involves a lateral homonymous hemianopsia of the opposite side; in other words, a lesion of the tract, of the radiations, or of the left cuneus involves a lateral homonymous hemianopsia of the right side, while a lesion of the same regions of the right side involve a lateral homonymous hemianopsia of the left side. These facts are easy to understand when looking at the following diagram.

To assure human vision, whether binocular or monocular, the two cunei have to come in action simultaneously. That simultaneous action is due to the presence of the anastomotic fibres which connect the two cunei and pass the corpus callosum, but, until now, neither the existence nor the pathway of those fibres is known.

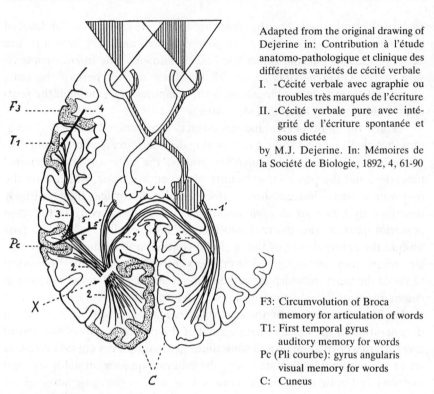

Adapted from the original drawing of Dejerine in: Contribution à l'étude anatomo-pathologique et clinique des différentes variétés de cécité verbale
I. -Cécité verbale avec agraphie ou troubles très marqués de l'écriture
II. -Cécité verbale pure avec intégrité de l'écriture spontanée et sous dictée
by M.J. Dejerine. In: Mémoires de la Société de Biologie, 1892, 4, 61-90

F3: Circumvolution of Broca
memory for articulation of words
T1: First temporal gyrus
auditory memory for words
Pc (Pli courbe): gyrus angularis
visual memory for words
C: Cuneus

1, 1':	Radiatio optica of Gratiolet
2, 2', 2'':	Fibres connecting Pc with C of the left hemisphere, and via the corpus callosum (2' and 2'') with C of the right side
3:	Fibres connecting Pc with the Circumvolution of Wernicke
4:	This black line represents the connections between the area of Wernicke and the area of Broca.
5, 5', 5'':	This black bifurcating line represents the connections between left Pc and left motor cortex (5') and right motor cortex (5'')
	* in pure motor agraphia it is probable that only fibres (5') are concerned
X:	the lesion intersects fibres (2, 2', 2'') and causes a right homonymous and hemianopsia and a verbal blindness without disturbance of writing

Figure 1: Diagram of the intra-cerebral pathway of the optic nerves and of the connections of the left angular gyrus.

Thus, while looking at an object with either one eye or both eyes, we are seeing it with both hemispheres. The same goes for letters, we see them with both occipital lobes, but we see them with the help of those common visual centers just like any pattern, as we see characters of a language which is strange to us (as I see, for example, Russian or Hebrew characters). In order to recognize a letter, in order for the *idea* of a word to be awakened by the combination of specific letters, it is necessary that these cortical centers of common vision be linked to the language zone; actually, this zone is represented only in the left hemisphere, at least for the right-handed, and the pathology shows that the center for visual memory of letters is at the level of the angular gyrus.

Therefore, the angular gyrus has a strong connection to the left occipital lobe and to the right occipital lobe. By what fibres are these connections made? Is it a matter of connections being made by the gray cortex here or, as is more probable, of connections being made with the help of the white matter? We can only suspect the fibres to be there, not yet being able to show their pathway or even their existence.

But the visual center for letters (angular gyrus) is also linked to the auditory center of words and through this with the motor center of articulation. The two latter centers are connected by one of the strongest cerebral connections there is, for in fact it goes back to earliest childhood and it is very probable, I propose that when we learn to read or later to read fluently, the visual image of the letters awakens simultaneously the auditory image and the motor image of articulation.

The angular gyrus, moreover, corresponds with the motor center of the upper limb and in particular with that of the hand. These connections are bilateral like those of the occipital lobes. If we have the habit of writing with our right hand, in other words with the motor center of the left hemisphere, we can still manage to write, as Wernicke already indicated, with our left hand or even with our foot. We can even manage to write by holding a pencil between the teeth and communicating the necessary movement to the head.

Therefore it is not necessary for writing to postulate existence of a so-called special graphic center, still less to localize it at the foot of the left second frontal convolution, for if this center existed, it had to extend at least to the whole motor zone of the limbs, not only of the left hemisphere, but also of the right one.

The pathology shows that the lesion of the visual center for letters (angular gyrus) results in agraphia as one of its consequences. I believe, as I said before, that the agraphia depends in this case upon the actual loss of the optimal image of letters (Dejerine, 1891). But agraphia can be observed in motor aphasia or in word deafness every time the meaning of the word itself is more or less damaged whenever the cortical zone of language is involved. The connection of the visual center of letters with the motor zones of the two hemispheres is also shown by the very interesting observation of Pitres (1884). His patient showed, as a result of motor aphasia, a hemianopsia of the left side with agraphia of the right hand. He wrote perfectly with his left hand, spontaneously, from dictation, and copying, but with his right hand he could write neither spontaneously nor from dictation, and he could only copy what he had just written with his left hand. For him, only an interruption between the zone of the superior limbs of the left hemisphere and the angular gyrus need be postulated, while the connections of the angular gyrus with the motor zone of the right hemisphere were intact. At this point I completely disagree with the opinion of Wernicke on this case. For the rest, as I said before while referring to the case of Henschen, it is difficult to understand, in the case of Pitres, the lesion of the so-called graphic center which permits copying, while writing from dictation or spontaneous writing is impossible.

These data being established, let us try to determine the symptoms resulting from lesion of those different parts and let us try to explain the symptoms of word blindness, then of hemianopsia and of hemiachromatopsia shown by the patient whose observation I described above.

A lesion of the left cuneus results in a lateral homonymous hemianopsia of the right side; lesion of the two cunei, complete word blindness called cortical; lesion of the left angular gyrus, word blindness with strongly marked problems in writing or total agraphia.

In my patient, the lesion of the left cuneus and the secondary degeneration of the optic radiations are sufficient to explain the hemianopsia of the right side. How to explain the pure word blindness here? As a result of the hemianopsia of the right side, this man did not see the characters with his left hemisphere anymore, he only saw them with the *right half* of each of his retinas, relating to his *intact right hemisphere*.[3] Therefore, he saw the letters as well as any other pattern and he copied them as such, but they meant nothing to him because the connections between these two common visual centers and the visual center of words (angular gyrus of the left side) were interrupted. The latter was not lesioned, as is shown by the study of his inner speech, the perfect integrity of his writing, either spontaneously or from dictation, and the fact that the optical images of letters could be revived by using his muscle sense to trace the contours of the letters in the air, either with the left or with the right hand. As for the defectiveness of copying, that is easily understood by admitting the interruption between the angular gyrus and the two occipital lobes.

The lesion of the underlying white matter in the left occipital lobe was fairly extended since it reached the ventricular ependyma, so that we can recognize that the fibres which connect the angular gyrus with the two occipital lobes are involved and without needing a second lesion, the little lesion found in the ply of the corpus callosum. The symptoms which depend on the lesions of the corpus callosum are indeed too obscure and there is still too little known about them, so it does not seem opportune to me to stress them.

As for the hemiachromatopsia, its cortical localization has not yet been determined with certainty, but the lesion of the little lingual lobes and the fusiform lobes might produce this symptom, as the observation of Verrey, reported by Landolt (1888), tends to prove.

Thanks to the completeness of the angular gyrus this man, struck by total word blindness, was able to write in a normal way for four years, either spontaneously or from dictation. For the same reason he never showed any problems in articulated speech, and inner speech remained intact. On the contrary, starting the day his angular gyrus was altered, ten days before his death, the man became immediately and totally agraphic; at the same moment he was struck by paraphasia. So the two known clinical forms of word blindness appeared one after the other, each depending on a different location.

In sum, today we must recognize two different clinical varieties of word blindness, each depending on a different location.

The first variety is produced by a lesion found in the language domain (angular gyrus of the left side), the second one by a lesion found in the common visual domain and separating the angular gyrus from the latter.

In the first variety — *word blindness with agraphia or strongly marked disturbance of writing* — the optical images of the letters are destroyed and the word blindness is accompanied either by total agraphia or by strongly marked disturbances in the different modes of writing. That lesion reaches the language domain; it is easy to understand why the patients show, in general, a certain degree of paraphasia. The destruction of the optical center of letters explain why, in this sense, optical images of letters cannot be aroused with the help of the muscle sense.

In the second variety — *pure word blindness with intactness of spontaneous writing and writing from dictation* — the center of optical images of letters, the angular gyrus, is intact, but the lesion divides it, isolating it from the common visual center. As a consequence the angular gyrus cannot become operative with visual stimulation anymore. On the contrary, it can become operative through voluntary stimulation, like spontaneous writing; through auditory stimulation, like writing from dictation; or even through the muscle sense (letters traced in the air by hand or foot). So spontaneous writing and writing from dictation are intact; only the act of copying is defective. As the lesion is totally beyond the domain of language here, patients do not show any trouble in speaking and their inner speech is intact.

With the help of the preceding data it will now be easy to clinically distinguish one form from another, each corresponding with completely distinct locations, as I have established.

Notes

1. Berkhan (1891). This case, in which a lesion was found at autopsy in the left angular gyrus, is wrongly regarded by the author as a case of subcortical alexia. On the contrary, it is a case of cortical alexia, as is demonstrated by the very marked deficits in this patient in writing under the three modalities. This last patient in fact presented the same problems with writing (paragraphia) as with speech (paraphasia). I would like to mention that one observes rather frequently a certain degree of paraphasia in cases of alexia due to destruction of the angular gyrus (Dejerine, Sérieux), a phenomenon which is absent in pure alexia.

2. This case concerns a woman with alexia and agraphia; her spontaneous writing and writing from dictation are severely disturbed, while her capacity to copy was relatively intact. At autopsy a focus of destruction is found in the left angular gyrus, explaining the alexia, and another lesion would have destroyed the entire posterior part of the second frontal gyrus on the same side — the center of writing movements according to Exner and Charcot. — Well, if the foot of the second frontal gyrus on the left is the center for the memory of writing movements, its destruction should result in a loss of all modes of writing (spontaneous writing, writing from dictation, and copying), just as destruction of Broca's convolution leads to loss of all modes of speech (spontaneous speech, repetition of words, singing). The destruction of the angular gyrus in Henschen's case suffices to explain the writing problems presented by the patient.

3. I would like to remark with Landolt, that in this patient the right-side hemianopsia was not a completely negative hemianopsia, because there was no absence of vision in each of

the visual fields on the right side, but a sensation of vague vision. In reality he was more hemiachromatopsic than hemianopsic.

References

Berkhan, O. 1891. "Ein fall von subcorticalc⁻ Alexie (Wernicke)". *Archiv für Psychiatrie und Nervenkrankheiten* 23: 558-564.

Bernard, J. 1885. "De l'aphasie et de ses différentes formes". *Thèse inaug.* Paris.

Dejerine, J. 1891. "Sur un cas de cécité verbale avec agraphie suivi d'autopsie". *Mémoires de la Société de Biologie* 3: 197-201.

———. 1891. "Contribution à l'étude des troubles de l'écriture chez les aphasiques". *Mémoires de la Société de Biologie*, 3: 197-201.

Dufour (de Lausanne). 1889. "Sur la vision nulle dans l'hémiopie". *Revue médicinale de la Suisse normande* 4: 455.

Henschen, S. 1890. "Observation. Avec autopsie, de Margaretha Anderson". *Klinische und Anatomische Beiträge zur Pathologie des Gehirns*, Erster Theil. Stockholm: Nordiska Bokhandel.

Landolt, E. 1888. *De la cécité verbale.* Travail publié dans l'ouvrage dédié à Donders à l'occasion de son jubilé. Utrecht, 27 Mai 1888.

Pitres, A. 1884. "Considérations sur l'agraphie à propos d'une observation nouvelle d'agraphie motrice pure". *Revue de Médicine* 4: 885.

Sérieux, P. 1892. "Sur un cas de surdité verbale pure." *Revue de Médecine* 13: 733-750.

Wernicke, C. 1885. "Einige neuere Arbeiten über Aphasie". *Fortschritte der Medizin* 3:824-830; 4 (1886) 371-377; 463-469. Reprinted in C. Wernicke. Gesammelte Aufsätze und kritische Referate zur Pathologie des Nervensystems. Berlin: Fischer, 1983.

Pierre Marie

Introduced by

YVAN LEBRUN
Dept. of Neurolinguistics, University Hospital,
Vrije Universiteit Brussel (V.U.B.), Belgium

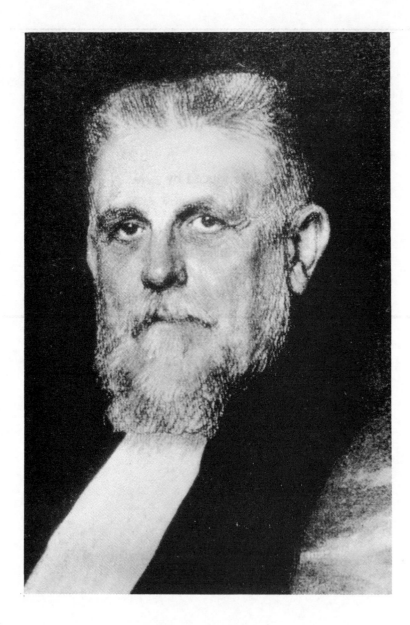

Pierre Marie
1853-1940

Biography

Pierre Marie was born in Paris in 1853. He first studied law, then turned to medicine. He was an intern in Broca's and in Charcot's departments and assisted Charcot in his private practice. Charcot was a witness at his wedding. In 1888 Marie became physician to the Paris hospitals. The next year the title of agrégé *was conferred on him. With Brissaud he founded the* Revue Neurologique *in 1893 and the* Société de Neurologie de Paris *in 1899. In 1895 he was appointed head of the* Infirmerie de Bicêtre. *In 1907 he became professor of pathological anatomy at the University of Paris, and in 1917 he succeeded Dejerine as professor of clinical neurology (The first occupant of this chair had been Charcot). Marie retired in 1925 and died at Pradet near Cannes in 1940.*

Selected Bibliography

Marie, P. 1906a. "Révision de la question de l'aphasie: la troisième circonvolution frontale ne joue aucun rôle spécial dans la fonction du langage". *La Semaine Médicale* 26:241-247.

———. 1906b. "Que faut-il penser des aphasies sous cortiales?" *La Semaine Médicale* 26: 493-500.

———. 1906c. "L'aphasie de 1861 à 1866. Essai de critique historique sur la genèse de la doctrine de Broca". *La Semaine Médicale* 26: 565-571.

———. 1926. *Travaux et Mémoires*, 2 vols. Paris: Masson and Cie. [Most of Marie's papers on aphasia which appeared between 1906 and 1912 have been reproduced in this book.]

——— and Ch. Foix. 1917. "Les aphasies de guerre". *Revue Neurologique* 25: 53-87.

———. 1922. "Existe-t-il chez l'homme des centres pré-formés ou innés du langage?". *Questions Neurologique d'Actualité* pp. 527-551. Paris: Masson et Cie.

Introduction

It is not often that a scholar leaves his mark on a branch of science by way of a number of papers which were, for the most part, published within a single year. A case in point is Pierre Marie. In May 1906 Marie published a first article on aphasia which stirred up a controversy that has never completely settled since (Lebrun & Hoops 1974). Reactions to this first paper were so fierce that the author felt obliged, as he told Alajouanine (mentioned in Alajouanine, 1952) many years later, to write a second and then a third article (Marie, 1906b and c) to clarify, explicate, and further substantiate his point of view. These three publications having been inaccurately interpreted by one of his opponents, Marie wrote yet a fourth paper, which appeared in 1907 (a), to put things straight. In the meantime, together with his disciple François Moutier he had published three case studies (1906d, e, and f) which, he thought, supported his views on Broca's aphasia and the third frontal convolution. At the end of 1906 (g) and in 1907 (b, c, and d) four more papers appeared which further illustrated Marie's conception of aphasia. This series of articles, which saw the light in a little more than 12 months time, caused a great commotion in French neurological circles, as a consequence of which the Société de Neurologie in 1908 decided to debate the issue of aphasia. The discussion lasted for three meetings (11 June, 9 July, and 23 July 1908), which were dominated by Marie and his main opponent, Jules Dejerine. Neither of them won the contest, it would seem, nor could they come to an agreement. Indeed, at the end of the last meeting, Marie stated that Dejerine's views and his own were diametrically opposed. After the memorable discussions in the Société de Neurologie in 1908, Marie did not make any further significant contribution to the field of aphasia.

What did the theory of aphasia which Marie propounded at the beginning of the century consist of?

The nature of aphasia

According to Marie there was only one aphasic syndrome, Wernicke's aphasia, which was characterized by oral comprehension difficulties and paraphasic speech. Written language was equally disturbed. The disorder of comprehension was sometimes severe and sometimes less pronounced, but it was never absent.

Aphasia was the consequence of a special intellectual impairment: a reduction of all knowledge and competence acquired didactically. Because of this mental deficit, aphasics also had difficulty in playing music, reckoning, reading the time, imitating series of gestures, mimicking, and even performing a number of professional tasks.

Aphasia could not be subdivided into different syndromes, as its various symptoms were always present. However, the severity of the symptoms varied in different patients, as it depended mainly on the extent and localization of the causal lesion in Wernicke's area, which comprised the posterior two thirds of the first two temporal convolutions and the supramarginal and angular gyrus on the left. Broca's aphasia was not a homogeneous syndrome but a combination of genuine aphasia (i.e. Wernicke's aphasia) and anarthria.

Marie rejected the possibility of pure verbal deafness because he could not believe that someone would lose the ability to understand speech while retaining his other verbal skills. In aphasia all aspects of language were disturbed because aphasia resulted from an intellectual impairment that of necessity affected all linguistic abilities. Marie, however, admitted the existence of pure alexia, which he considered a special form of visual agnosia. He also called it an extrinsic aphasia because the causal lesion lay on the margins of Wernicke's area.

In 1917, after he had examined a large number of soldiers with traumatic aphasia, Marie somewhat revised his theory of aphasia, allowing that Wernicke's aphasia could be subdivided (clinically) into temporal aphasia, aphasia due to a lesion of the supramarginal gyrus, posterior aphasia, and what he called a limited aphasic syndrome. His description of these forms of aphasia remained, however, vague and unspecific.

The nature of anarthria

Anarthria was a disorder of articulate speech, that is, a disturbance of the complex movements of respiration, phonation, and articulation in speech. This condition usually combined with Wernicke's aphasia to form Broca's aphasia. However, it could also occur in isolation, in which case inner speech, oral comprehension, reading, and writing were preserved.

According to Marie, anarthria was the same as pure motor aphasia, which was also called sub-cortical motor aphasia. He objected to the use of the latter two nomenclatures, however, as they suggested that the condition denoted was a form of aphasia, which it definitely was not.

Although he repeatedly stressed that anarthria was not aphasia, Marie was never clear as to what it really was. In the first of his 1906 papers he suggested that anarthria was akin to pseudo-bulbar palsy. However, in his second 1906 paper he claimed that anarthria was a disorder of coordination of speech movements and was completely different from pseudo-bulbar or paralytic deficits. One year later (1907b), he disclaimed any knowledge of the pathophysiology of anarthria. In May 1908, at an ordinary meeting of the Société de Neurologie he agreed with Gilbert Ballet (1908) that anarthria was a form of apraxia. During the meetings which the Société de Neurologie devoted to aphasia in June and July of the same year, he repeated that he did not know what the mechanism underlying anarthria was. Ten years later his conception of anarthria had not improved, as is shown by the hazy and unspecific description he gave of the condition in the paper he published with Foix in 1917.

In his 1906 papers Marie stated that Broca's aphasia was a combination of Wernicke's aphasia and anarthria. He repeated this at the meeting of the Société de Neurologie on 11 June 1908. He also said that in his opinion Broca's aphasia could never evolve into anarthria, as Broca's aphasia was an aphasic condition while anarthria was not. In 1908 then, he rejected the possibility that in Broca's aphasics the aphasic component might clear up while the arthric component remained. In the paper he published in 1917 with Foix, however, he mentioned patients who at first had aphasia and anarthria and later on only anarthria.

The localization of Broca's aphasia and of pure anarthria

Marie attacked what he regarded as the dogma of the third frontal convolution. In his view the foot of the third left frontal gyrus could not be considered to be the localization of Broca's aphasia, as there were cases of destruction of the posterior part of this gyrus in righthanded individuals without ensuing aphasia, and conversely there were cases of Broca's aphasia in which the third left frontal convolution had been found to be intact. With François Moutier, Marie reported a few such cases in 1906 (d,e,f). According to Marie, Broca's aphasia always resulted from a lesion simultaneously destroying part of Wernicke's area and part of what he called the lenticular zone. This zone was a quadrilateral extending between the island of Reil and the lateral ventricle and including the insula, the claustrum, the external and internal capsule, and the caudate and lenticular nucleus. The third frontal convolution and its underlying white matter explicitly lay outside this zone.

In Broca's aphasia the true aphasic component resulted from damage to the cortex or white matter of Wernicke's area, while the articulatory component had its origin in the lenticular lesion. Re-examining the brain of Broca's first patient Leborgne (Broca 1861), Marie (1906c) pointed out that the lesion far exceeded the limits of the third frontal convolution and extended well into the temporal lobe, reaching as far as the supramarginal gyrus. This case, therefore, did not show Broca's aphasia to be localized in the foot of the third frontal convolution on the left but on the contrary supported the claim that aphasia always corresponded to a lesion in Wernicke's area.

In pure anarthria, the lesion lay in the lenticular zone. Indeed, the condition could result directly from damage to the lenticular nucleus. Moreover, the causal lesion could be in either hemisphere, in contrast to injuries entailing aphasia, which were always confined to the left hemisphere.

The iconoclast

In his historical essay which opens the first of his two volumes on *Aphasia and Kindred Disorders of Speech*, Henry Head (1926) called Marie an iconoclast because he denied the existence in the brain of something like auditory, visual, or motor images of words. Marie also refused to allow that there were separate centers for the understanding of spoken and written language. He was particularly emphatic about this during the third meeting which the Société de Neurologie devoted to aphasia in 1908. He claimed that 'verbal images' was a rhetorical expression devoid of meaning, and he maintained that the cerebral language zone could not be subdivided into specialized language centers, the lesion of which would entail a distinct form of aphasia.

In what was probably his last contribution to aphasiology, a lecture delivered at the Faculty of Medicine in Paris and published in *Questions Neurologiques d'Actualité* in 1922, Marie contended that the language zone was not innate. In contradistinction to the motor and sensory cortex whose functions appeared predetermined and invariable, the cerebral area which subserved language could be used for other purposes in case the individual did not acquire language. In short, there were, according to Marie, no pre-formed verbal centers and no verbal images to be stored.

Marie also warned against diagram-making in aphasiology. Such diagrams were gross oversimplifications of the clinical reality. Moreover, they represented their author's prejudices and biases too much to be of any use. The stance adopted by Marie after 1906 was, in fact, a conversion, for at the beginning of his career, when he was working as Charcot's assistant, he himself drew a chart supposedly depicting the neurobiology of language. This drawing became known as Charcot's bell schema. It is often reproduced in historical essays on aphasia.

Examination of aphasia

In several of his publications Marie insisted that aphasics should be extensively examined, and he pointed out that some deficits would only show if the patients were given special tasks. He specifically recommended that comprehension be tested otherwise than by just asking the patients such customary questions as "Close your eyes" or "Cough". He himself devised several clinical tests, one of which is still occasionally used: the Three-Paper Test.

Conclusions

Marie, it would seem, should be given credit for having fought against an undue atomization of aphasia and for having insisted that every aphasic has comprehension difficulties. And he was right in objecting to aphasic syndromes being derived from theoretical constructs rather than from clinical observation. On the other hand, he did not succeed in defining with clarity the forms of aphasia he had recognized. He did not manage to depict disorders of language as accurately as he did a number of other, non-verbal, diseases. He must have realized this, for in a letter to Alajouanine (mentioned in Alajouanine, 1952), which he wrote shortly before his death in 1940, Marie stated that he had never intended to work out a theory of aphasia. All he wanted to do when he published his first paper in 1906 was to show that the third frontal convolution could not be considered the localization of Broca's aphasia. He had not anticipated that his article would evoke such fierce reactions. The violent criticism which his views on Broca's zone elicited caused him to write a second, then a third, and finally a fourth paper, all in a short period of time, to defend himself and explicate his conviction. He felt pressed to put forward a theory of aphasia which he had not yet had time to develop. He then, as he himself explained to Alajouanine, took refuge "in the fortress of anarthria". He knew this condition existed but he had no clear notion of it. He never had. Nonetheless the disorder is often called *l'anarthrie de Pierre Marie* in French aphasiological literature.

References

Alajouanine, Th. 1952. "Pierre Marie et l'aphasie". *Revue Neurologique* 86: 753-764.
Ballet, G. 1908. "Apraxie faciale (impossibilité de souffler) associée à de l'aphasie complexe (aphasie motrice et aphasie sensorielle) Apraxie et aphémie". *Revue Neurologique* 16: 445-447.
Broca, P. 1861. "Remarques sur le liège de la faculté de langage articulé, suivie d'une observation d'aphemie". *Bulletins de la Société d'Anthropologie* 6:330-357.
Head, H. 1926. *Aphasia and Kindred Disorders of Speech*. Cambridge: Cambridge University Press.
Lebrun, Y. and R. Hoops. 1974. *Intelligence and Aphasia*. Lisse: Swets and Zeitlinger.
Marie, P. 1906a. "La troisième circonvolution frontale gauche ne joue aucun rôle spécial dans la fonction du langage". *La Semaine Médicale* 26:241-247.
———. 1906b. "Que faut-il penser des aphasies sous cortiales (aphasies pures)?". *La Semaine Médicale* 26: 493-500.

————. 1906c. "L'aphasie de 1861 à 1866. Essai de critique historique sur la genèse de la doctrine de Broca". *La Semaine Médicale* 26: 565-571.

———— and F. Moutier. 1906d. "Nouveau cas d'aphasie de Broca sans lésion de la troisième frontale gauche". *Bulletins et mémoires de la Société médicale des Hôspitaux*, session of 23 november, reprinted in P. Marie, *Travaux et Mémoires*, 2 vols. Paris: Masson and Cie, 1926.

———— and F. Moutier. 1906e. "Sur un cas de ramollissement du pied de la troisième circonvolution frontale gauche chez une droitier sans aphasie de Broca". *Bulletins et mémoires de la Société médicale des Hôspitaux*, session of 16 november, reprinted in P. Marie, *Travaux et Mémoires*, 2 vols. Paris: Masson and Cie, 1926.

———— and F. Moutier. 1906f. "Nouveau cas de lésion corticale du pied de la troisième frontale gauche chez une droitier sans trouble de langage". *Bulletins et mémoires de la Société médicale des Hôspitaux*, session of 14 december, reprinted in P. Marie, *Travaux et Mémoires*, 2 vols. Paris: Masson and Cie, 1926.

————. 1906g. "Un cas d'anarthrie transitoire par lésion de la zone lenticulaire". *Bulletins et mémoires de la Société médicale des Hôspitaux*, session of 14 december, reprinted in P. Marie, *Travaux et Mémoires*, 2 vols. Paris: Masson and Cie, 1926.

————. 1907a. "Sur la fonction du langage. Rectifications à propos de l'article de M. Grasset". *Revue de Philosophie*.

————. 1907b. "Présentation de malades atteints d'anarthrie par lésion de l'hémisphère gauche du cerveau". *Bulletins et mémoires de la Société médicale des Hôspitaux*, session of 19 july, reprinted in P. Marie, *Travaux et Mémoires*, 2 vols. Paris: Masson and Cie, 1926.

————. 1907c. "A propos d'un cas d'aphasie de Wernicke considéré par erreur comme un cas de démence sénile". *Bulletins et mémoires de la Société médicale des Hôspitaux*, session of 1 february, reprinted in P. Marie, *Travaux et Mémoires*, 2 vols. Paris: Masson and Cie, 1926.

———— and F. Moutier. 1907d. Sur une cas d'atrophie sénile du cerveau présentant au niveau du pied de F_3 à gauche une dépression qui aurait pu farie penser à une lésion en ce point. *Bulletins et mémoires de la Société médicale des Hôspitaux*, session of 12 july, reprinted in P. Marie, *Travaux et Mémoires*, 2 vols. Paris: Masson and Cie, 1926.

————, Ch. Foix and I. Bertrand. 1917. "Topographie cranio-cérébrale". *Annales de Médecine* 4, No. 3.

———— and Ch. Foix. 1917. "Les aphasies de guerre". *Revue Neurologique* 25: 53-87.

————. 1922. "Existe-t-il chez l'homme des centres pré-formés ou innés du langage?". *Questions Neurologique d'Actualité* pp. 527-551. Paris: Masson et Cie.

N.B. The discussions at the Société de Neurologie on 11 June, 9 July and 23 July 1908 were published in *Revue Neurologique* (1908) 16: 611-635, 974-1023, 1025-1047.

Selection from the work of Pierre Marie

The Third Left Frontal Convolution Plays No Special Role in the Function of Language*

The nature of aphasia

II**

One fact dominates the study of aphasia, and it is the following: *in the case of all aphasics there exists a more or less pronounced difficulty in comprehension of spoken language.* The degree of deficit can, however, be very variable. In very severe cases of aphasia the patients are entirely unable to understand what is said to them. In less severe cases the patients understand simple questions very well and can execute simple orders. But if the questions or the orders become more complicated, one immediately sees the characteristic deficit of aphasia. Thus it is necessary to do more than to say to the patient: "Cough, spit, stick out your tongue, close your eyes". One must gradually increase the complexity of the commands. Then the patient who appeared to execute simple commands so well reveals the gaps that exist in his comprehension of spoken language. Usually the commands to be executed need not be too complicated. There is hardly an aphasic who is capable of successfully executing one of the following commands, provided he is hearing them for the first time, so that no learning experience

* Translated from "La troisième circonvolution frontale gauche ne joue aucun rôle spécial dans la fonction de langage." Semaine Médicale 26: 241-247 (1906) Reprinted in P. Marie *Travaux et Mémoires*, Paris: Masson & Cie, pp. 3-30 (1926)

** The Roman numerals refer to the corresponding sections in Marie's original paper.

has taken place. These are the ones at present most in use in my practice:

A. — "Of the three unequal pieces of paper placed on this table: you will give me the largest one, you will crumple the middle-sized one and throw it down, and as for the smallest, you will put it in your pocket".

B. — "You will stand up, you will tap three times on the window with your finger, then you will return in front of the table, you will walk around your chair and you will sit down".

It is up to the individual, at his discretion, to vary the complexity of commands of this type. Some patients actually would have great difficulty in executing a single act. In order to confuse other patients one must order two acts consecutively or even, but more rarely, three or four.

Is this a question of word deafness? According to the classical definition, this would mean that the sense of words used in a particular way is not understood, that the patient hears these words but does not know what they mean and perceives them only as a simple, undetermined noise. Such an attitude is absolutely erroneous. In order to prove this one can repeat to the patient the same complicated command, taking care to break it down into successive and isolated acts. Then one is surprised to see that each act is perfectly executed. Thus it is not the words of which the given commands are composed which are incomprehensible to the patient, since he understands these same words perfectly when he is freed from the complication of remembering a series of acts.

There is, moreover, another way to prove that if aphasics do not successfully execute a series of commands, it does not mean that they fail to understand the sense of the words. The physician must pantomime the different parts of the order, and then tell the patient to reproduce the series of acts which he has just seen. In severe cases the patient is generally incapable of carrying out this task in full. No one can maintain that this incapacity to execute an order given without words may be caused by word deafness.

In the case of aphasics there is something much more important and much more grave than the loss of the meaning of words; it is a *very marked diminution in intellectual capacity* in general.

This concept of the intellectual diminution of aphasics ought, in my opinion, to dominate the doctrine of aphasia; having neglected this, authors have misunderstood the true nature of aphasic disorders. In describing aphasia, most clinicians declare that *"the intelligence is intact"*. Although this fits completely with prevailing concepts, it is impossible for me to accept this definition.

If, for my part, I were to give a definition of aphasia, the factor which I would be compelled to stress would be the *diminution of intelligence*. Certainly most authors, while declaring that intelligence is intact, recognize the existence of this intellectual diminution and even mention it in their works; but it is for them an accessory phenomenon and they do not attach any importance to it. They are very wrong in not taking this diminution into account when building a theory of aphasia.

III

In order to obtain proof of this diminution of intelligence, however, it is not sufficient for the doctor to remain for a few minutes with the aphasic, or even to watch his behavior. There must be a methodical examination. Then one learns that there is a deficit, not only in language but especially in the supply of *things learned by didactic processes*. Is it because of a simple language deficit that aphasic musicians find their musical faculties altered? Not only may their ability to compose or read a piece of music be affected. They may also be unable to play from memory pieces with which they had been familiar. Is it because of a simple language deficit that patients find themselves incapable of recognizing the time on a clock or of setting the hands of their watch to a given hour? Is it because of a simple language deficit that many aphasics are incapable of completing even a simple problem of addition or subtraction? Often they begin the problem on the left, showing that they have not the slightest idea of the simplest laws of arithmetic. And certainly it is not because of a simple language deficit that global aphasics find it impossible to reproduce correctly a series of simple acts performed before them without any use of speech.

Some time ago in our practice, we had a very curious experience in regard to this subject. It involved one of my patients who had been stricken several years earlier with an aphasia of moderate intensity (which, however, did not impede him from taking part in normal life). He was a cook, a good cook who, without doubt, knew his trade very well. One day I asked him to prepare for me a fried egg. So we all went into the kitchen, with the supervisor to function as the expert. There, in front of the stove, the patient was given the necessary ingredients: a pan, an egg, butter, pepper, salt, and he was told to exercise his talents. The man hesitated a moment, then committed the following mistakes. These were pointed out to us by our supervisor, who was quite scandalized to see how badly a cook did with a test that even for a simple housewife would be nothing at all. He began by breaking the egg in a very clumsy manner and he emptied it into the pan without taking any precaution to avoid breaking the yolk. Then he put some butter in the pan on top of the egg, covered it with salt and pepper, and put the whole thing in the oven. This was obviously wrong and the supervisor remarked to us that it had been done inverse to the way it should have been done, the butter put in before heating the pan and the egg added afterwards. Needless to say the dish was utterly unacceptable, which, however, did not seem to bother our patient particularly. Here again, evidently, it was not a question of a difficulty with language but of an intellectual loss.

IV

In sum, the question of language apart, there is an incontestable intellectual deficit in the case of aphasics and, as I said above, it is often necessary to make a methodical examination in order to discover it. At first glance, the mentatism of these patients presents no striking deficit. At home they take part in family life; at the hospital they come and go, visit with their friends, eat, go to bed at the same hours and under the same conditions as their neighbors in the room. In short, they conduct themselves normally in communal life. However, the extent of their cerebration is very noticeably restrained; they lack initiative and restrict themselves to the execution of simple acts of existence and especially to material acts.

There is one other factor which creates an illusion and strengthens the impression that the intelligence of aphasics is intact. It is the preservation and sometimes even the exaggeration of their emotional reactions. These patients love and hate, suffer or rejoice, in the same way as their companions. In brief, aphasics live a moral life completely similar to our own and it is for this reason that we have been led to consider their psychic faculties as normal by virtue of our instinctive tendency to declare "intelligent" those who feel and think as we do. I could give many examples of emotional preservation in aphasics. I have known those who love women and choose them for the same reasons and with the same diverse aspirations as the rest of humanity.

The observance of social distinctions is an element of their moral life which leaves little to be desired. One of my patients, a global aphasic, was a former notary clerk. Because of this, rather than because of his education (he could no longer even read) he considered himself socially superior to his comrades in the room. Indeed! He was never seen to condescend to the least familiarity with them. He kept apart and at a distance from them. In contradistinction, another of my global aphasics from a very humble condition, made himself, for a meager salary of a few sous a week, the devoted domestic of a more fortunate friend. He served very conscientiously an office analogous to that of valet of the sick room.

A similar case can be made for violent emotions previously undergone. Aphasics conserve the faculty of experiencing emotion as they remember it. One of my patients had been abandoned by his wife in very painful circumstances; the slightest allusion to the name of the *wife* put him immediately into a state of violent anger. His face became red, sweat formed on his forehead, and the patient clenched his fist in a tragic way. It was apparent to what degree the memory of an injury many years old could still move this poor man. To conclude this category I would like to recall the voluntary politeness of these aphasics as additional proof of the conservation in their case of the affective and moral sphere.

Above are some of the reasons why the mentality of aphasics is often considered to be normal. There is still another: their air of satisfaction, and the vivacity and exuberance of their mimicry certainly appear to reflect the integrity of their mental faculties. Well, this supposed richness of mimicry actually hides a great poverty. In this regard I must remark that *I include in the word "mimicry" acts which are very diverse*. "*Emotive*" *mimicry*, that which is expressed instinctively and which our fathers used to call "movements of the soul", is incontestable in the case of aphasics. It is exuberant, somewhat like that of children. However, it is completely different for "*conventional*" *mimicry*, a well-understood abstraction, either negative or positive; signs which are so habitual that they become in time instinctive and no longer conventional. If a "global aphasic" is told to perform certain acts dependent upon conventional mimicry, such as to make a sign of disgust, to show that he wishes to go to bed and sleep, to shake a finger, to give a sign of contempt — it is quite rare that the patient executes the given order. If he succeeds, it is only after he has hesitated and looked about for some minutes.

As for "*descriptive mimicry*", the incapacity is still more marked. I do not believe that I have ever seen a global aphasic try to use mimicry to explain an event which has happened to him. I have never seen any of them capable of explaining his trade through use of gestures. This lapse in the exercise of descriptive mimicry is a new and important argument in favor of a deficit in the intellectual faculties of these patients, for we must keep well in mind that here too, the psychic alterations noted are entirely independent of the exercise of speech.

The localization of aphasia

VII

Since aphasia is *one*, its localization ought equally to be *one*. And so it is in reality. The only cerebral area whose lesion produces aphasia is the so-called Wernicke's area (gyrus supramarginalis, gyrus angularis, and feet of the two first temporals). One must be careful to remember that this area is also one of those which Flechsig considers as a very special center of association, and indeed when one examines the psyche of aphasics without preconceived opinion, one notes that inability to associate ideas plays a large role in their speech disorder. Thus our conclusions regarding Wernicke's area agree with those of the classics, but they differ from the classics in another way, as shown by the following declaration:

It is an error to attempt, at least by the anatomico-clinical method, to separate this area into different centers, some of which would be predisposed to audition of words (word deafness), others to reading (alexia), etc. etc. Nothing authorizes us from a clinical point of view to attempt such a dissociation; Wernicke's aphasia is a syndrome which appears with all its elements where there exists a lesion, even a limited lesion, in Wernicke's area in any one of its points. Here is a new application of the law which Dr. Guillain and I established for the pyramidal tract (1902). We showed that a lesion limited to this tract in the motor region of the internal capsule, far from causing this or that monoplegia according to its location, as is taught, simply determines a *hemiplegia*. And the intensity of this hemiplegia is directly proportionate to the extent of the lesion in the pyramidal tract. This law of *the global production of cerebral hemisyndromes by lesion of only one portion of the zone which gives rise to them* is a general law; thus a lesion of a portion of the cerebral zone which presides over pain perception gives rise to a *hemianesthesia* of an entire half of the body; thus the lesion of one portion of the visual zone gives rise to a *hemianopsia* affecting half of the visual field. It is by the same law that the lesion of one portion of Wernicke's area gives rise to the syndrome of global *aphasia*.

To return to this last topic, we have said that clinical study does not authorize us to isolate in Wernicke's area diverse centers ruling this or that special act of the function of language. One of the reasons why this dissociation is impossible is that the lesions which determine aphasia always produce a more or less extensive destruction of the white matter subjacent to Wernicke's area. If (as is far from having been proven) there existed at this level in the cortex special centers for this or that operation of language, the lesion of the white matter would cause a considerable difficulty in evaluating and distributing troubles of this sort. I have said that the intensity of the hemiplegia was proportionate to the extent (in width) of the lesion of the pyramidal tract; it is the same for aphasia in proportion to the involvement of the white tracts emanating from Wernicke's area. If the alteration of this cortical zone is very extensive or if the lesion of the subjacent white matter is such that this zone becomes isolated from the bundles of condensed fibers along the external wall of the occipital horn of the ventricle (the inferior longitudinal tract, etc.), one observes a very marked aphasia. If the alteration of the cortical zone of Wernicke and the subjacent white matter is not very extensive, the aphasia will be slight, sometimes even very slight and difficult to discover if one does not see the patient in the first days following the ictus. In a word, *the intensity of the aphasia is proportionate to the extent of the lesions in Wernicke's area or in the fibers of origin.*

Anarthria

VI

The anarthria which is in question here is certainly anarthria due to a focal lesion in the cerebrum. It is characterized by the fact that the speech of the patient is either almost gone or at least incomprehensible; in this regard anarthria might be confused with Broca's aphasia. But the characteristics separating these two syndromes are numerous and decisive. Unlike aphasics, anarthrics understand perfectly what is said to them, even when it is a question of complicated sentences. They can read and write, and are even capable of indicating by signs how many syllables or letters compose the words they are unable to articulate. With these different characteristics one will easily recognize the clinical pictures described in the classical treatises under the name of *subcortical motor aphasia*. The term was proposed by Dejerine, but at the Congress of Medicine at Lyon, Pitres (1894) showed that it is necessary to separate this language disorder from the group of aphasias, in order to associate it with the pseudobulbar paralyses. This opinion of the distinguished professor from Bordeaux deserves to be adopted completely: *anarthria is not aphasia.*

It is essential to agree which deficits of language will be placed in the category of aphasia and which will not. According to what we have said about the characteristics of the Broca's and Wernicke's aphasias, it is evident that from the point of view of a sensible nosological classification, what must constitute true aphasia is not the mere fact of speaking badly or the fact of not speaking at all; what constitutes aphasia is the condition of insufficiently understanding speech, of presenting the intellectual loss which we stressed in the first part of this article, and finally, a very important factor, of having lost the faculty of reading and writing. But none of these deficits occur in anarthria. Therefore we agree with Pitres that anarthria can and should be carefully distinguished from aphasia.

The localization of anarthria

VII

For *anarthria*, there is no difficulty, and everyone agrees in localizing its lesion in the region of the lenticular nucleus, either in the nucleus itself or in the anterior part and the knee of the internal capsule, or in the external capsule. One fact must be noted: that anarthria does not belong exclusively to the left hemisphere and can be seen also when the lesion is situated in the right hemisphere at the level of the zone of the lenticular nucleus. Here is a major difference between it and aphasia, which does belong exclusively to the left hemisphere.

One other fact can be noted: that when anarthria is due to a lesion of only one hemisphere, it can present a spontaneous tendency to heal or at least it may become considerably attenuated, due, no doubt, to the substitution of the healthy hemisphere. On the other hand, even a moderate aphasia hardly ever improves, because there can be no question here of a similar substitution. In cases where anarthria is due to a lesion of the lenticular nuclei in the two hemispheres it can remain persistent, and then it often coincides with the syndrome of pseudobulbar paralysis.

Since we are discussing anarthria, we must emphasize the fact that we are dealing here not only with motor deficits affecting the control of all the very complex mechanisms which combine in the exteriorization of language. These mechanisms have already been very well analyzed by P. Raugé (1894), in a communication at the Congress of Medicine at Lyon.

The mechanical elaboration of speech is made up of at least three essential acts: (1) the production of a current of expired air whose force, speed, and rhythm are controlled by the nerve centers; (2) the placing into vibration of this current at the level of the vocal cords which renders it sonorous and modulates it by intonation; (3) the elaboration of this current which has become sonorous into vowels and consonants, that is to say, the production of speech properly formed by articulation. Not only articulation, as has been generally and wrongly thought, but all these different mechanisms are often found to be simultaneously altered in anarthria. Brissaud, in his lessons, has already insisted on troubles of intonation, etc., in pseudobulbar paralyses.

This question of anarthria has led us a bit far, but rightly so, for it is fundamental. To sum up the anatomico-pathological definition of anarthria, we must limit ourselves to recalling that it has its localization in the zone of the lenticular nucleus and that it can be determined by the lesion of this zone in either hemisphere.

Broca's aphasia

VI

In Broca's aphasia patients can no longer read or write and they have trouble understanding what is said to them. In a word, the clinical picture is very analogous to that of Wernicke's aphasia, but with an important difference: *they are no longer able to talk*. So the essential difference which exists between a Wernicke's aphasic and a Broca's aphasic is that one can talk and the other cannot talk; but for all the rest, they resemble one another. These are facts which have been noted by every author.

"Word deafness" in Broca's aphasia has been the subject of many studies, among which one must reserve a particular place for the work of Thomas and Roux. And it is a very curious thing that most of the authors who clearly noted the existence of "word deafness", alexia and agraphia, seemed to be reluctant to note it in Broca's aphasia, because in their way of thinking this constellation of symptoms common to the two forms of aphasia was susceptible of blurring the lines differentiating them. It is just this constellation of symptoms which we wish to emphasize, for it gives the key to the enigma. The following formula: *the aphasia of Broca is the aphasia of Wernicke with speech missing*, would at least present, within lines which are doubtless a little too rigid, a formula which is in large part the truth.

The localization of Broca's aphasia

VIII

As we said above: Broca's Aphasia = Aphasia + Anarthria. This simple definition is sufficient to indicate to us what lesions will give rise to Broca's aphasia. It is an aphasia, therefore there will be lesion of Wernicke's area or of the white fibers which give rise to it; it is an anarthria, thus there will be a lesion in the zone and in the vicinity of the lenticular nucleus. The thing is so simple that it appears diagrammatic, and yet it is really true. [...]

The third left frontal convolution

V

Let us now consider the localization of Broca's aphasia in the foot of the third left frontal convolution. In question here is the sort of dogma adopted without contest by numerous generations of physicians. To attack such a dogma can seem reckless, yet the results of my anatomico-clinical studies are such that I feel compelled to oppose this universally upheld localization. The dimensions of this article do not permit me to quote at length from the documents on which my conviction is founded, but these documents will be published at a later date with all the necessary information, either by myself or by one of my students. At present I can only present a summary analysis and furnish some of the figures on which it is based.

The arguments which I invoke against localizing Broca's aphasia in the third frontal convolution fall into two categories:

1. There are cases in which isolated destruction of the posterior region of the third left frontal convolution in right-handed individuals is not followed by aphasia. The number of these cases is small, it is true, and I will explain why further on. But it is quality rather than quantity which is important here. And provided that the observations are precise, their demonstrative value leaves nothing to be desired. For my part, I have had occasion in my

practice at Bicêtre to do an autopsy in a case of this type. The lesion at the foot of the third frontal convolution was completely manifest and yet the patient, who was right-handed, had presented no difficulty with speech.

2. There are very clear-cut cases of Broca's aphasia in which there is complete integrity of the third left frontal convolution. A number of cases of this type have been published by different authors, notably by Touche and by Bernheim in his important publications on motor aphasia inspired by Dejerine. I myself have observed several cases of "motor type" aphasia with integrity of the third frontal convolution; the description of these brains with histological examination of the convolutions will be published eventually.

In summary, these two types of evidence show:
1. that one can talk, and talk without any difficulty, even if the third left frontal convolution is destroyed; 2. that in a good number of cases of Broca's aphasia, there exists no lesion of the third frontal convolution.

Obviously the results of this inquiry into the role of the third left frontal convolution lead immediately and naturally to the conclusion that *the third left frontal convolution plays no special role in the function of language*.

It might be argued that the localization of language in the third left frontal convolution rests upon material too solid to be shaken by a few contrary observations. Are there not an enormous number of cases in which aphasia has coincided with a lesion of the third frontal?

I will not contest the fact that in a great number of cases of Broca's aphasia one finds a lesion of the third left frontal convolution. I have noted it in about half the cases of Broca's aphasia which I have observed in my practice at Bicêtre. The fact is undeniable, but still one must interpret it correctly.

We must remember this: aphasia is usually due to cerebral softening. Therefore, when destruction of the Sylvian artery occurs upstream of the point where this artery branches off to irrigate the third frontal, there will naturally occur a softening of this convolution as well as of the other perisylvian convolutions. In such cases the resultant softening of the third left frontal convolution would be an unimportant factor, since the best characterized aphasia can be observed without any lesion of this convolution. When this lesion is found, it is purely and simply a coincidental factor due to the extension of the obliterated vascular territory and nothing more.

On the Function of Language:
Corrections concerning the Article of Grasset* (excerpts)

In the January issue of the *Revue de Philosophie* there appeared an article by Grasset on the function of language and the localization of psychic centers in the brain. This article was, in large part, dedicated to the examination of recent works which I published in *Semaine Médicale* reviewing the question of aphasia. Grasset's interpretation of my opinions on aphasia was entirely incorrect and I was especially surprised at this inexactitude since the talent of Grasset as a popularizer is with reason universally appreciated. I fear that in this article his purpose was not the thorough examination of my doctrine, but rather the belittlement of opinions directly contrary to those expressed in his own books.

Thus I find myself obliged to re-establish the facts for the readers of the *Revue de Philosophie.* I will not attempt a methodical refutation of the assertions of Grasset; that would carry us too far and would not have much interest for anyone. I will limit myself to reviewing my doctrine of aphasia, leaving to my readers the task of comparing this review with the version published by Grasset. Unfortunately, since I am not a psychologist, I must content myself with speaking here as a physician who has medically observed medical facts, and I will attempt to avoid overly technical explanations.

I had the great honor of serving as intern to Broca and Charcot: I was thus brought up to believe in cerebral localizations. At the time when I was at the Salpêtrière my teacher Charcot was giving his memorable lectures on aphasia; it was to me that he assigned the task (and even today I am proud of this choice) of preparing a critical review of all his opinions. On that occasion I composed a diagram which has become almost classic, showing the different centers of language and their functions (this diagram is found on page 295 of the *Centres nerveux* of Grasset).

---

* Translated from "Sur la fonction de langage. Rectifications à propose l'article de M. Grasset" Revue de Philosophie, 1907, Reprinted in *"P. Marie: Travaux et Mémoires"*, Paris: Masson & Co, pp. 93-113 (1926)

This is reported here in order to demonstrate that nothing in my origins would lead me to conceive the slightest doubt on the subject of cerebral localizations, especially those which deal with language.

When in 1895 I was in charge of the practice of the infirmary of Bicêtre, one of the topics to which I dedicated myself with the most interest was aphasia. I had occasion to perform frequent autopsies on aphasics or anarthrics, for the number of such patients in this practice was always very considerable (according to a recent survey made by my intern, Moutier, during the last month in my practice there were thirty-four living aphasics). Under these particularly favorable conditions my studies on aphasia were carried out.

As a faithful disciple, I began by striving to arrange my cases according to the different classic categories. But as my methods of clinical examination became more minute and precise, I noted to my great astonishment, and also to my great displeasure, that the patients whom I observed did not correspond to the descriptions of the authors, or they corresponded only partially.

The clinical picture of aphasia proved to be very different, depending upon whether one studied it in books or observed it in nature. During this time the anatomico-pathological examination of the autopsies did not give very encouraging results. Thus it happened that I sometimes found cases of aphasia without lesion of the third left frontal convolution, and also cases of lesion of this convolution without the production of clinical aphasia. On the other hand, when the third left frontal was altered in the case of aphasics, it was never isolated; always other lesions existed, notably in Wernicke's area.

Year after year I refused to admit that these facts, so manifestly contradictory to the classic teachings, could be anything but errors of observation on my part, and for this reason I resolved not to publish anything in regard to aphasia. But little by little as I became more convinced of having methodically and carefully studied my patients during their lifetime, I became more confident in the results furnished by examination of their brains after death. Thus I found myself slowly and progressively led to doubt the truth of the classic doctrines. Soon my doubts became more precise and I acquired the formal conviction that the dogma of aphasia was only a false dogma.

Thus in May 1906, I proposed in an article in the *Semaine médicale* that I would review the question of aphasia. Since then I have had occasion to repeat this proposal in two other articles in the *Semaine médicale* and I have made several communications on this subject to the medical society of the hospitals of Paris, undertaking to present to this society all the autopsies on aphasics carried out in my practice. Up to the present time these autopsies have always confirmed my opinion. I will try to give a quick sketch of the arguments contained in these diverse publications.

But first of all it is necessary to summarize the classic opinions. From the anatomical and physiological point of view, the authors distinguish, in the left hemisphere of the human brain, a certain number of centers to whose activity would be due the function of language.

For the enumeration and localizations of these different centers I could not do any better than to quote the books of Grasset, which describe current ideas about these centers.

For language there are *sensory* centers of *reception*. One is the *auditory center* A, which is "the auditory center of symbols or the center of auditory symbols. Accumulated there are the auditory images of words, of songs, of music." This center is found in the posterior part of the first temporal convolution. The other *sensory* center, or center of reception, is the *visual center* of words V, which is located in the gyrus angularis.

Beside these centers of reception there are *centers of transmission* or of *emission*, which are: 1. the *motor verbal center* M, "the center of motor images, of words, of spoken symbols" which is located "in the gray matter of the foot of the third frontal"; 2. the graphic motor center E, *center of writing*, which is found in the foot of the second left frontal convolution.

Such is the classic doctrine adopted by Grasset, who used it as the basis of his explication of the function of language.

With this doctrine of the classic centers of language let us compare the opinion to which my anatomical clinical studies have led me. I *deny* that there exists in the left hemisphere a *verbal auditory sensory center* localized either in the foot or in the middle part of the first temporal (center A in the description of Grasset).

I *deny* that there exists a *visual verbal sensory center* localized in the gyrus angularis (center V in the description of Grasset).

I *deny* that there exists a *center of writing* localized in the foot of the second left frontal convolution (center E in the description of Grasset).

I *deny* that there exists in the foot of the third left frontal convolution a *verbal motor center* (Broca's center — center M in the description of Grasset).

In a word, *of the four centers of language described by Grasset I do not admit one.*

How, after that, will the readers of the *Revue de Philosophie* judge the following sentence of Grasset: "Well then, the old classic formula appears to be slightly modified and supplemented, but not at all refuted by the works of Pierre Marie"; or, again, this totally hilarious sentence: "But we should not believe however that the conclusions of Pierre Marie *entirely* conform to the classical doctrine of aphasia"?

Let us speak frankly. The conclusions of my work disturb Grasset, and I can understand why when he clings to his diagram of the "polygon". But if I am right and if I succeed in proving that the four centers of the classic authors on which he based his diagram do not really exist, it becomes a polygon resting on air, and Grasset, all unawares, will have done geometry in space.

But instead of doing his best to pretend that my modifications of the doctrine of aphasia are only "slight modifications" (we have just seen that they in fact do nothing less than overthrow the four classic centers of language), why does Grasset not simply provide facts, new facts with anatomical evidence, which disagree with my point of view? Would not a scientific discussion, objective and clear, be infinitely preferable to all the skills of dialectic which can fool no one, as they are in opposition to the truth?

The best response I can make to the errors of Grasset's article is to set forth my theories for the readers of the *Revue de Philosophie*.

We have just seen that I refuse to admit the four centers of verbal auditory images A, verbal visual images V, verbal motor images M, graphic motor images E. It is nonetheless true that certain focal lesions in the left hemisphere of the brain determine more or less serious problems of language of an aphasic character.

It is these aphasic troubles which are going to guide us and which will permit us, not to penetrate the mechanism of language (we are very far from that, alas!) but at least to gain an approximate idea of some details of this mechanism.

Here I am obliged to have recourse to some clinical descriptions; my non-medical readers will just have to excuse me.

First we must recall the teaching of the authors. Taking as a point of departure the centers of language enumerated above, they attribute to the lesion of each of these a special form of aphasia: *the lesion of the cortical center of motor images of articulation* (the cortex at the foot of the left frontal) will produce CORTICAL MOTOR APHASIA, characterized by the following symptoms: spontaneous speech is abolished or extremely difficult and limited; reading and writing are equally abolished or very noticeably reduced; comprehension of spoken language is also affected.

The isolated lesion of fibers of the white matter subjacent to the third frontal (the cortex of this convolution remaining intact) would bring about PURE MOTOR APHASIA, characterized by the fact that the articulated word alone is altered, the patient cannot talk, but his internal language is conserved; also he can read and write and understand spoken language with no difficulty.

The lesion of the center of graphic motor images (foot of the second left frontal) would bring about AGRAPHIA. This form, however, is not accepted by all authors.

The lesion of the center of verbal auditory images (foot of the first or of the first two left temporals) would give rise to WORD DEAFNESS, a sensory variety of aphasia (due to the alteration of a center connected with the sense of hearing). The word deafness would consist of the fact that the patient hears words as simple noises, but is unable to recognize meaning, because he has lost his verbal auditory images. However, according to the authors, in *pure word deafness* intelligence would remain intact as well as producing spoken language, reading, and writing: only the psycho-sensory reception of spoken language would be missing.

The lesion of the center of verbal visual images (gyrus angularis of the left hemisphere) would produce WORD BLINDNESS, a sensory variety of aphasia (due to the alteration of a center connected with the sense of sight). Word blindness consists of the fact that the patient sees written words as complicated designs, but cannot recognize their meaning because he has lost his verbal visual images. In pure word blindness there is almost complete conservation of intelligence, as well as of articulated language; only reading is missing. Let us take these different varieties of aphasia and examine them one by one without preconceived theoretical formulas, simply in the light of anatomico-clinical facts.

I must declare, first of all, that I have never encountered cases of *pure word deafness* (the impossibility of comprehending spoken language with conservation of spontaneous speech, reading, writing, and integrity of intelligence).

Not only have I never seen a case of this type, nor any which approached it (although lesions of the temporal lobe are far from rare), but

I can affirm that my fellow-physicians will never encounter this. My firm conviction is that *pure word deafness* is a simple myth and that the observations published, in very small number, are found to be full of error. The most frequent of these errors, the easiest to commit, is to neglect certain simple troubles of auricular transmission (labrynthine deafness of Freund or other deafness).

The existence of word deafness is linked to that of the so-called center of the verbal auditory images, the *verbal auditory sensory center*. We know the centers of the human brain only by the phenomena of deficit which are produced on the occasion of their destruction. Therefore, in order to affirm the existence of a verbal auditory sensory center, the isolated destruction of a certain region of the brain (first temporal convolution) would have to bring about the phenomena which the classic authors have described under the name of word deafness. This, however, never happens.

Thus I admit neither *pure word deafness* nor the *sensory center of verbal audition*.

And yet it is incontestable that certain aphasics understand spoken language badly or not at all, and that this lack of comprehension is produced following injury to a region in the left hemisphere of the brain. This region is the *Wernicke's area*, named for the author who first studied the form of aphasia linked with lesions of the posterior part of the territory of the Sylvian artery. Wernicke's areas is, grosso modo, made up of the gyrus supramarginalis, the gyrus angularis, and the foot of the first two temporal convolutions; we are not yet in a position to make a more precise delineation, just as we are not ready to say whether the symptoms which accompany the lesions of this zone are due to the alteration of the cortex rather than to that of the subadjacent white matter. As may be seen, it is a far cry from here to dividing ex professo Wernicke's area into distinct centers, each having a special function, as the classic authors have done.

But clinical observation clearly demonstrates that when this zone is stricken by a lesion (a lesion which affects the white matter) there is produced a group of symptoms constituting the syndrome known as *Wernicke's aphasia*. The patient can speak, sometimes he even speaks too much, but his words, although well pronounced, are often not understandable (jargon aphasia) or they are completely deformed (paraphasia). Reading and writing are partially or totally abolished; the patient understands spoken language badly or not at all.

On the point of this lack of comprehension of spoken language the interpretation of the classicists and my own interpretation differ completely, whatever Grasset has to say about it.

For the classicists, as we have seen, there exists a center of the audition of words, a *sensory* center in which auditory images are arranged, stored, and compared. When this center is stricken by a lesion, these auditory images are destroyed and disappear; the patient can no longer receive the words into his auditory center, and thus cannot compare them with the auditory images which would have been gathered together and catalogued there previously. The patient is unable to understand what is said to him; it seems as if he is hearing a strange language spoken.

In my opinion, when individuals are stricken with a lesion in the region of Wernicke's area, their lack of comprehension of spoken language must be interpreted differently.

I believe this aphasia is not due (as the *sensory* theory of the classic authors would have it) to a lack of functioning of only one auditory center. I have remarked that except in rare cases where the inability to comprehend spoken language is absolute, the patient with Wernicke's aphasia understands isolated words, brief phrases, simple orders. Thus, one cannot say that there is complete impermeability of intracerebral auditory paths. But when the phrases are enlarged, when the number of words is augmented, and the order is made more complicated, the patient ceases to comprehend. If, on the other hand, each word is pronounced separately, if the sentence is subdivided, if the order is given step by step, one notes that the patient is once again able to understand. In summary, what confuses the patient the most is the *complication* of language.

I have tried to describe in the broadest terms the divergence of opinion between the classic authors and myself. I have said that Wernicke's area is not a *psychosensory* center, but an *intellectual* center. I have recalled that loss of intelligence in the case of aphasics is considered a constant or very nearly so, by the great majority of authors. But while I maintain that there is an *intellectual* loss, I have tried to emphasize the fact that the whole range of intelligence is not affected in the same way as comprehension of spoken language. These losses of intelligence of aphasics constitute a specialized deficit bearing especially on the stock of things learned by the didactic processes. I have cited the case of one of my aphasics, a former chef, who was intelligent enough to take a normal part in daily life, yet was incapable of frying an egg.

*
* *

In his article in the *Revue de Philosophie*, Grasset raised still another question on which we are not absolutely in agreement; it is that of the *diagrams*, which Grasset makes a personal issue.

He accuses me of having, in my first article in the *Semaine médicale*, actively attacked the diagrams which he dedicated to the centers of language. If such had been my intention I would have no reason to hide it and I would acknowledge it frankly.

Quite to the contrary, I can give formal assurance that I did not have Grasset in mind at all, but rather Lichtheim, Wernicke, and several foreign authors, when I wrote the following sentence which has annoyed the gentle professor at Montpellier: "*To arrive at constructing the doctrine which today includes all the diverse aphasias*, authors have relied almost exclusively on theoretical ideas; several have even taken for a point of departure a diagram of a complicated graph and from it they have drawn a long series of deductions".

Should Grasset desire to take the time to re-read this sentence, he will see that I speak only of authors *who have* CONSTRUCTED *the doctrine which* TODAY INCLUDES *all the diverse aphasias*; I do not believe that it would occur to anyone to count Grasset among them.

Taking me to task on this point, the distinguished professor at Montpellier challenges me to give my opinion on the use of diagrams in neurology. I will do it dispassionately, for it is long since I repudiated my last diagram.

Certainly, diagrams can render service in teaching and it would be unjust to condemn all of them, but there is a condition: that we demand of diagrams only what they can give and that we reserve them almost exclusively for *anatomical facts* or for theories derived directly from anatomical facts.

To claim to translate psychology into diagrams of an anatomical order when we are completely ignorant of the physiology and even of the fine anatomy of the brain, this we cannot allow! It is unfortunately what Grasset has too often been glad to do. How is it that he has not felt the truth when eminent psychologists have reproached him on this subject? Did not someone even say that in order to represent psychic phenomena, no one should be permitted to use terms or diagrams borrowed from the anatomy of the nerve centers, such a vocabulary seeming "antiscienfitic, dishonest, and hypocritical"? Certainly it is not a question of applying these rather severe epithets to the work of Grasset, for whom we all profess the greatest esteem. But how can we not regret that too often he combines in his diagrams a very controversial physiology with conventional anatomy? This is the case especially for his delicate psychological speculations and, thanks to his great talent, he succeeds at times in rendering them almost credable.

Arnold Pick

Introduced by

A. D. FRIEDERICI
Dept. of Psychology, Free University of Berlin
Berlin, Germany

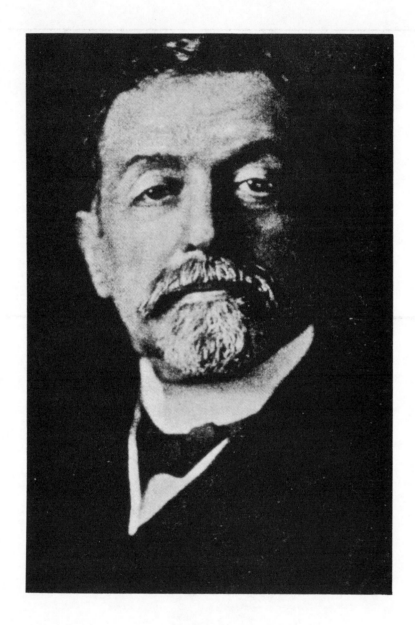

Arnold Pick
1851-1924

Biography

Arnold Pick was born in a small town in Moravia (Czech Republic) in July 1851. He grew up bilingual; he received his school education in Czech but his parents, who identified with German culture, spoke German to him. After the Gymnasium *Pick went to the University of Vienna in 1869. He worked with Meynert, who had also been the teacher of Wernicke and Freud. He received his doctorate at the University of Vienna in 1875. After that he went to Berlin to work in the well-known Charité under Westphal. There he met — among others — Wernicke. After two years of residency as "Sekundararzt" in a psychiatric clinic in north Germany near Oldenburg, Pick accepted a similar position in Prague. There he received the academic title of* Dozent *and with it faculty membership in Psychiatry and Neurology (1878). In 1880 he was appointed director of the psychiatric hospital at Dobrzan. Six years later he was appointed to the chair and the professorship of Psychiatry and Neurology at the German University of Prague (at the age of 35). He held this position for 35 years, which was not always easy, because of the political animosities between the German and the Czech Universities in Prague. Although he retired in 1921, he continued his active scientific life and published several of his most important papers on aphasia. He died in 1924. During his lifetime Pick contributed 260 articles and 16 books to the fields of neurology and psychiatry, 145 of these after the age of 50.*

Selected Bibliography

Pick, A. 1891. "Neue Beiträge zur Pathologie der Sprache". *Archiv für Psychiatrie und Nervenkrankheiten* 28: 1-52.

———. 1905. *Studien über motorische Aphasie*. Wien: Deuticke.

———. 1913. *Die agrammatischen Sprachstörungen*. Berlin: Springer.

———. 1923. "Sprachpsychologische und andere Studien zur Aphasielehre". *Schweizer Archiv für Neurologie und Psychiatrie* 12: 105-135, 179-200.

——— and R. Thiele. 1931. "Aphasie". *Handbuch der normalen und pathologischen Physiologie*. Bd XV, ed. by A. Bethe and G. Bergmann. Berlin: Springer.

Introduction*

The psychological framework

Pick tried to integrate the contemporary psychological thinking as propounded by Karl Bühler, William James and Wilhelm Wundt in his writings on aphasia. Pick recognized two major areas of interest within the field of the psychology of language. One area concerns the conversion from mental content to spoken expression, the path from *thought to speech*. A second deals with the path from *spoken language to thought*, the different stages between hearing and understanding.

Language Comprehension

In his handbook article "Aphasie" (1931) Pick first described the stages of normal language comprehension. He believed that a description of the different levels of the comprehension process may serve as a guide to the understanding of different comprehension disorders. Pick distinguished (1) *perception* and comprehension of the sound of words, on the one hand, from (2) *understanding* of words and sentences, on the other hand.

In speech perception sound and noise sensations will first combine into "patterned forms" (Gestalten) with the assistance of the speech melody; then the word begins to differentiate, and on the basis of some previous knowledge it will be recognized as a phonetic unit, as an "auditory pattern", and thereby as a unit of a particular language. He stressed that these "auditory patterns" can be recognized in spite of an insufficient recognition of the individual phonemes. The more familiar the word is, the more likely this is to happen.

* This work was supported by the Alfred Krupp von Bohlen und Halbach Stiftung.

Comprehension of the sounds of words is primarily based on an acoustic-motoric speech reflex that adjusts the speech apparatus to what is heard. The identification of a particular pattern is supported by the covert or overt repetition of what has been heard. Pick interpreted this motoric speech reflex as a remnant of the infantile acoustic-motor speech reflex, which is prominent in an earlier stage of language development and inhibited in later stages. The confrontation with complicated linguistic material may, however, cause a disinhibition of this reflex in normal adults so that these basic procedures can be used again.

The understanding of words and sentences requires more than just the process of word perception, which could be described as a *reactive* (automatic) emergence of word meaning from memory. Since *the meaning of a sentence is more than the sum of the meaning of the individual words*, Pick, therefore rejected any explanation of the process of understanding that is based on the assumption of fixed connections between words and concepts. The meaning of a word sometimes only emerges from the meaning of the sentence. His description of this process is not always very precise: he stated that the understanding of words and sentences is mediated by the emergence of a "general meaning-awareness" which is guided by the intention to interpret the perceived elements. In the next step — and here it becomes clearer — word category and the grammatical form of the word are recognized. The comprehension of the first word initiates the understanding of the sentence in that a preliminary structure is built on the basis of the intonational and syntactic information given.

The preliminary structure plays a role in differentiating names for things and actions, those items which carry the meaning in simple sentences, whereas those words expressing relations (function words) can be dismissed. The listener understands by developing a content pattern by analogy formation. This is achieved through successive meanings applied to words, whose occasional ambiguity is compensated for by the meaning of the whole sentence. The development of the thought in the listener may take place by completion of the syntactic pattern, or the thing described itself may serve to clarify the content.

Pick stressed that the different stages he describes are not necessarily serial. Instead, he proposed the different stages are interactive (*durcheinander verschränkt*) such that word meanings may be accessed even before the word is fully auditorily perceived or the meaning of the sentence can be represented before the meanings of all individual words are accessed.

He was quite aware of the incompleteness of his description of the comprehension process. For instance, he did not address the problem of how connected sentences are processed in a normal listener. The psychological analysis and the pathological data at hand did not allow him to make more concrete claims about this process.

The description of language production is much more detailed than that of the comprehension process. This may be due to the fact that Pick had a greater variety of relevant data from normal and aphasic language use (e.g., speech errors) to base his description on.

Language Production

The different processing stages from thought to speech are classified into two groups: that of thought formulation and that of linguistic formulation. In his handbook article "Aphasie" Pick described the different stages less clearly than in his earlier book *Die agrammatischen Sprachstörungen*. What follows will, therefore, be based on this earlier text.

As a first stage Pick assumed what his contemporary Marbel called "*Bewußtseinslage*" (level of consciousness). He also referred to Messer (1906), who assumed that "wordless thinking" is prior to verbalization. A second stage, which he called "*Bewußtheit*" (awareness), is described as "conscious of content, but without adequate verbal description". With reference to Bühler (1908) he described the subject as being in a state of "condensed thinking". The next step now is the transition from the structure of thought to the structure of sentences. Pick assumed that the thought schema gives rise to a *sentence schema*. This schematic formulation — which also implies syntactic formulation — precedes the selection of words. Since the meaning of the individual word is determined by its position, the grammatical relations of the mental construction must be completed *before* word selection occurs: "the plan must be fixed before the individual elements can be inserted". He describes the insertion of words as follows: the selected content words are first inserted, then function words are inserted and content words are "grammaticalized", that is, inflected. These processes are all automatic, not conscious. The different stages described here show some relation to process models proposed in contemporary psycholinguistics. Perhaps the most striking feature of Pick's theory of language production is its close resemblance to those psycholinguistic models, which postulate independent levels for processing syntactic structure on the one hand, and lexical items on the other hand (e.g., Fromkin, 1973; Garrett, 1975, 1980).

Aphasia

Although Pick provided this rather detailed description of the different sub-processes involved in both language perception and production, he failed to explain the different aphasic syndromes within this framework. He distinguished several clinical forms of aphasia. On the basis of Wernicke's schema he divided them into (a) motor (frontal) and (b) sensory (temporal) aphasia. He considered the transcortical motor and transcortical sensory aphasia only as stages of recovery from their cortical counterparts (frontal and sensory aphasias) but not as qualitatively different types. Thus the only other established form besides Broca's and Wernicke's aphasia is total or global aphasia (with lesions in both frontal and temporal areas). Amnestic aphasia may be an additional form of aphasia, which is, however, not explicable in Wernicke's schema.

Pick concentrated on the two classical aphasias, motor and sensory aphasia. He devoted the whole of his 1913 book to the phenomenon of agrammatic speech disturbances, *Die agrammatischen Sprachstörungen*. The subtitle indicates that the primary goal of this book is to provide a psychological foundation of the agrammatic deficits. Having laid out a general theory of language production, his explanation of the agrammatic syndromes appears to be only loosely related to it. Pick distinguished *motoric* and *sensoric agrammatism*, being associated with, respectively motor and sensory aphasia. Note that this does not mean that agrammatic speech is paralleled by agrammatic comprehension in frontal aphasia — a notion which has been put forward recently by Caramazza and Zurif (1976) and by others — but (rather) it means that there are two different forms of expressive agrammatism; one is called *quantitative agrammatism* (i.e., agrammatism), the other is referred to as *qualitative agrammatism*. The latter is synonymous with what Kleist (1916) called paragrammatism. This form is characterized by an incorrect use of auxiliary words, word inflections, and incorrect prefixes and suffixes. The former case is mainly characterized by omission of these elements. He observed that the expressive sensory (temporal) agrammatism (paragrammatism) coincides with paraphasic speech. Any account of these two forms of expressive agrammatism must begin, according to Pick, with the clinical fact of a loss or defective command of the grammatical devices.

The genesis of frontal or motor agrammatism is explained by the principle of economy. Pick started off with the observation that in these patients the word order in simple sentences is mostly preserved. He took this to indicate that these patients are sometimes still able to produce a sentence schema and that the lack of bound and free morphemes has to be explained by speech economy. "The patient attempts to produce the best possible result (a "Notsprache", which makes him most understandable) with the least expenditure of effort, utilizing the optimal but still automatic application of his linguistic resources". He assumed that adjustment to a telegraphic style will gradually influence the formulation of the thought. The paragrammatic syndrome, the temporal form of expressive agrammatism, brings to bear the fact that the use of grammar is by no means a unified process, but contains many factors which may be affected separately. Pick thought that in paragrammatism the disorder could be attributed to a deficit which precedes the motor function. Frontal agrammatism, in contrast, has to be viewed as a disorder of the motor function itself. The two forms of expressive agrammatism are thus different in nature.

Thus, although Pick provided, for the first time, a psychological model of language production in which the major process levels are already described to explain aphasic deficits, he did not really advance the explanation of agrammatism as compared to earlier descriptions.

References

Bühler, K. 1908. "Tatsache und Probleme der Denkvorgänge." *Archiv für die gesammte Psychologie* 9:1-92.
Caramazza, A. and Zurif, E. 1976. "Dissociations of algorithmic and heuristic processes in language comprehension." *Brain and Language* 3: 572-582.
Fromkin, V. 1973. *Speech Errors as Linguistic Evidence*. The Hague: Mouton.
Garrett, M. 1975. "The analysis of Sentence Production". *Psychology of Learning and Motivation*. Vol. 9, ed. by G. Bower. London: Academic Press.
———. 1980. "Levels of processing in sentence production". In *Language Production*, Vol. 1, *Speech and Talk.*, ed. by B. Butterworth. London: Academic Press.
Kleist, K. 1916. "Uber Leitingsaphasie and grammatischen Störungen". *Monatschrift für Psychiatrie und Neurologie* 48: 118-199.
Messer, A. 1906. "Experimentell-psychologische Untersuchungen über das Denken." *Archiv für die gesammte Psychologie* 8: 1-224.
Pick, A. 1913. *Die agrammatischen Sprachstörungen*. Berlin: Springer.
——— and R. Thiele. 1931. "Aphasie". *Handbuch der normalen und pathologischen Physiologie*. Bd XV, ed. by A. Bethe and G. Bergmann. Berlin: Springer.

Selection from the work of Arnold Pick

From thinking to speech*

The author would like to illustrate his point of view by using the same analogy which he used to illustrate how a certain stage in formulation is accomplished. From everywhere he wants to gather large and small building blocks from which, gradually, the complete design of the road to be examined will emerge, once they are placed in their naturally or environmentally determined place. Although in the beginning certain parts will be outlined only vaguely, others will show more or less clear contours. But even if we do not make progress at the moment, a kind of network (in a geographical sense as well) will be achieved, whose mesh can gradually be filled in.

The author has conceived a notion, bearing a special relation, to the example put forward by W. James while paying careful attention to the pathology in the process of formulation discussed in this paper, which points particularly toward a more exact distinction between two stages, i.e. mental formulation vs — and preceding — formulation in speech.

Mental formulation is fundamental for the distinction — which comes from the Würzburg school — between thought as the content of consciousness and the faculty of thinking as prior to judgment and conclusion; it is the latter faculty which is expressed in the formal components of the sentence.

This definition has two characteristics: first, in ignoring 'images' in the

---

* Translated from "Die agrammatische Sprachstörungen", Berlin: Springer pp. 228-235 (1913).

process of thought, one assumes a kind of thinking or knowing that has no object; second, in assuming that the process of thinking takes place prior to the formulation of speech, one assumes that there is a prespeech stage of formulation, corresponding to the scheme of W. James; thus the complex of objective and subjective-objective relationships referred to as mental formulation is included. In emphasising these latter relationships, the meaning of emotions as fundamental to emotional acts of thought is already defined; their meaning for the formulation of sentences, especially in their function of "viewpoint", reaches far beyond a purely intellectual factor; this is then definite in determining at which point in time the image of a word occurs, even if it could be subsumed accordingly under the mental formulation. The mental scheme and especially its emotional character is ready before the linguistic formulation (including, of course, the choice of words) has its onset;[1] if this occurs at an earlier point in time, which is the case when affective factors prevail, then speech is not or not completely formulated (interjection or a one-word, interjectional sentence; cf. earlier explanations, especially after Pilsbury).

The conceptual operation whose job is to make the content of consciousness capable of being expressed could naturally not escape the attention of those concerned with these questions, but regarding the transition which thereby takes place, the author believes himself in general to have gone further; if he believes it justified to speak of a formulation which immediately precedes the linguistic formulation and which is for that reason independent of it, he also believes it so with reference to the syntax of deaf-mutes.[2] The presence of this syntax, despite the absence (albeit for external reasons) of actual speech, shows that the distinctive images to which we first reduce the "total image" — to use Wundt's terminology — are not just thrown together, but are the result of an ordering that obeys certain psychological laws: we can in fact speak of a formulation, a "bringing together according to a specific formula".

We can interpret those forms of innate agrammatism in which linguistic development stops at the stage of psychological formulation, a stage in which grammatical formulation is either not accomplished or, in different ways, only poorly developed, in the same way. A separate discussion will show that in modified form this also applies to various forms of disorders or illness-caused destruction of fully developed grammatical formulation.

Further evidence for the concept presented in this article can be gathered from the speech of children. It has been known for a long time that even a child in its first stage of linguistic development does not lack the beginning of mental structure. Repeatedly, statistical studies have tried to establish which words develop soonest and oftenest in the speech of children. Recently, however, it has been pointed out that the words most frequently used by children, the nouns, fulfill quite varied functions; we conclude that such differentiation cannot really be possible without at least a very simple mental structure, because what Owen has previously said about the mental structure of an adult is, mutatis mutandis, true for the child as well. O'Shea (1907:43) is quite right to say: "Too easily we overlook the pronominal, verbal adjectival function of first words,... unconsciously we infer these words from the attitude, the facial expression, the intonation of the child".[3]

These factors, in relation to single words, give further justification for assuming that, already at this stage of speech development, there is a certain degree of mental formulation; this is why even with a child, we speak of one-word sentences or sentence-words, insofar as, in the combination of a one-word sentence with gestures, the first signs of relation and formulation emerge, though not in a grammatical (as interpreted by Romanes 1893:297) but in a mental sense.

As for assuming the likelihood of logico-mental organization, the author would like to put forward another argument, one that also touches upon the pathological field. In his tachystoscopic experiments Messer (1906:77) has demonstrated the existence, as a phase of understanding that precedes full comprehension, what he calls "spheres of consciousness," of consciousness of the overarching sphere in which the word inheres.[4] This is accounted for by the associative coherence out of which a superordinate or coordinate concept emerges. The author (Pick 1909:37) has described an analogue in cases of damaged or recovering speech comprehension. There he also indicates that the same observation can often be made in disturbances of the expression of speech. Similarly it is not unusual to observe that, at the onset of apraxia, aphasic patients who suffer accompanying apraxic symptoms, when asked to show the tongue, will respond with an incorrect but similar movement despite good understanding of the question. This can be linked to the observation that something of the same kind occurs in slips of the tongue: instead of, With the left ear? one asks, With the left eye? Very interesting, and showing even more clearly the phenomenon under discussion, is the observation made by a private teacher, Dr. Sträussler, only recently heard by the author: on being asked his age, a paraphasic patient replies: "I can't remember how long I am old". When we notice processes of super-ordination, organization, and subordination influencing speech, the development of which, after all, we have learned especially from the "normal" slip-of-the-tongue phenomenon, we now know to reside in the mental, we may take this as support for the assumption that this influence takes place at the stage of mental formulation.

Indications of such a mental formulation can also be found in several older articles, e.g. Vignoli (cited by Jodl) speaks of an "articulation of thought" preceding articulated language. Lotze also expresses a similar notion, in almost the same form as the author; this cannot be mere coincidence.[5] Of course, the idea of mental formulation has not always been clearly expressed, but can be inferred from the full context. O. Dittrich's "syntactification of meaning" can be interpreted in this manner; for when in this context he speaks (Wundt:95) of images of sounds, which are already heard as reproducing parts of inner speech during the syntactification of meaning (we will say more about this well-known phenomenon later on), it seems that this syntactification of meaning is something like mental formulation.[6] It even does not seem far-fetched to look upon it as a bridge for the attempt to combine the notion represented in this paper with Wundt's notion of synthesis (apperceptive analysis of a state of affairs and synthesis of the thus successively achieved layers into a final apperception).

Something similar has been described by Moskiewicz (1910:347); among the principal concepts directing the course of imagery he finds some "that appear to me as schemata(!) that still should primarily be filled with images ... only hints of directions ... a series of hypotheses".

The possibility of what is here called a mental scheme, a mental structure, is also considered by Sheldon (1907:248) in his explanation of the use of the linguistic method with questions of logic. We refer to his explanation here because it clarifies the object of discussion quite well, be it in part only in a figurative sense.[7] His argument appears latently[8] in several places in philologists' explanations; Wunderlich (1901:xxviii) emphasises in the discussion of complex sentences the consideration of the laws of thought and adds that "the inner vehicles (probably meaning the laws of thought) usually guide the person who is speaking without the person being aware of this".

In attempting to clarify the trajectory along which the dawning thought must travel until it reaches its complete linguistic formulation, the explanations coming from the Würzburg school will also be helpful, especially regarding the processes ranked according to degrees of clarity. To begin with, there is Marbe's "conceptual state", of which we have given a description before, and which comes close to what is described by B. Erdmann as intuitive thinking, a thought in the beginning of its dawning and therefore not yet clearly formulated.

We have stated that W. James (1890:251), regarding the well-known tip-of-the-tongue phenomenon, assumes an adaptation of the missing word to a schema, even before the word is actually found; it seems quite probable that the moment of occurrence of this feeling of fitting or non-fitting comes close to the moment of the state of consciousness.[9] It has been demonstrated by Messer (1906:177) that this is what actually happens in mental formulation; he has been able especially to demonstrate the "conceptual state" in this form in his experimental-psychologicy studies on thinking. This is the state "in which an opinion, a thought is present, which can only be adequately formulated in a sentence, while no words can be detected in consciousness". In this way the temporal localization of the conceptual state" in this form in his experimental-psychology studies on The attempt to compare the occurrence of a state of mind in this stage to what happens when one is searching for a forgotten word appears to be justified by Messer's observation (p. 183) "that the ensuing opinion on the quality of the emerging content of thought is partly prepared, but partly replaced by the 'conceptual state' of the fitting (non-fitting), the meaningful (meaningless), the right (wrong, faulty or ineffective)."

If in Messer's conception wordless thinking comes to the fore and so far the share of emotions has been stressed here, the conclusions that demonstrate the existence of "mental levels" of numerous logical relations ("in which relations between objects or concepts in the mind appear to full advantage" (Messer)), appear to be more relevant here, where we are talking about mental formulation. We will discuss these conceptual states more fully later on, so for the moment we will just point out that for the physician study of them appears to be important for two reasons: First, because contrary to its aforementioned occurrence as the first stage in the development of mental content, in symptomatologically similar conditions, H. Jackson's so-called "dreamy states" are to be observed in cases of psychic dissolution during the precursor of the epileptic attack as being the last stage just before unconsciousness. Second, considering the question of localization, it is important that the aforementioned observations, including especially the "tip-of-the-tongue phenomenon", also point to relationships with the temporal lobe.[10] Exactly what meaning is to be given to the explanation of these relationships becomes clear when we take the view of the author concerning the localization of agrammatism in the temporal lobe and try to localize the processes, that correspond to linguistic formulation in almost the same manner as now happens with finding words.

The assumption we make here, namely that the "conceptual state" is a first stage in the ordering of the path from thought to speech, corresponds to Messer's view, who states directly (p. 188), "but we believe that in the complete linguistic formulation of the content that has been thought (or meant) in this conceptual state we will find only a more developed, richer form of what was given only rudimentarily". We must conceive of this development as proceeding in different stages, especially in the direction of increasing clarity of thought content that exist in consciousness only dimly and rather emotionally. Such a second stage of organization might correspond to Achs's notion of consciousness, in which "the contents exist consciously, however without adequate linguistic meaning". In any case, we believe that we may conclude from Achs's article that he is also inclined to assume a mental organization preceding the linguistic one.

What is being said here with respect to the succession of states of mind and consciousness during linguistic formulation also corresponds to Bühler's view (1908:346). Thus when he hears the subject describe the first stage as "formal overview of extensive lines of thought", while another subject calls it exactly analogous to the well-known descriptions of what happens just before drowning, Bühler compares them with the "poetic way of thinking" of Lazarus.

A further step in the line of thought developed here poses the question: How shall we imagine the transition from thought structure to sentence structure in the practice of speaking? Perhaps it will be permitted to employ an image. One might imagine that the mental schema, achieved by thought processes energizes a linguistic schema. We can think of this schema as analogous to the basic linear outline of a mosaic picture.[11] In the next stage, in which word selection takes place, the words are "inserted" into the compartments of this mosaic design. The syntax can be analogized with the localization in this basic design and with the simultaneously commencing process of grammatizing, including its modifying influences, which the components of the word undergo partly from the basic design, partly from each other. If the words follow each other according to the sense of the thought and adapt to each other in form and order, then this can be pictured by way of two such schemas. Just to avoid misunderstandings, we especially emphasize, in view of the arguments against the parallelism of thought and speech, that the assumption of two such schemas does not, of course, lead to the assumption of a correspondence between those schemas; that the schematic formulation of the sentence precedes the choice of words, as well as the syntactic and the portion of the grammatical functions that corresponds to it, is shown by the fact that the meaning of a single word, whatever it may be, is determined only by the position it takes or interacts with; therefore the mental framework should in principle be ready in a grammatical sense as well: before the choice of words ensues, the plan has to be determined before the different pieces are put together.

It would remain, however, the most uninteresting schema in the full sense of the word,[17] if we did not at least try to interpret the transition to grammatical formulation in terms of a series of processes in the sense of the functional psychology which we have taken as a model in this article, meanwhile searching for those factors that effectuate them.

It must be assumed that the psychological schema hitherto produced and put forward as the analogue for the complex of objective and subjective relations of the content of thought creates first of all a grammatical sentence schema which is supposed to reflect that mental formulation that subsequently is to be developed by the listener. The development of this sentence-formulation schema may also be pictured according to a kind of overall picture in Wundt's sense, being active in the gradual analysis into its parts and finding in this its fulfillment through the automatic, habitual process of grammatizing words.

Agrammatism*

Among the phenomena of motor aphasia, some have been discussed which are manifested in the loss of or disturbance in the use of those linguistic devices which in a general way serve to grammaticize speech. We shall now discuss this form together with some others.

The descriptive terms which have been applied to these various forms are derived partly from anatomical and partly from functional considerations. They have only gradually become known, having been initially grouped together under the designation agrammatism. To eliminate the obscurities which arise from this fact we must add a few remarks on the nomenclature.

The term was first used in a general way for agrammatism of presumably frontal origin. When it was found to occur with a lesion of the temporal (sensory) portion of the speech field, a *sensory agrammatism* was distinguished from what had been termed *motor agrammatism* because of its association with motor aphasia. Following this, it was observed that in the *impressive* part of speech, in speech comprehension, defects in the comprehension of grammatical form occur which deserve to be included in agrammatism and are thus designated sensory.

Moreover, the recognition that temporally determined expressive agrammatism is characterized primarily by erroneous grammatical constructions (paragrammatisms) in contrast to the frontal type with its *telegraphic style* led Kleist to distinguish the temporal form as *paragrammatism*.

Since we have already discussed the symptomatology of motor agrammatism let us now, with regard to pathogenesis, approach the pertinent defects of the expressive side with a comparable description of paragrammatism.

This temporally determined form is characterized, in pure cases, by disturbances in the use of auxiliary words, incorrect word inflections, and erroneous prefixes and suffixes. In other words, it concerns all those lin-

* Translated from "Aphasie" In: "*Handbuch der normale und pathologische Physiologie*", edited by A. Bethe and G. Bergmann, Bd XV, Berlin: Springer, pp. 1469-1477 (1931)

Reprinted with permission from Jason W. Brown "*Aphasia by Arnold Pick*", Springfield: Charles C. Thomas, pp. 76-86 (1973)

guistic devices which serve to express *relationships* between objects and which differ widely and quantitatively from one language to another. According to the localization, other temporal symptoms are found in the early stages which may later disappear. In contrast to motor agrammatism, the tempo of speech is not retarded, tending rather to logorrhea with intact sentence pattern and intonation. Occasionally, some motor phenomena are found, such as the dropping of inflections, with juxtaposition of the words that compose the skeleton of the sentence.

In rare cases which, with respect to other symptoms, show complete recovery, and more rarely as an introductory stage in progressive cases, an isolated grammatical disorder may represent the only symptom; e.g. confusion of genders, finally followed by exclusive use of the feminine form.

The patient commonly notices his errors, without always being able to describe or correct them. Occasionally the correct grammatical structure emerges via the feel for the language (*Sprachgefühl*) evoked by partially saying it aloud to him. The influence of emotions may also have a salutory effect in this case as in others. The frequent coincidence of temporal (expressive) agrammatism with paraphasia, due to the common localization, may result in unintelligible speech, with defects which may be hard to classify. The linguistic formulation plays a guiding role in preparation for writing as well, and accounts for the similar occurrence of agrammatism in writing. Also of importance in evaluation is the presence of linguistically justifiable agrammatisms, this being more common in colloquial language than generally supposed, even in highly developed languages (e.g., English).

Any account of the two forms of expressive agrammatism must begin with the clinical fact of a loss or defective command of the grammatical devices of the language (syntax and grammar in the restricted sense). With regard to precise definitions, we must determine how far these phenomena are due to disorders in the speech field and how far they represent secondary phenomena due to disorders in other regions, though surely little can be said about the latter at this time.

Initially, processes of mental and inner-speech formulation preliminary to the speech fields do not appear to be affected by the lesion under consideration. However, we may infer on the basis of observation that disorders which affect the course of these processes can impair syntax and grammar. Gross disorders of thought in confusion or twilight states, such as mild flights of ideas or thought contamination in manic states, can have such an effect. A manic patient said "Ich war tödlich Bronchialkatarrh gewesen" (I had been deathly bronchial catarrh). A Czech housemaid unfamiliar with German writes (what has been said of spoken agrammatism also applies to writing) in a hysterical twilight state, *"Kucharko!* (cook). Ich bin (inserted later) *klinika* (the clinic in the nominative) Pick *prijata* (admitted, no inflection), *chci vam* (I want you), unintelligible word marked out *wünschen a* (and) *isst* (eats, apparently for *ist* "is") *zavreli"* (they have locked in).

These factors can obviously also affect word order in different ways. Whether this is also true of organic lesions sparing the speech field is the subject of a study undertaken by Head. It is, for example, probable that disorders of the linguistic representation of spatial relationships may be due to spatial disorders, as in defects of orientation, which because of defective formulation of thought entail a defective use of the corresponding auxiliary words. Also we must consider the fact that the patient stresses significant words reflecting his emotional state and not the situation as seen by the listener, and this may make speech unintelligible to the listener.

These factors fall outside the strict field of aphasia, and it is not always possible to determine whether their influence also concerns or involves the speech field processes under consideration. However, there may also be factors within aphasia proper which are active in the process of thought and speech formulation. Among those already mentioned as more frequent are the narrowness of the perspective of awareness, in part the purposeless scattering of attention (regarded by Kussmaul as the sole cause of agrammatism) and incongruences between formulation in thought and formulation in language (with resultant thought and speech contaminations). Nor is it unlikely that the above speech production could be secondarily impaired by other disorders of the speech field. Thus, defective verbal memory may impair the syntactic structure, since another word put in the place of the missing one may have a damaging effect on sentence construction.

Regarding telegraphic style of primary origin, discussed in relation to motor agrammatism, in which word order is not appreciably disturbed, alterations of word order have occasionally been reported as due to a discrepancy between the normal order (most important element first) and the grammatically required order (final position of the verbs as in the language of children). However, a thorough investigation of this question, based upon linguistics, the language of children, deaf-mute language, and sign language, is not yet available. As in normals, the condition is due to the fact that the intention is chiefly directed towards that meaning which is expressed primarily by nouns and verbs, so that the words which form the skeleton of the sentence are stressed while the accompanying auxiliary words, which are thought or felt in addition to these, remain unuttered. We see this in the situation where the patient strongly believes he has spoken the omitted words. With regard to word order, we must also consider the opposing influences of emotion and the preserved feel for the language. Certain disturbances of this kind (e.g. verb at the end of the sentence) represent the reversion to a childish mode of speech. In discussing defective processes of grammatization in the strict sense of the word, we must consider prepositions, word inflection (prefixes and suffixes), articles, and pronouns which serve this purpose. We must also consider the aforementioned effect of practice on these processes, even in the preschool period, which creates a feeling for the language (*Sprachgefühl*). Consequently, we speak of the analogy of acquired typical linguistic patterns. This feel for the language surpasses the influence of later grammatical schooling, even in educated persons. (Consideration of this difference is essential in the pertinent examinations.) Laboratory grammaticization of given words and grammaticization in ordinary discourse are by no means the same (grammar and *Sprachgefühl*!), as observed clinically. In this regard, it should be mentioned that the agrammatical speaker often has superior writing. Both the time factor of the possibility of prolonged formulation and the mental attitude play a part, since for most individuals writing is a considered act. This difference also appears in talking with the doctor and with the family and colleagues. It is readily apparent here that the factor of better education is not insignificant.

In certain cases it must be assumed that auxiliary words, especially prepositions, corresponding to a certain external speech formulation are also lacking in inner speech. More frequently it is not their absence but their inadequate evocation that is responsible for this disorder.

A similar situation applies to word inflection, which is omitted in accordance with the law of economy. This corresponds to normals; the existence of essentially formless languages of high standing (e.g. English) indicates that the corresponding form components in other languages provide an extra that is superfluous to comprehension (cf. also the ordinary telegram!). Conversely, inflection is lacking because it does not adequately or properly respond to the stimulus, leading in the latter case to corresponding errors. In multilinguals the disorder will appear uniquely or mainly in (most often) the latest acquired language.

Testing with single improperly conjugated or declined words, apart from the meaning of the single word as sentence, is chiefly an examination of knowledge gained in school and usually of very brief retention. This appears mostly when, in the face of poor test performance, the patient's actual discourse indicates adequate feel for the language; also, the "formulation of sequences" (*Reihenbildung*) can be preserved with incorrect word inflection.

A distinction should be made between the above-mentioned telegraphic style and pidgin (so-called 'Negersprache') characterized by a simple succession of *uninflected* nouns and verbs. While this form shares with telegraphic style the absence of auxiliary words which characterize relationships, in the dropping of inflectional devices (in certain languages the prefixes and suffixes as well) it represents a still further regression to an infantile stage of speech. It also shares with telegraphic speech the fact that relationships are conceived along with the nouns and verbs, or in advance of the utterance, but it shows further regression than telegraphic speech.

Regarding the *genesis* of the two forms of expressive agrammatism, a distinction must be made, with reference to *frontal (motor) agrammatism* (the *telegraphic style*), between its immediate onset after a lesion and its slow development with a gradual increase in vocabulary from an initial one-word sentence stage. In the latter instance, because of the linguistic poverty, a gradual adjustment takes place such that only the skeleton of the sentence is produced. The former instance concerns the factors discussed above: emergence of the skeleton of the sentence alone, during the mental formulation in thought or inner speech; absence of or defect in the auxiliary words which are normally produced in automatic fashion. It is probable that the patient with motor agrammatism at times retains the sentence skeleton since he may not comprehend the prepositions nor be able to write them. We may assume that adjustment to a telegraphic style, which makes the prepositions appear superfluous, will gradually influence formulation in thought. The lack of inflection in juxtaposed words may be explained by speech economy, due to the fact that speech is difficult to produce at all and inflection requires even more energy. The patient attempts to produce the best possible result (that which makes him understood best) with the least expenditure of effort, utilizing the optimal but still automatic application of his linguistic resources. Of the ideas that are inchoate and ready for transmission to the executive apparatus, only the essential components are selected. (This represents a pathological intensification of what is termed "brachylogy" in linguistic psychology, speech in which the obvious is omitted.) Another likely factor is the attention fixed on the effortful production of speech. If the prepositions are either not automatic or only incompletely so, attention will not suffice for their voluntary production.

This whole line of thought is consistent with the fact that this aphasic disorder concerns an intensification of the normal tendency to agrammatism.

Sentence rhythm will often be intact in cases of advanced recovery, so far as it is subordinate to the retained sentence skeleton. Disturbed rhythm is probably secondary to defective language, though a primary impairment may be present due to simultaneous involvement of the corresponding (musical) functional region.

In addition to our previous comments, it should be emphasized that the situation will influence word order: not only the speaker's appraisal of the situation, but what he takes to be the listener's appraisal as well. As a result of his linguistic poverty, the agrammatic patient utilizes the situation far beyond the norm. The relation between spoken and written agrammatism will vary, depending on the mental attitude, according to whether the patient tends more to the one or the other. Agrammatism may be entirely lacking in writing in spite of the greater difficulty of this activity.

Difficulties will also arise from the conflict between the persistent but ineffectual feeling for sentence form and the forceful influence of emotional factors. This opposition of imitation and spontaneity corresponds to the same phenomena in the linguistic development of the child.

Isolated words produced in the initial period can be termed agrammatical only, as in the normal case, insofar as they take the place of a sentence. This is evidenced chiefly by observations in which patients speaking in such a manner can modify the few words at their disposal, not only in accent but also in articulation (lala, dada, etc.) to express different thoughts.

Parenthetically, we see in the patient's inability to linguistically express the relations of things that disorders directly involving morphology refer back to semiological defects (semantics).

In re-education, the feel for the language which results from years of practice plays a part insofar as its remnants can be built upon. Even if one begins grammatical instruction this will not build up a rote sequence, but is effective only as an extension or reconstruction of the feel for the language.

Awareness of one's defect is commonly lacking in motor agrammatism. As in the normal individual, the patient devotes his attention to the meaning of the utterance. Accordingly, awareness will vary depending on whether he is attending more to speaking (which may lead to further impairment) or trusts to his presumably intact feel for the language to carry him to success. In many cases the feel for the language is apparent in the course of the function, and the patient will notice his error. Sometimes he is still unable to specify it, while at other times he hesitates without coming to a conclusion. To some extent this is related to the fact that the patient speaks better with the doctor than in ordinary communication; in the latter case he depends on the established automatism, while in the former the urge toward better speech has a positive effect.

Infantile or *native agrammatism* is an arrest of speech development due to defective brain development or a cerebral disease at a pregrammatical stage. It is characterized by both frontal and temporal phenomena. In cases of permanent arrest, which may occur independently without other mental defects, proper feel for the language does not develop, a deficiency which is compensated by later schooling only inadequately if at all. In mentally retarded states the disorder may be due to defective thought formulation, the child not having entered into the "relationship stage", so that relations of things do not properly enter his awareness.

In *paragrammatism*, the *temporal* form of expressive agrammatism, it must be remembered that grammar is by no means a unified process, but contains many factors which may be affected separately or in combination. In this form, the disorder lies one stage deeper than telegraphic style. It is also of a different nature; in the latter, functions corresponding to the inner speech form, which ordinarily are accomplished through the sentence framework, are not carried out (the reasons for this are given above). In the paragrammatic patient, this process, automatized even to the feel for the language (which is all that is still effective) is accomplished but in a defective manner, since the individual processes occur either improperly or not at all. With regard to the opposition between volition and automatism and the disturbing influence of attention directed toward a function, voluntary intervention in these processes will not be helpful in most cases. Even in normals, as we have shown, grammaticization that relies simply on feel for the language often succeeds better than that directed by the will.

The various paragrammatical errors also concern functionally differentiated degrees of defects in certain forms of activity. This is definitely proven by such observations as isolated confusion of pronouns and more so by the use of *du* retained after an illness in a patient who had evidently used it dialectally in his youth. [By this is meant the use of the German familiar pronoun *du* in addressing persons with whom the patient was not on sufficiently familiar terms.] Such facts — confusion of *haben* and *sein* [auxiliaries each appropriate to specific verbs], forms of the article — also show that this is not a disorder of motor function, but a defective application of motor effects. In the normal, these have become automatic through analogies from the feel of the language and are not carried out on the basis of knowledge of the corresponding grammatical rules. Of course, certain mental processes to which these motor processes are subordinated do come into play.

There is a discrepancy between poor agrammatical speech and better appraisal of ungrammatical sentences presented to the patient. This is explained by the contrast between defective or absent feel for the language and the fact that the patient recognizes what he sees as incorrect, but is incapable of putting it into correct grammatical form.

This example of a dynamic interpretation clearly demonstrates the advantage over an extremely anatomical view based on assumed "elements" or functions. The assumption of a fixed localization of single words and even parts of words in the neural elements, in explanation of phenomena of the type discussed here, requires us also to assume partial destruction of specific types of discrete ganglion cells by the lesion.

It is unlikely that temporal expressive agrammatism is an expression of inadequate functioning of the right hemisphere, since it occurs with a small lesion. One should be cautious even in the presence of bilateral lesions. Agrammatism due to previous lesion of the left side may reappear or be intensified by symmetrical lesion of the right side. Certainly, the extent to which impairment in interhemispheric relationships is involved must remain in doubt.

The close bounds between the functions affected in amnesic aphasia, paraphasia, and sensory agrammatism are apparent in the frequent concurrence of the three forms and their common localization. Detailed clinical and anatomical research is needed to clarify the relationships and differences between these forms.

Although sensory agrammatism and paraphasia appear to have a common pathogenesis, as suggested by their coincidence and by localizational factors, this does not appear certain, since even in severe paraphasia, components of the sentence form are undisturbed. Moreover, no transitional forms exist between seemingly ungrammatical segments of jargon aphasia and segments with defective forms corresponding to true temporal agram-

matism. Therefore, it seem probable that just as paragrammatism is produced by other disorders (thought contamination and sentence contamination), this applies to jargon also as a result of disinhibitions, perhaps reinforced by perseveration. Of course, the topographically determined coinci-
·dence of the two syndromes implies their interpenetration. Also, amnesic
factors, resulting from the same localization, may have a disturbing effect.
This is due to an absence of the pertinent word in the formulation, which is
thus retarded and requires modification (Lotmar).

Some general comments and interpretations might be added here concerning the localization of the various types of agrammatism. With regard
to the expressive forms, it should not be thought that the grammatical
knowledge or the feel for the language is localized to a precise area. The
relationship is rather to be explained in terms of functional impairment in
those regions corresponding to stages in verbalization in which the syntactic
and especially the grammatical processes are applied and so serve to match
what is to be said to the thought pattern. It should be emphasized that the
preexisting sentence pattern is decisive in word order, while in grammaticization the processes are applied to the words as they emerge. Similarly but
with modification according to the course of the process, this also applies to
sensory agrammatism. This, together with the fact that agrammatism is
often secondary in nature, makes it clear that lesion and locus of function
need not coincide. At least, this appears to be the case with regard to large
lesions with their abundance of secondary phenomena.

Beyond the frontal or temporal localization, little can be said with certainty. For motor agrammatism as a secondary phenomenon, Broca's area
is of causal significance. With regard to temporal paragrammatism, it is
often obscured by severe paraphasia with lesion of Wernicke's area. It most
likely has a functional correlation with the second and third temporal convolutions, for as the paraphasia diminishes, it may be clinically observed
that both grammaticization and selection of words are closely related. This
is also in agreement with occasional findings at autopsy. The coincidence of
paragrammatism and sensory agrammatism suggests also that identical processes and substrata are involved in the origin of their symptoms. The
localization of these disorders in the second and third temporal convolution
of the left hemisphere (even with localization elsewhere, the same
mechanisms may be involved) suggests involvement in the acoustic portion
of inner speech, in its participation in processes underlying the grammaticization of speech; also, there may be involvement of those higher psychic

processes which are obstructed at the stage of their intervention in grammaticization.

Naturally, in the "localization" of agrammatism, the same reservations expressed in the discussion of "centers" must be taken into account.

It would be premature to attempt to fully explain the various forms in this manner. Little is known of the linguistic-psychological basis, and perhaps it is not yet possible to even approach these questions.

As a suggestion concerning these factors, it might be pointed out that the occurrence of certain small parts of speech, such as *but, because, nevertheless*, etc. depends on emotional state. Thus, we should investigate why these words are lacking, or their effect on sentence formation does not occur.

While these considerations must remain tentative, they nevertheless provide a starting point for further research on this central problem of aphasia theory.

If we consider these forms of expressive agrammatism from the functional and localizational points of view, we may see the following sequence: paragrammatism as the first in the sequence of processes subsequent to word choice; defective grammaticization of words; absence of such grammaticization; and, depending on the degree of speech difficulty, telegraphic style or pidgin. After this comes linguistic puerilism as a still higher degree of linguistic poverty, impairment of the phonological side of speech (apparently occuring regularly with involvement of grammaticization). Clearly, this interpretation is in harmony with what we know of the localization of the temporal and frontal forms, as well as the similar effects upon these mechanisms emanating from higher psychic centers.

Sensory (impressive) agrammatism is discussed under the heading of word deafness.

Notes

1. We will hear a lot about the influence of this factor upon word order — which is also an important part of linguistic formulation — in the chapter in question, which will support the line of thought that is alluded to here; for now, we will only point to what v.d. Gabelentz called the psychological subject, a term not used by others, meaning the word which is by interest receives the most emphasis and therefore is put in the first place; it is clear that "interest" also belongs among the factors of mental formulation. In this context we may point to the way in which especially the emotional factor is thrown together with the linguistic formulation, which emerges much later. Wunderlich (1901) expresses it

directly "the affect and the unconscious production of speech of the naive human being forms sentences before he becomes conscious of the words".

2. If we follow Wundt in ascribing syntax to the sign language of the uneducated deaf-mute person, in spite of contradiction from Delbrück and Sütterlin, thorough illumination is to be found in the chapter about word order.

3. Logical arguments against this interpretation may be put to rest by this discussion from the logician Bosanquet. "The grammatical analysis classifying words as substantives, adjectives, adverbs, verbs, and so forth, cannot be interpreted as if it would tell us what these words are in themselves; it is rather the other way around: it teaches what they mean in the context of a meaningful sentence. For reasons of convenience they are considered separately, like parts of a machine, but the performance which grants them their names, comes about only when they are put together" (Bosanquet, 1897).

4. Delbrück (1886) already characterized the phenomenon, recently described as sphere of consciousness, as follows: even with an uneducated person words belong in more or less understandable groups, demonstrated by the fact that members of separate groups are confounded much more often within each group than two members of different groups.

5. "The objective elements of thought have to be brought into certain shapes, according to the peculiarities of human thinking. Then just as for a construction project in which forces are supposed to operate in a certain manner, the building blocks have to be cut in mutually determined shapes first — out of merely spherical elements only a heap of stones of that shape can be made — so our thinking has to place each of the elements, which in the beginning are no more than conditions in our arousal, in a form which assigns to it in the later connection the type of application and the given means in which it is connected to others" (Lotze ——, 2:243)

6. This is also suggested by the fact that Dittrich (p. 118) speaks of an interval between the conception of meaning and the external production of sounds during which the production of the oncoming external articulation takes place (the conception of meaning also precedes this articulation).

7. "Judgement may be an indivisible instantaneous whole and yet have a complicated internal structure, similar to that of the sentence. And curiously enough Bosanquet himself believes that it has. The map we see at one glance, has the same structure as the map we draw slowly. The discrepancy between logical (or psychological) and grammatical subject and predicate is admitted by most linguists, who nevertheless avowedly pursue linguistic method. And further the inner thought might have a general correspondence in form to the verbal expression, without the same order or emphasis of parts, or without a one-to-one correspondence throughout".

8. In the following utterance by Stern about the form of what is to be said, one can observe as well the onset of a mental formulation: "Each human being wanting to produce a sentence — be it a child or an adult — has to anticipate in his mind the essential content of what he is going to say already in advance in some hazy form. If one would agree with Wundt in calling this an "overall picture" or if the anticipation is more emotional and volitional in character, is not important for our study" (Cl. and W. Stern 1907).

9. Later on we will hear that the conceptual state also includes emotional conditions and that therefore also the second side, the psychological formulation, which was formerly emphasized, the individual viewpoint of the speaker, his opinion, can be given in this

state; this seems to be necessary because we have to assume that these personal factors expressed in the formulation are the original ones and precede the judgmental ones.

10. With this cursory remark — a more detailed discussion can only be given in the appropriate place — we do not mean to say that everything associated with "dreamy states" can be located in the temporal lobe; but it agrees with careful localization to say in view of the clinical phenomena and pathological-anatomical determinations that the temporal lobe is involved.

11. It must be noted that such an explantion has nothing in common with the mosaic structure of psychic life found in the older reflex psychology. H. Sachs (1905:68), in one of his expositions dedicated to the meaning of the sentence, rejects a "mosaic image" in the sense of the construction of thought out of separate elementary parts, but this rejection does not apply, according to his earlier presentations, to the assumption under discussion, the assumption that an already outlined picture will be filled with mosaic tiles. It does not fit the facts, however, when Sachs (ibid.) apparently lets the meaning of the sentence emerge only when all the phrases have been said; for it has been shown by Marty (1908:149f.), in his discussion of the inner constructive form of speech, how "the overall meaning of a sentence is prepared by tentative images and expectations about the function of its separate elements". W. James (1890:254) expressed himself similarly at an earlier time and developed very elegantly from that the right emphasis on this reading. Bühler (1912:895) speaks of a "preconstruction" that aims at the content as well as at the form of what follows (Bühler 1912).

12. Whenever it has been noticed before that what is offered to us from the linguistic side as a clarification of these questions does not extend itself beyond a "programme" most of the time, it can be pointed out here that philologists are working hard to fill the programme with content; as when Methner (1911) tries to explain how in many kinds of relative clauses and *cum* clauses, even if they contain undisputed facts, i.e. given connections of concepts, the same mood is used that otherwise only expresses self-produced or free connections of concepts (i.e. the subjunctive).

References

Bosanquet, B. 1897. *Essentials of Logic*. London: Macmillan.
Bühler, K. 1908. "Tatsache und Probleme der Denkvorgänge." *Archiv für die gesammte Psychologie* 9:1-92.
———. 1907. "Tatsachen und Probleme zu einer Psychologie der Denkvorgänge: I. Uber Gedanken." *Archiv für die gesammte Psychologie* 9: 297-365.
———. 1913. *Gestalt-Wahrnehmung. Experimentelle Untersuchung*. Stuttgart: Spermann.
Delbrück, B. 1886. "Amnestische Aphasie." *Jenaische Zeitschrift für Naturwissenschaften* 20: Supplement II.
Dittrich, O. 1903. *Grundzüge der Sprachpsychologie. Vol 1. Einleitung und Allgmeine Grundlegungen*. Halle: M. Niemeyer.
Gabelentz, G.v.d. 1901. *Die Sprachwissenschaft*. 2. Auflage, Leipzig: Tauchnitz.
James, W. 1891. *The Principles of Psychology*. London: Macmillan.

Marty, A. 1908. *Untersuchungen zur Grundlegung der allgemeinen Grammatik und Sprachphilosophie.* 1. Band Halle: Niemeyer.

Messer, A. 1906. "Experimentell-psychologische Untersuchungen ber das Denken". *Archiv für die gesammte Psychologie* 8: 1-224.

Methner, R. 1911. *Bedeuting und Gebrauch des Konjunktivs in den lateinischen Relativsätzen und Sätzen mit* cum. Berlin: Weidmann.

Moskiewicz, G. 1910. "Zur Psychologie des Denkens: I." *Archiv für die gesammte Psychologie* 18: 305-399.

O'Shea, M.V. 1907. *Linguistic Development and Education.* New York: Macmillan.

Pick, A. 1911. *Uber das Sprachverständnis: Zwei Vorträge.* Leipzig: Barth.

Romanes, G.J. 1893. *Die geistige Entwicklung beim Menschen.* Leipzig: Günther.

Sachs, H. 1905. *Gehirn und Sprache.* Wiesbaden: Bergmann.

Sheldon, W. 1907. "Methods of investigating the problem of jugdment". *Psychological Bulletin* 4: 243-255.

Stern, Cl. and W. 1907. *Die Kindersprache: Eine sprachtheoretische und psychologische Untersuchung.* Leipzig: Barth.

Wunderlich, H. 1901. *Der Deutsche Satzbau.* 2. Auflage Stuttgart: Cotta.

Henry Head

Introduced by

PATRICK HUDSON
Department of Experimental Psychology, University of Leiden
The Netherlands

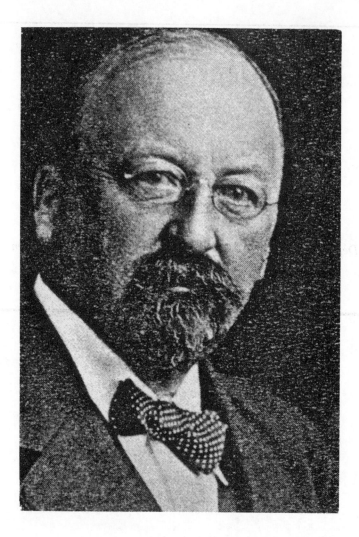

Henry Head
1861-1940

Biography

Sir Henry Head was born in 1861. Before going to the University of Cambridge in 1880 he spent some time at the University of Halle. From 1884 to 1886 he studied under Hering at the German University of Prague. His first appointment was at University College Hospital in London. In 1896 he was appointed to the London Hospital for the first time. He became a Fellow of the Royal Society in 1899 and later served on the council, becoming vice-president of the society in 1916. From 1905 to 1921 he was editor of the Journal Brain. *He was knighted in 1927, one year after the publication of his last and most famous work,* Aphasia and Kindred Disorders of Speech. *As well as Studies in Neurology he also published a volume of verse, including his own work and translations from the German. While in Czechoslovakia he is reputed to have introduced Association Football (soccer) to the country. Head died in 1940.*

Selected Bibliography

Head, H. 1920. "Aphasia and kindred disorders of speech". *Brain* 43:87-165.

———. 1920. "Aphasia: An historical review". *Brain* 43:390-411.

———. 1923. "Speech and cerebral localization". *Brain* 46:355-528.

———. 1926. *Aphasia and Kindred Disorders of Speech*. Cambridge: Cambridge University Press.

Introduction

Henry Head is best known today for his attack on the "diagram-makers". These were aphasiologists such as Wernicke and Lichtheim, who had made their reputations based upon diagrams relating centers in the brain to the effects of damage to those centers and the connections between them. The chapter selected here, from Head's major work on aphasia, is reprinted to give the flavor of the actual attack which was launched. As Head has himself been attacked for the later production of what was effectively a diagram (cf. Geschwind, 1964), it is interesting to see exactly how he attacked the diagram-makers. Head did not, however, make his name on that one chapter, even though it had a considerable influence on the history of aphasiology after its publication. He is also remembered as one of the first researchers to attach an importance to the higher levels of mental functioning which he assumed to underly the performance of language and which he believed to be impaired after local damage to the brain.

Head represents a link between a number of influential individuals and streams of thought spanning the nineteenth and early twentieth centuries. On the one hand he was clearly influenced by Hughlings Jackson. Head had many a conversation with Jackson after Jackson had given up all hope and interest in promulgating his ideas to a wider world. These conversations were not, however, about Jackson's views concerning disorders of speech. As Head said in the preface to his book *Aphasia and Kindred Disorders of Speech*, "Many were the talks we had together on evolution and dissolution as manifested in the functions of the nervous system ... but he seemed to have lost heart with regard to his papers on aphasia, in consequence of the complete neglect into which they had fallen. After his death, when I read them through in order, they came as a revelation, and not only explained the observations I was making on patients with war injuries but also indicated the route of further advance". Head republished Jackson's aphasia papers in *Brain* in 1915 and, reading Head's own writings, it is possible to see that he considered his work as a natural extension of Jackson's ideas.

Head's attack on the diagram-makers stemmed not from a dislike of diagrams as such, but from his feeling that the simplistic notions derived from the application of diagrammatic models led to a serious underestimation of the clinical picture. Even this would not have been so bad had he not felt that some patients' symptoms were being ignored for the sake of the convenience which a diagram offered when performing diagnosis at the bedside. It was his experience as a clinician, together with his application of Jackson's ideas, which led him to lose his "robust faith" in the efficacy of the diagrams.

Along with Pick and Goldstein, whose work he admired, Head represented a movement toward the conception of neurological disorders in psychological terms. He may be seen as an early proponent of the cognitive approach to mental functioning. Hidden in the foreword to his book is a note of thanks to a young member of the Cambridge Psychology department, Frederick Bartlett. It should come as no surprise that Head used the word 'schema' in his theoretical constructions. Today we still find 'schemata' or 'frames' occupying a central role in artificial intelligence.

Head proposed four basic types of aphasia. He called these 'verbal', i.e. a defective power of forming words, whether for internal or external use. He viewed this as being more a productive than a receptive disorder, except in severe cases. Syntactical defects are characterised by the talking of jargon. This is not, however, the production of neologisms, which may be found in other cases. Syntactical disorders show short jerky sentences, slurring or omitting altogether many of what he called "junction" words. "Even when they are present, it is difficult to hear the articles, conjunctions and other components necessary to a perfectly formed sentence". Nominal disorders are not, for Head, a difficulty in shaping words or phrases, but a disturbance of their nominal significance. This "depends essentially on inability to designate an object in words and to appreciate verbal meaning". What Head wished to stress with this categorization of deficits was the essential centrality of the disorder, in both production and understanding, apart from specific manifestations in either speech or writing. Semantic defects are, for Head, subtly different from nominal ones. He wanted to convey, in contrast to the specific loss of nominal aphasia, the fact that patients with this type of aphasia were incapable of grasping the greater whole, even though they could faultlessly produce the parts. It is not the meanings of individual words (which loss is what he called nominal), but the ability to combine them further which is lost.

The semantic loss is the one most obviously related to the problems of symbolic formulation and expression which Head felt were central to aphasia. By these he wanted to convey "a purely descriptive term for the various forms of behaviour which are found by experimental observation to be affected in conjunction with disorders of speech". The processes that were necessary for these are assumed to lie above the more basic language processes. Head understood that a disturbance of speech was a disturbance of the harmony of the various processes which commonly act together. "Each response is a fresh reaction to abnormal conditions: it is a morbid phenomenon due to an attempt of the organism to adapt itself to a new situation created by the defects of the function which result from the lesion".

Head also stresses that no one disorder was solely perceptual or expressive. Because he viewed language processing in terms of a higher order of psychological and symbolic functioning, each individual act of speech might show more or less of particular types of disorder. He selected the four types he did, not to define distinct categories, but to "indicate their most salient features". Furthermore, he stressed that "each variety of aphasia comprises defects in excess of those which can be deduced from its name".

Finally, in this brief description of Head's ideas on aphasia, it is interesting to note that he felt strongly that a study of the symptoms could not lead directly to the categories of speech. His view was that defects arise from an interaction between many different processes attempting to adapt dynamically to the effects of a lesion. There "is no point to point correspondence between physiological processes and the constituent elements of an act of speech". On this basis, and armed with a strong belief in the importance of clinical observation, Head attacked the diagram-makers.

Geschwind (1964), while discussing the paradoxical position of Kurt Goldstein, actually devotes some considerable space to a criticism of Head. He notes that Head's otherwise comprehensive review misses out Dejerine's paper, which itself had such an effect on Geschwind. More importantly, however, Geschwind criticizes Head for first attacking the diagram-makers and then, effectively, coming up with a diagram himself. The standard criticism which Geschwind so rightly makes of other authors, of ignoring primary sources, may be leveled at himself here, rather than at Head. Head certainly attacked the diagram-makers, but what he proposed in place of diagrams was quite clearly a different sort of object, qualified in just those areas where he attacked the diagram-makers. It was, also, not the activity of diagram-making he objected to, but the way such diagrams were used.

Whether or not one agrees with Head's specific analyses or criticisms, and whether or not one finds his own model of the cognitive and linguistic processes and their interrelation convincing, Head's own words represent a refreshing, and readable, blast of fresh air. Perhaps the most convincing test of his ideas, and of his approach, would be to replace the specific models and data attacked in his chapters with models and data drawn from today's work on aphasia. If there is a certain resounding sense in such a retranslation, and resounding it will certainly be, then perhaps we should consider carefully just what sort of traps and errors of thought we are propagating today.

References

Geschwind, N. 1964. "The paradoxical position of Kurt Goldstein in the history of aphasia". *Cortex* 1:214-224.
Head, H. 1926. *Aphasia and Kindred Disorders of Speech*. Cambridge: Cambridge University Press (Reprint: New York: Hafner, 1963).

Selection from the work of Henry Head

Cerebral Localization*

We have already seen that the usual conceptions of localisation of function are not only unsupported by experiment, but are entirely inadequate to explain the phenomena of aphasia and kindred disorders of speech. The so-called "centres" in the cortex are not conglomerations of cells and fibres where some particular and more or less exclusive function is initiated, to be abolished by their removal. They are points where the progress of some mode of action can be reinforced, deviated or inhibited; in fact they are foci of integration.

A destructive lesion of one of these "centres" throws some highly organised function into disorder. Vigilance is lowered at that point and the tissues of the brain can no longer carry on those high-grade physiological processes necessary for the consecutive development of some particular somatic or psychical activity. This is hindered or blocked and a new adjustment occurs, which results in what we call the abnormal response.

So far as the loss of function or negative manifestations are concerned this response does not reveal the elements out of which the original form of behaviour was composed. Like all such pathological reactions it is a new condition, the consequence of a fresh readjustment of the organism as a whole to the factors at work at the particular functional level disturbed by the local lesion.

Should inhibition or control of some lower neural activity form one of the normal results of integration in the higher "centre", the abnormal

---

* From *Aphasia and Kindred Disorders of Speech*. London: Cambridge University Press, 1926. Chapter 11, p. 498-512.

response may comprise positive manifestations due to release of this function. This phenomenon, so common amongst the psychological and pathological activities of the central nervous system, plays comparatively little part in the disorders of speech produced by organic lesions of the brain, which are to a preponderant degree manifestations of functional loss.

According to the older view of cerebral localisation, various functions generated in different areas of the cortex are brought together like fragments of a mosaic to produce some higher form of activity. Should this be disorganised by a lesion of the brain, it was assumed that the elementary processes out of which it was composed must be revealed in their primary character. Thus the phenomena of aphasia were supposed to discover the motor, auditory and visual elements of normal speech.

I have shown that such a conception is completely untenable and is not justified by the facts either of experiment or of clinical observation. No function is "localised" strictly in any part of the cortex and no form of activity, somatic or psychical, is built up into a mosaic of elementary processes which become evident when it is disturbed by a lesion of the brain.

On the other hand, local destruction of tissue prevents the normal fulfilment of some form of behaviour and the reaction which follows expresses the response of the organism as a whole under these changed conditions. Moreover, the abnormal manifestations can be described only in terms of the act which has been disturbed, and do not reveal the supposed elements out of which it has been synthesised.

In the light of such conceptions the term "cerebral localisation" must be employed in a strictly limited sense. Firstly, it signifies determination of the site of the lesion associated with disturbance of some function, such as the use of language; secondly, it implies discovery of the exact nature of the functional disorders which follow injuries to different parts of the brain.

1. Suggested explanation of the site of the lesion in the various forms of aphasia

That lesions situated in different localities of one hemisphere can produce specific changes in the power to employ language is one of the most remarkable facts which emerge from the study of aphasia. The material at my disposal is in no way sufficient to determine this relation with precision. Moreover, in all attempts to correlate the site of structural changes with defects of function it must never be forgotten that the severity and acuteness of the lesion exert an overwhelming effect on the manifestations.

But in spite of these deficiencies, I think we are justified in drawing the following conclusions from the cases cited in this work. The more definitely the injury destroys the lower portion of the pre- and postcentral convolutions and the parts beneath them, the greater the probability that the defects of speech will assume a "verbal" form. A lesion in the neighbourhood of the upper convolutions of the temporal lobe tends to produce "syntactical" disorders. Destruction round about the region of the supra-marginal gyrus causes those defects in the use of language which I have called "semantic"; whilst a lesion centred around the angular gyrus, in a somewhat more posterior position, seems to disturb the power to evoke and to understand names or other "nominal" expressions.

Thus, lesions in certain parts of the left hemisphere tend to be associated with more or less specific disorders of symbolic formulation and expression. It is impossible to deduce the various forms assumed by an aphasia from any logical or a priori analysis of the structure and use of language; but I think some light can be thrown on the peculiar relation between the nature of the defects of speech and the site of the injury by considering the physiological functions exercised by cerebral structures in the vicinity of these foci.

Verbal aphasia is more particularly associated with injury to the foot of the precentral and neighbouring gyri and the parts beneath them. A lesion within this area, either in the right or the left hemisphere, is liable to produce some loss of power in the opposite half of the tongue and lips, which interferes with perfect articulation. With the gradual acquisition of capacity to use words, this mechanism on the left side becomes associated with the more definitely verbal aspect of the new function; yet a disorder or speech which follows destruction in this region is not "motor", "effector" or "expressive", nor is it purely articulatory, even in the slighter cases of aphasia. The act as a whole is disturbed, but the greatest incidence of this loss of function affects the formative aspect of words and phrases rather than the power to appreciate their significance.

Syntactical aphasia is associated with lesions in and around the upper temporal gyri and the parts beneath them. This is the neighbourhood of the so-called "auditory centre". But the defects of speech which are the subject of this investigation are in no way due to auditory imperception or to a disturbance of auditory images; they are principally shown by defects of rhythm and inability to form coherent phrases. Hearing and the interpretation of sounds may remain intact; thus, No. 14, when playing the piano clumsily, was able to recognise and correct the wrong notes he struck. Moreover, all the patients of this group understood and executed oral commands. They showed, it is true, some difficulty in appreciating what was said to them in conversation; but this was due to want of power to reproduce exactly the phrases they had heard, rather than to lack of auditory perception.

There is no difficulty in thinking logically without syntax. If I say to myself "Cat...grass...window...mat...fire", I recognise that the cat, walking on the grass, sprang in at the window and lay down on the mat by the fire. Should this "agrammatical" formula be reinforced by visual images of the cat in the act of carrying out these movements, no more is wanted to insure full registration of the facts. But it would be difficult or impossible in many cases to convey to another person the full meaning of a series of nouns or nominal expressions without combining them by means of syntax. A phrase is not solely the conjunction of distinct words; it is thought expressed with a view to appreciation by an auditor (see Gardiner, 1922). This need not always be another individual; for in silent or internal speech we are often our own listeners. Speech is a mental process which we may or may not exteriorise. "We speak", as Jackson says, "not only to tell other people what we think, but to tell ourselves what we think". As our own auditors we demand a certain normal rhythm together with the power to formulate and emit words arranged syntactically, duly stressed and accentuated. Much silent thought is incoherent, jerky and linked together by non-logical processes. But on certain occasions, especially when writing spontaneously, internal speech is elaborated by means of syntax into strictly coherent phrases.

All speech contains elements that subserve the rhythmic purposes of the phrase, rather than its actual meaning. Syntactical defects increase the difficulty of producing a progressive flow of articulated sounds. Like a running jumper, who is unsuccessful in taking off, the aphasic of this group cannot correct himself: he may go back to his starting-point and try again, but finally gives up in confusion. He usually dashes on hoping that his jargon will be understood; he cannot go slowly and does not as a rule deliberately return to a word wrongly pronounced in the hope of correcting his faulty articulation.

In the course of the development of speech the parts around the upper temporal gyri on the left side become necessary for rhythmic phrasing and a lesion in this portion of the brain tends to disturb more particularly perfect execution of this aspect of speech. The morbid manifestations are not due to primary lack of perception of the meaning of sounds, but to disorders of rhythm, stress, syntax and those factors in speech which are so necessary to weld isolated words into a coherent expression of the speaker's ideas, or to convey them to the comprehension of an auditor.

It is worthy of note that the temporal lobe is one of the last portions of the brain to reach full development in the history of man. Speech was originally evolved out of cries of fear, joy or anger intended to express the feelings of the speaker. Powers of oratory were acquired when it became necessary to persuade other members of the tribe of the utility and rectitude of these emotions.

A lesion situated in the left hemisphere between the post-central fissure and the occipital lobule tends to affect more particularly the meaning and categorial use of language. One of the main differences according to Elliot Smith between the brain of man and that of gorilla lies in the enormous development of this region, particularly the supra-marginal and angular gyri.

When the lesion lies in the neighbourhood of the angular gyrus and the parts beneath it, the defects of speech are liable to assume a nominal form. The patient is unable to name objects, or to choose them with certainty to oral and to printed commands.

If I am asked to name an object placed before me, I recognise that it possesses certain characteristic qualities and attempt to find the verbal symbol which expresses them adequately. Now, in daily life the recognition of these qualities is mainly dependent on sight; detailed meaning, form, colour, place and relation to other objects are largely based on visual impressions. Touch, and to an even less degree smell and taste, play little part in determining the name of an object; for these senses require contact, whereas vision gives information concerning objects at a distance.

The angular gyrus, where a lesion produces more particularly loss of power to evoke appropriate names, is situated just in front of the area striata, where destruction of tissue produces definite localisable distrubance within the visual field. I wish, however, carefully to exclude the idea that perfect vision is necessary for the integrity of symbolic formulation and expression, or that nominal aphasia is directly associated with defects in the visual field. I suggest only that, during acquisition of the power to speak

and understand spoken words, certain anatomical structures became necessary for the due performance of these acts. Such topographical associations
came about because particular parts of the brain were already required for
some lower function, which played a part in the evolution of one of the
many aspects of the use of language.

It is less easy to explain the association between semantic aphasia and
lesions in the vicinity of the supra-marginal gyrus; for capacity to understand the deeper significance of words and the wider meaning of a whole
sentence seems to be dependent on the integrity of this region in the left
half of the brain. Injury to this portion of the right hemisphere may be
associated with local disorders of somatic sensibility, consisting mainly of
inability to recognise differences in the physical qualities and relations of
external objects, such as their form, weight, size, texture, together with
want of power to appreciate differences in degree of tactile and thermal
stimuli.

With the acquisition of speech this area on the left side of the brain
became associated with the complete categorical comprehension of relations. Man was not only able to differentiate objects by means of names,
but to understand the remote meaning of a logical series of verbal, pictorial
or other symbols. Thus, the activities of this region became of profound
importance for comprehending and recording the march of events; this
resulted in the realisation of space and time as a guide to the aim and intention of action.

Semantic defects consist more particularly in want of recognition of the
ultimate meaning of a logical and consecutive statement together with
incapacity to keep in mind the intention of the act originated spontaneously
or to command. These disorders are manifested in want of orientation and
power to comprehend the aim and purpose of speech, thought and action.
Can it be that ability to carry out these processes was acquired as a higher
development of interest in recognition of mutual relations, qualitative, spa-
cial and temporal, between objects in the external world?

All such attempts to explain how a lesion in a certain part of the brain
came to be associated with defects of symbolic formulation and expression
are purely hypothetical syggestions and do not form an inherent part of my
general thesis. Moreover, these disorders of speech are not necessarily
accompanied by any other loss of function. Verbal aphasia may exist without paralysis of the lips and tongue; syntactical defects do not require auditory imperception; nominal aphasia is not of necessity associated with loss of

vision, nor the semantic form with disorders of somatic sensibility. Nor is it possible by analysis of the phenomena of aphasia to discover any elements which can be attributed to disorders of motion, sensation, hearing or vision.

2. The nature of the disorders of speech produced by a local lesion of the brain

"Symbolic formulation and expression" is a purely descriptive term for the various forms of behaviour which are found by experimental observation to be affected in conjunction with disorders of speech. It is in no sense a definition: because some form of psychical activity cannot be logically included under this term there is no reason why it should not suffer in fact, and conversely there are many symbolic processes which escape. Moreover, the use of a symbol in one way can be disturbed, although it may be employed with ease in some other manner.

I am not attempting to set up a new human "faculty", an elementary class of conscious processes, or even a primary and coherent group of psychical aptitudes. I use the term "symbolic formulation and expression" as a convenient designation for the various actions, which are manifestly disturbed as the result of certain organic lesions. In the same way "verbal", "syntactical", "nominal" and "semantic" are employed to indicate the diverse forms that may be assumed by the defective use of language in consequence of destruction of different portions of the brain.

Although I do not believe that disorders of speech reveal the elements out of which it is composed, I have habitually employed the term "integration" in the following sense. I do not intend to imply that a series of factors are summed algebraically. At each physiological level the organism reacts anew to its environmental conditions, and the character of the response depends not only on the reactive significance of the impulse but on the state of the receptive centre. This is best seen by tracing the fate of sensory impressions from the periphery to the highest functional levels. A multitude of impulses pass into the spinal cord by way of the posterior roots, grouped to a great extent according to whether they originate in superficial or deep structures. These reach their first synaptic junction somewhere between the cells of the posterior horn and those of the posterior column nuclei. Here occurs the first functional integration: the organism reacts to form a fresh pattern of afferent impulses and in this form they are transmitted to the receptive nuclei of the optic thalamus. From this point they pass to act upon the cortex and the essential centres of the thalamus itself. Each of these organs responds in an appropriate manner to produce what we call a normal sensation. But, should some morbid condition exist on either side of this mechanical system, remarkable reactions appear unlike any manifestations which can otherwise occur.

So, when speech is affected, the various processes which commonly act in harmony are disturbed. Each response is a fresh reaction to abnormal conditions: it is a morbid phenomenon due to an attempt of the organism to adapt itself to a new situation created by the defects of function which result from the lesion. No two cases are exactly alike: for the manifestations depend not only on the site and severity of the destruction of tissue, but on the mental characteristics and aptitudes of the patient.

In every instance the names chosen for these specific defects are intended solely to indicate their most salient features. It is a mistake to suppose that, even with the most definite varieties of aphasia, every test yields a distinctive result. One task may suffer diversely with each form of disordered speech, whilst another is affected more or less uniformly throughout. Thus, the abnormal behaviour of patients belonging to the various classes of aphasia is characterised in part only by mutually distinctive responses.

It is of fundamental importance that these names should be understood and employed in an indicative sense only. They are useful labels and not exclusive definitions. Having determined empirically what functions are affected, we can then speak of them as disorders of symbolic formulation and expression. Closer examination may show that still further differentiation is possible. Certain tasks, necessitating articulated speech or the understanding of spoken words, are found on examination to be disturbed in a peculiar manner and to each such class of disorder we are justified in applying a distinctive designation.

But each variety of aphasia comprises defects in excess of those which can be deduced from its name. Verbal and syntactical aphasia consist of more than a disturbance of articulated words and phrases, whilst the nominal and semantic forms interfere with wider aptitudes than the appreciation of verbal or general meaning. The power of setting the hands of clock to command, of imitating movements made by the observer, of drawing to order or constructing a ground-plan, orientation, and many other actions may suffer in association with more directly linguistic tasks.

Moreover, the loss of power is relative and not absolute. A man who is unable to read or to write under certain conditions can do so if the task is presented to him in some other way. For example, it may be impossible to read aloud or to write to dictation the simple words of the man, cat and dog tests; yet the patient can both find the correct names and transfer them to paper in response to pictures. Visual images may still be available for use in spontaneous thought, although they cannot be employed to command in a normal manner for recalling and registering relations.

This strictly observational method and purely indicative nomenclature makes it possible to correlate the defective psychical aptitudes with the degree of loss of function and so with the extent and situation of the organic lesion. This is entirely impossible if the names given to any specific variety of aphasia are supposed to correspond to some pre-existing psychical category, or if the clinical manifestations are thought to reveal the elements out of which speech is composed. For instance, alexia and agraphia are nothing more than expressions for inability to read and write. Reading and writing signify solely that a human being is behaving in a certain manner connected with the use of language; they are useful descriptive terms corresponding in conceptual rank with the words walking and eating. They cannot be employed as categories of physiological activity; still less can want of capacity to read or to write be associated specifically with destruction in some limited area of the brain.

Such terms as "aphasia", "amnesia", "apraxia" and "agnosia" are even more abstract and still further removed from the actual phenomena. Yet, at one time or another, attempts have been made to correlate each of the morbid conditions designated by these terms with the topography of brain lesions. But aphasia, or inability to speak, does not correspond to any self-contained disorder that can be discovered by examination. Amnesia signifies no more and no less than loss of memory, and there is no memory apart from things remembered; "general memory" is a misnomer. Apraxia is employed to designate a form of behaviour in which the patient cannot perform at will certain high-grade actions prompted without or in his own initiative; but these form a widely heterogeneous group belonging to various psychical categories. Finally, agnosia comprises conditions so different as visual, auditory or tactile imperception and defects of language characterised by loss of appreciation of symbolic meaning.

So long as we clearly recognise that these words are purely abstract terms corresponding to no constituent groups of phenomena, psychical, physiological or anatomical, they may be employed as summary indications of different varieties of abnormal behaviour. But they can never be correlated in a distinctive manner with the site of any anatomical lesion.

Thus, throughout my work I have used the words aphasia and amnesia solely as shortened indicative expressions to avoid detailed description. But I have avoided the terms agnosia and apraxia in connection with the high-grade disorders of speech which form the basis of this research. As I have already shown, both imperception and that loss of power to execute certain acts at will, known as apraxia, can interfere materially with the use of language; but the defects so produced are of a different order from those with which I am concerned. Moreover, nothing could be more deceptive than attempts to explain the phenomena of aphasia and amnesia in terms of verbal apraxia and agnosia. All such expressions must be employed solely as descriptive of certain forms of abnormal behaviour. Used in any other sense they belong to that deceptive class of clinical terms, which, although they explain nothing, produce a fictitious feeling that an absolute classification of the phenomena has been attained.

The progress of medical knowledge has been profoundly hampered by failure to bear these principles in mind. Time, place, quantity and intensity have been inextricably confused in so-called "diagnosis". Disease is an event which manifests itself in certain ways, and our business as practical physicians is to select from the morbid phenomena those which we consider to be important as a guide to our subsequent conduct. Since no two examples can ever be identical, we choose out certain features as significant and, collating them with our previous experience of similar or diverse signs in other cases, we conclude that the patient is suffering from a certain disease. But this entity, which we have erected by conceptual abstraction from the events that are happening before us, has no existence apart from our own intellectual activities and those of persons whom we can persuade to think like ourselves. No disease can be defined exactly; its boundaries are always hazy, and the more closely we limit its characters the less does the final result correspond to actual experience.

All names of diseases and formal collections of signs and symptoms are counters which help us to represent to ourselves what is happening to the patient. This power of intellectualising the observed facts and erecting conceptual categories is a useful aid to action; but these so-called "diagnosis" have no absolute value. Names, such as "angina pectoris" or "epilepsy", cannot be translated into equivalent anatomical terms. Directly we behave as if they possessed any validity other than descriptive, we are liable to fall into the fallacious mode of reasoning which has been so prevalent in the study of aphasia and kindred disorders of speech.

The power to employ language is acquired by every individual in the course of his life-time and is improved and widened by practice and conscious effort. At first it consists solely of capacity to speak and to comprehend spoken words; the majority of human beings progress no further in the art of using these vocal symbols. But civilised man invented writing to perpetuate his utterance and to transmit them to his fellows distant from him in space and time. In order to understand these arbitrary signs and to interpret their significance into action, he learnt to read. Out of simple acts of enumeration sprang arithmetic and higher mathematics, the purest form of symbolic thinking. Pictorial representation, a lowly form of intellectual statement, became refined until it became possible to construct more or less elaborate diagrams, such as a ground-plan.

Education steadily improves the power of employing these procedures for intellectual operations of ever increasing complexity. But essentially they are all developments of simple acts of speaking and comprehension of spoken words. It is here that we must look for the evident diversity in the manifestations caused by organic lesions of the brain.

On the other hand, less primitive, more recently acquired and highly abstract forms of symbolic formulation and expression are liable to be disturbed in a more massive way. Should the patient fail to solve a problem in arithmetic, there may be nothing in the actual record to betray the nature of his defects of speech; yet, from his difficulties in speaking or in understanding what is said to him, it is at once evident to what class his disorder belongs.

Acts such as writing stands in an intermediate position. When the written material is examined from the point of view of formulated thought and expression of meaning, it is liable to show distinct abnormalities corresponding to the various forms of aphasia. But its more structural characters, the formation of letters and spelling of words, tend to suffer in a less specific manner.

The effects produced by an organic lesion of the brain on the more primitive acts of language fall naturally into disorders of verbal formulation and defective recognition of meaning. But it would be a fundamental fallacy to divide aphasia into two exclusive groups according to these categories, as erroneous as the analogous classifications into aphasia and amnesia, or apraxia and agnosia.

So long as the disturbance of function is of slight degree, or the task set extremely easy, the defects of speech may appear to consist almost entirely of want of power on the one hand to formulate, or on the other to understand, spoken words. But, even in such cases during the severer stages of the malady both aspects of speech are definitely affected. A verbal aphasic is misled by the wrong words he has enunciated, either aloud or to himself, and it is difficult to avoid the intellectual consequences of such false formulation. In the same way, syntactical defects prevent accurate silent reproduction of phrases heard by the patient and so reduce his power of comprehending exactly what has been said to him.

Conversely, want of appreciation of meaning spoils verbal formulation. The nominal aphasic cannot find the right word, whilst the semantic is unable to complete his sentence or to bring thoughts and actions to a logical conclusion.

In every instance we are dealing with an abnormal reaction evoked by morbid physical conditions; one form of intellectual behaviour cannot be abstracted from the other and treated as if they were separable and completely dissociated activities of the mind.

Speech, examined introspectively, appears to be a progressive act, which may be analysed into events appearing at separate moments of time. As a gun is aimed, the trigger pulled and the cartridge explodes, so it would seem as if we first think of what we want to say, then select the terms in which to express it and finally embody them in words and phrases.

But this is certainly a misleading and fallacious method of stating what actually occurs. An act of speech comes into being and dies away again as an alteration in the balance of psycho-physical processes; a state, never strictly definable, merges into another inseparable from it in time. When this transition is interrupted and the evolution of a perfect response is prevented by physical causes, fresh integration becomes necessary and new phenomena appear. These in no way represent temporal elements in a series of normal events. Unimpeded symbolic formulation and expression cannot be analysed into a sequence of semantic, nominal, syntactical and verbal processes which normally follow one another in time. Each specific disorder of speech is an abnormal reaction, manifested in some particular way throughout the whole duration of those acts, which take on a fresh form in consonance with the physical disability. Had these reactions corresponded to the constituent parts of an orderly sequence in normal speech, disturbance at some definite point of time would have prevented the development of all those processes which followed later in the series. This is certainly not the case; these disorders of speech do not reveal the normal order of psychical events. They disturb in certain ways the progressive development of language processes as a whole and so produce the different varieties of aphasia.

Habitual acts, which have been become almost automatic, may be prevented altogether if a task is presented in some unfamiliar manner. Thus, a man who can write his name and address correctly is unable to do so if he is asked to put down those of his mother with whom he lives; the unusual beginning has increased the difficulty and made it impossible to write the words that would otherwise have come easily to him.

Moreover, it is often easier for the aphasic to arrive at a result by following a sequence than by direct recognition of a single word or unit. Individual symbols, such as the days of the week, the months, the letters of the alphabet and numbers can be more readily comprehended and manipulated as part of a series than when they stand alone.

Such a method of using progression is a reversion to an earlier type of response, and is employed when the more highly developed method breaks down. It then becomes easier to arrive at a correct answer by saying over the series until the required word or number is reached than to recognise it without this procedure. Some normal persons, especially when adding up low numbers, count to themselves, a relic of the finger counting habitual in childhood.

That form of behaviour which we call the use of language has a history, and many of the phenomena of disordered speech resemble the stages by which the complete act was developed in each individual. The patient describes an object or mentions its use instead of giving it a name; he spells the words he is reading instead of recognising them directly; he counts on his fingers when he should add or substract. In fact he falls back in many ways to more infantile modes of response.

But the mechanism underlying symbolic formulation and expression is not a palimpsest from which, when the more recent writing is removed, an earlier text is revealed in a primitive form. The aphasic may return to the less exacting methods of solving a problem which resemble those adopted in childhood; but his mind differs fundamentally from that of a child. In the earlier days, when he was acquiring the use of language, he gradually refined and extended his verbal aptitudes and power of employing symbols of all kinds. When these are disturbed in consequence of physiological defects, he falls back on methods of arriving at the desired result corresponding to the steps by which he acquired the art of using language. Thus, he describes a colour by comparing it to a concrete object, although he cannot give its name; blue is like the sky, red is blood and green resembles grass. Apart, however, from this adoption of a form of response more prevalent in childhood, the phenomena of disordered speech do not strictly correspond to stages of its historical development.

Nor do they represent complementary portions of the psychical process itself. Normal acts of speech cannot be analysed into verbal, syntactical, nominal or semantic elements. I have chosen these terms solely to indicate that amongst a group of morbid phenomena the most distinctive loss of linguistic capacity fell mainly on some one of these grammatical features. Each specific form of aphasia is accompanied by disorders of function too extensive to correspond with any constituent element of speech, and the various abnormal manifestations cannot be combined like the pieces of a puzzle to compose a coherent whole. Each group of morbid reactions far exceeds the due proportion of an integral part of the total psychical process.

Every disorder of speech is manifested in psychical terms; but in no instance can the nature and extent of the disturbance be deduced from a priori consideration of the normal use of language. Each particular variety of aphasia represents the response of the organism under the changed conditions produced by physiological defects, and we cannot discover the form it assumes from logical conceptions with regard to the processes of the mind. The morbid phenomena must be determined solely from observation of the actual facts. However unlikely the conclusions may appear at first sight, they must be judged by experimental evidence only. Moreover, it is well to remember that if any two hypotheses equally explain a set of observed facts, there is no inherent reason why the simpler one should lie nearer to the truth. Biological processes do not of necessity conform to the logical demands of the human intellect.

A disturbance of speech represents physiological defects manifested in terms of a psychical act. Let us imagine that, whilst my attention is fixed on the eyepiece of a polariscope, the constituents of the solution under examination are changed without my knowledge in such a way that the rotation they produce shifts from left to right. I am at once aware that the polarity has been reversed and make the necessary adjustments which can be read off on the scale. The alteration in chemical constitution of the fluid becomes evident to me in terms of polarised light. So the physiological changes responsible for disorders of speech can be recognised solely by psychological tests.

Thus the various forms assumed by an aphasia do not correspond to any elementary categories of the act of speech. Although expressed in terms of the defective use of language, they cannot be deduced logically and must be discovered by observation. As the result of defective physiological activity a certain form of behaviour is thrown into disorder; the consequences appear as a morbid psychical reaction, which does not reveal or correspond to any normal group of mental processes.

There is no point to point correspondence between physiological processes and the constituent elements of an act of speech. At one time it was supposed that a certain part of the brain A exercised a certain function A^1 which was directly associated with a psychical process A^2. Destruction of A was followed by manifestations corresponding to loss of A^2. But I have been able to show that this is not the case. An aptitude such as the use of language is gradually acquired during the life of each individual and a high level of physiological activity is required for the performance of these complex acts; should vigilance be diminished from any cause they will fade out and cease to be possible. Simpler, lowergrade activities can still be exercised, and other psychical reactions do not suffer apart from those which stand in direct relation with highly purposive physiological processes normally exercised by the injured structures.

A local lesion produces a limited loss of physiological capacity determined by the site and severity of the injury. This in turn interferes with the efficient performance of those psychical acts which can only be exercised and developed at a high level of vigilance. But the loss of function is determined by a failure of physiological potency, although it is expressed and can alone be recorded in psychical terms.

The Diagram Makers*

1. The English School

Jackson's earlier papers excited universal interest amongst that band of young Englishmen who were attracted to the novel study of the structure and functions of the nervous system. In 1862, he had been appointed to the National Hospital for the Paralysed and Epileptic, which had been recently founded, and came under the influence of Brown Séquard, then practising in London. Here, those who worked in the wards became familiar with the most recent advances in French medicine, not only from the teaching of this renowned physiologist and clinician, but in daily intercourse with his relative and famulus, Victor Bazire, the translator of Trousseau's lectures, then in charge of the electro-therapeutic department.

At first, Jackson's insight and clinical industry caused his name to be cited by all the writers on aphasia, alongside that of Broca; but gradually they began to complain that he was obscure. They failed to comprehend why he denied the existence of a centre for the faculty of speech, and why he contended that the loss of function consisted in failure to formulate a proposition. For after all no one could deny the categorial existence of speech, reading and writing; and if anatomical localisation were a fact, these various human aptitudes must be disturbed more or less independently by lesions of specific centres and their commissural fibres.

In 1869, Bastian published his famous paper, which had so profound an influence on the subsequent development of the questions (Bastian, 1869a). His whole work was founded on the axiom that "we think in words", and that "these words are revived as sound impressions in the auditory perceptive centres of the cerebral hemispheres". He believed "that words become nascent in consciousness primarily and perhaps principally as revived auditory impressions (Bastian, 1880)". Based upon this conception he divided the higher forms of the disorders of speech into two main groups, amnesia and aphasia proper. In the former condition the thinking power of the individual is impaired almost in direct proportion to the loss

---

* From *Aphasia and Kindred Disorders of Speech*. London: Cambridge University Press, 1926. p. 54-66.

which he experiences in his power of expression. There is a distinct defect in the memory for words, not only for use in articulate speech, but also in silent thought. True aphasia, on the other hand, is a condition in which silent thought is possible; the words are revived as sound impressions in the auditory perceptive centres. But, when this thought has to be spoken articulately, impulses arising from these revived impressions must be transmitted to the more immediate motor centres for speech. In the same way, when the individual attempts to write, the revived sound perceptions call up visual impressions, which are transmitted to the motor centres for the hand.

In *amnesia* there is an inability to recall words, i.e. they cannot properly be revived in the auditory perceptive centres, and there is an almost proportional impairment of the thinking power. Now it would appear that this condition must be due either to some abnormal state of the auditory perceptive centre itself, where words have to be revived, or else to some defect in those portions of cortical grey substance, which have to do with the exercise of that marvellous power of voluntary recall of past impressions to consciousness, which occurs in the processes of recollection. In this condition we obviously have to do principally with defects of the cortical grey matter of the hemispheres, rather than with defects of afferent or efferent fibres connecting this with lower nerve centres. But in *aphasia*, as we have seen, the individual is able to think and understand what is said to him, though he cannot express himself either by speaking or writing. Now, we can well imagine that this will be precisely the condition of a person in whom those efferent fibres are damaged (and functionally inert) along which the motor stimuli are wont to pass that primarily incite those combined muscular contractions necessary, for speech on the one hand, and for writing on the other. There being no notable injury to the cortical or convolutional grey matter, the individual can carry on processes of thought as before, and the afferent fibres not being damaged, he can understand what is said to him. But he cannot translate this thought into articulate speech or into written language because the first part of the path along which the motor stimulus would have to pass, in order to incite the necessary combined muscular movements, is broken up or damaged. A lesion of both these sets of fibres in any part of their course between the cortical grey matter and the corpus striatum, or in this body itself, would therefore produce such a result. Just so, a lesion of either one of these sets singly, would produce the corresponding simple condition of which aphasia is compounded.

He then proceeds to explain that if the fibres emerging from the auditory centre were injured in any part of their course, the individual would be able to think and to write, but not to speak. If, on the other hand, the damage destroys efferent fibres from the visual centre alone, the patient would be able to speak, but could not express himself in writing.

Ogle (1867) had already described agraphia, and had laid down that the loss of power to write might belong either to the amnesic, or to what he called the "atactic group" of disorders of speech. In the former, the patient writes a confused series of letters which have no apparent connection with the words intended, whilst, in the latter case, all attempts to write result in mere succession of up and down strokes bearing no resemblance to letters. This view was woven by Bastian into the texture of his theory that all high-grade disorders of speech are due either to the destruction of the auditory and visual centres, or to some affection of the fibres transmitting impressions between them and the lower motor mechanism for the tongue and lips, or for the hand in writing.

Here we see the origin of the conception that disorders of speech can be classified as affections of independent centres, or of the paths between them. It inevitably led to the production of a diagram.[1] As each case arose, it was lopped and trimmed to correspond with a lesion of some cortical centre or hypothetical path. Bastian (1897a) early developed the idea that the so-called motor centres of the cortex were in reality sensory in function; they were occupied with the appreciation of the data of "muscular sense" and were therefore what he called "kinaesthetic". Thus, his well-known diagram showed not only an auditory and a visual word centre, but also one for the tongue and one for the hand, which he spoke of respectively as f "glosso-" and "cheiro-kinaesthetic".

By the time his book was issued, he and his followers had come to believe so firmly in this form of a priori explanation, that in any case of speech defect they thought it was possible to foretell the situation of the lesion with perfect assurance. Four pages are therefore devoted to a list of the clinical manifestations and the site and the nature of the lesion which produces them.

For eighteen years, at University College Hospital, Bastian had demonstrated to generations of students a man who had been seized with loss of speech in December, 1877 (Bastian, 1877b). On each occasion the famous diagram was drawn and we were told what commissural fibres were affected, and why the visual centre must be intact, although that for hearing

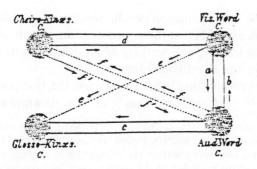

Figure 1. *A diagram illustrating different word centres and the mode in which they are connected by commissures. The connections represented by dotted lines indicate possible but less habitual routes for the passage of stimuli. From Bastian (1898, p. 106).*

was in a state of lowered vitality. But, alas, the post-mortem examination revealed unexpectedly profound changes. The whole of the area supplied by the middle cerebral artery, with the exception of that of its first cortical branch, showed the grossest destruction. The angular and supra-marginal convolutions had disappeared together with the superior temporal, excepting only its anterior third; the superior and inferior occipital convolutions were intact, but the atrophy had extended into the middle occipital convolution; the trunk of the middle cerebral and all its branches were blocked. Much of the posterior segment of the internal capsule together with the greater part of the thalamus had disappeared; anteriorly the atrophy had extended into the white substance up to the corpus striatum which was also much diminished in size. No wonder Bastian admitted that "the difficulties in reconciling the persistent and often-verified clinical condition with the post-mortem record are extreme". He did not recognize that what he called the "clinical condition" was nothing more than a translation of the phenomena into a priori conceptions, which had no existence in reality.

Moreover, all this school of observers believed that they could interpret the clinical manifestations directly in terms of anatomical paths and centres; each one added one or more cases to those that had already become classical. Thus, Bastian's first paper contained two original observations only. It was an era of robust faith and nobody[2] suggested that the clinical data might be insufficient for such precise localisation; still less could they believe that the conclusions reported by men of eminent good faith might be grossly inaccurate. In reading these admirably written papers, we are astonished at the serene dogmatism with which the writers assume a knowledge of the working of the mind and its dependence on hypothetical groups of cells and fibres.

But we must not forget that Bastian was the first person to describe "word-deafness" and "word-blindness"; in 1869, he wrote as follows:

> "Most aphasic patients can understand perfectly what is said to them, and can follow and feel interested when they hear others read aloud. In these cases we may presume that the afferent fibres connecting the auditory centres of the medulla with the auditory perceptive centres of the cerebral hemispheres and also these latter centres themselves are intact, so that the spoken sounds revive their accustomed impressions in the hemispheres, these being perceived as words, symbolic of things or ideas, which being duly appreciated by the individual as they are conjured up, suggest to him the thoughts which they are intended to convey. In certain of the severe cases of aphasia, however, as in that recorded by Dr. Bazire and in Dr. Gairdner's case, it is distinctly stated that the patient either did not gather at all, or with difficulty and imperfectly, the import of words when he was spoken to, although he could be made to understand with the utmost readiness by means of signs and gestures. Must we not suppose that in such a condition either the communication of the afferent fibres with the auditory perceptive centres is cut off, or that this centre itself, in which the sounds of words are habitually discriminated and associated with the things to which they refer, is more or less injured? In either of these cases, though the sound is not appreciated as a word having its definite meaning, we must not expect that there would be deafness; the sound would be still heard as a mere sound, only it does not call up that superadded intellectual discrimination, by the ingrafting of which upon it, it can alone be made to serve as a symbol of thought. Hence the individual does not adequately comprehend when spoken to, though he may be quite capable of receiving and appreciating fully the import of sounds and gestures, which make their impression upon his visual perceptive centres ...". (Bastian 1869a)
>
> "And, where the individual cannot read, I am inclined to think that this must be owing either to some lesion of the afferent fibres to the visual perceptive centre, of the visual perceptive centre itself, or of the communications between the cells of this centre and those of the auditory perceptive centre. If lesions existed in either of the first two situations, the visual impression could not receive its intellectual elaboration, and consequently it could not call up its associated sound (word) in the auditory centres, and hence no meaning would be conveyed by the hieroglyphic marks of the printed or written pages. They would be to the person mere meaningless strokes, just as we have assumed that if similar defects existed in the auditory perceptive centres, or in the afferent fibres with which they were connected, the individual could not appreciate the meaning of spoken words; these would be to him mere sounds". (Bastian 1869a, p. 484)

Broadbent accepted this view of the auditory and visual centres, insisting however on the dual aspect of word formation; words are not only articulate sounds, but also serve as symbols of an idea. In spite of his admiration for Jackson's teaching, he was constitutionally inclined to a mechanical view of disorders of speech. He held (Broadbent, 1872) that "if the nervous system is the instrument of language and of thought, then the objective aspect of the operations concerned in what are subjectively mental processes will be changes in cells and fibres, and we shall understand the physiology of intellectual operations only so far as we can represent them in terms of cells and fibres".

He restated the close functional relation of the act of articulate speech with "that part of the upper edge of the fissure of Sylvius, which forms the posterior end of the third frontal convolution of the left hemisphere", and asserted that he had never met with a single example of the opposite kind. This portion of the cortex is not the seat of a faculty of language, "but simply a part of the nervous or cell and fibre mechanism, by means of which speech is accomplished, which mechanism may be damaged elsewhere above or below this particular node". He insisted that to look for a lesion in precisely the same part of the hemisphere in amnesia and aphasia could ony lead to confusion. The formation of motor word or sound-groups and their intellectual elaboration are two entirely different and independent processes. The latter is the result of the convergence of impressions from the various perceptive centres upon an intermediate cell-area in the super-added convolutions, where they are combined and elaborated into an idea of which the word is a symbol.

In 1879, Broadbent reported a beautiful case of "jargoning" aphasia and accompanied his comments by a diagram. This contains an auditory centre and one for executive speech, united by a commissure. But the most remarkable feature is that "naming" and "propositioning" are separated from one another and to each is assigned a centre at a higher level in the hierarchy than that for hearing and for speech. He was led to this conclusion from the fact that his patient could formulate ideas but could not express them or name objects correctly.

As the result of his beautiful dissections, Broadbent (1872) had already arrived at the conclusion that "the convolutions which are not in immediate relation with crus, central ganglia or corpus callosum by means of fibres are those of the island of Reil, those on the under-surface of the temporo-sphenoidal lobe and of the orbital lobule, those on the flat inner aspect of the hemisphere, and those along the middle of the convex surface of the hemisphere from the occipital extremity as far forwards as the first ascending parietal gyrus".

Now these convolutions, he argues, are the latest in order of development, and "on this ground alone might be supposed to be concerned in the more strictly mental faculties, which are the latest in their manifestation... It would, moreover, seem to accord with the general plan of construction of the nervous system and with what we know of the mental operations, that these convolutions which are withdrawn, so to speak, from direct relation with the outer world, should be the seat of the more purely intellectual operations, receiving the raw material of thought from the convolutions on which sensory impressions impinge, and employing for the transmission outwards of the volitional product those convolutions which are in communication with the motor ganglia and tract".

Thus, he mapped out by indirect means those portions of the cortex which must contain the perceptive centres for hearing and vision. But it was Ferrier's (1875) experimental researches that led the English school to place the auditory centre in the first temporal convolution, whilst that for vision was located in the supra-marginal and angular gyri. To Broca's area was assigned the glosso-kineasthetic centre, whilst that for writing was placed in the posterior portion of the second frontal convolution.

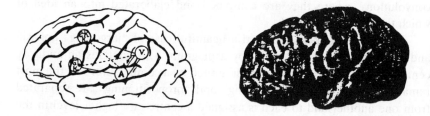

Figure 2. *Diagram showing the approximate sites of the four word centres and their commissures. From Bastian (1898, p. 19)*

2. The German School

Flourens taught that all parts of the cerebral hemispheres were equally endowed with those functions proper to them. Vision, hearing, memory and voluntary action disappear step by step with ablation of the cortex and, although no sense-organ is thereby totally deprived of sensibility, all specific perceptions are destroyed. Perceptions and the will depend on the integrity of the cerebrum exactly as coordination of voluntary movements is the result of cerebellar activity. As a corollary to this conception he held that any part of the hemispheres could carry on, to a greater or less extent, the general functions exercised by the whole; conversely, when the surface of the brain was gradually sliced away, all of them were more or less affected.

This doctrine has a profound effect on physiology and continental medicine for nearly fifty years; and in spite of Jackson's demonstration of the nature of those convulsive seizures which bear his name, the cerebral hemispheres were held to be an inexcitable mass of nervous tissue with uniformly distributed functions.

In 1870, Fritsch and Hitzig succeeded in producing isolated movements of various muscle groups by electrical stimulation of certain spots on the surface of the brain. Excision of these areas was followed by disorders of motion in the same parts of the body and they concluded that some, and probably all, psychical functions depend for their material existence on the activity of certain circumscribed centres in the cerebral hemispheres. From the very first they insisted that these were not strictly "motor", but were concerned with the mental aspect of the muscular act.

Ferrier (1873), instigated by Hughlings Jackson, entered the experimental field in 1873 and profoundly influenced the English school; he localised the site of Bastian's auditory centre in the temporal lobe, but unfortunately placed that for vision in the region of the angular gyrus. Munk followed in 1877, and determined the true position of the visual centre in the occipital lobes, adding the conception of "mind-blindness" ("Seelenblindheit").

Meanwhile Goltz asserted, as the result of his experiments, that the same disturbance of motion, sensation and vision followed extirpation of any part of the hemispheres; the more extensive the destruction the graver was the loss of function, and he believed that his observations were incompatible with the theory of specific cortical centres. Thus every school of clinicians could draw experimental support from the statements of one or other of these observers.

Germany had just emerged victorious from her war with France and the awakened national consciousness influenced even so remote a subject as cerebral physiology. In 1874, Wernicke published his pamphlet entitled *Der aphasische Symptomencomplex* based entirely on work of his fellow-countrymen. The names of Ogle and Jackson are cited, but in such a way that it is evident he had not read their papers; Bastian he consistently ignores.

Wernicke's theory of the nature of aphasia was the direct outcome of Meynert's researches on the projection systems of the cortex. This observer was able to show by tracing afferent tracts, particularly the visual fibres, to their expansion on the hemispheres, that the posterior part of the brain was "sensory" in function.[3] Conversely, by following centrifugal paths, the anterior portion appeared to be obviously "motor". But, since the cerebrum is essentially the organ of consciousness, these "motor" centres must be occupied with conceptions of movement, whilst the "sensory" areas are the seat of memory images of sense impressions. The actual cells of the cortex are neither motor nor sensory, but have one fundamental property, the power of receiving impressions; their diverse functions depend upon the nature of the apparatus with which they are connected by projection fibres, either centripetal or centrifugal. The vital process within them is in nature identical.

Following up this reasoning Wernicke placed the auditory centre, the seat of sound memories, in the first temporal convolution and the conceptual basis of articulated speech in Broca's area. He then proceeded to construct a diagram with commissures and incoming and outgoing paths, deducing from it the phenomena which should follow interruption at each point in this mechanical system. Every part of this hypothetical representation he endowed with profound and definite functional significance. A lesion of the first temporal convolution, by destroying the auditory centre, must abolish "sound-images" ("Klangbilder") and so lead to want of understanding of spoken words. At the same time the patient cannot name objects and shows aphasic defects in speaking because he cannot appreciate and correct his faulty utterances. This form of "sensory" aphasia can be recognised by the flow of words and lack of auditory recognition. It is accompanied by agraphia, but the educated patient can understand print though he cannot read aloud.

Destruction of the third frontal convolution, the seat of images of movement for articulated speech, leads to "Broca's aphasia". The patient is more or less dumb, but can understand all that is said to him both orally and in print. Should the commissure between these two centres be interrupted, he can understand everything in whatever manner it may be presented to him; but his choice of words is restricted, he cannot read aloud and usually is unable to write.

Ten cases are cited in support of these deductions; of these the first was a good example of auditory imperception that ended in recovery. There is nothing to indicate the situation of the lesion and yet Wernicke considers he is justified in "assuming a focal lesion in the first temporosphenoidal convolution" (Wernicke, 1874:46). Of the remaining examples it can only be said that the clinical records are inadequate, or the details of the post-mortem findings unconvincing.

In his text-book, published in 1881, Wernicke makes no attempt to justify his theory by an appeal to observation. The diagram with its two centres and commissural paths appear again and the clinical forms of disordered speech are deduced from it as from a figure in Euclid (Wernicke, 1881:205). These are now four in number: (1) Motor aphasia, equivalent to the aphemia of Broca, due to destruction of the third frontal convolution. The patient can utter at most a few words only, but can understand all forms of speech. (2) Conduction aphasia, due to interruption of the paths between the two centres. In this form there is no lack of words but they are misapplied; understanding is perfect. (3) Sensory aphasia,[4] produced by destruction of the auditory centre in the first temporal convolution. The number of words is unlimited and words are wrongly used, but the most important symptom is complete inability to comprehend oral speech. (4) Total aphasia; here both expression and comprehension of speech are destroyed in consequence of a lesion comprising both centres.

Wernicke was completely satisfied with his attempts to deduce the clinical manifestations from hypothetical lesions; every unprejudiced person will be convinced, he says, how firmly the facts support the theory. In 1903, he published "A case of isolated agraphia"; no better example could be chosen of the manner in which the writers of this period were compelled to lop and twist their cases to fit the procrustean bed of their hypothetical conceptions. Such a title can only mean that in this patient every other act of language could be perfectly performed, except that of writing. But the recorded symptoms show that the patient had much difficulty with spontaneous speech and in comprehending what she read. She was unable to understand some spoken words, nor could she carry out perfectly oral commands. She is said to have shown almost complete inability to write, and it was with great difficulty that she could be brought to make the attempt. She was unable to draw to command, although she could copy drawings and writing. She failed to say the days of the week or the months in their proper order and had forgotten the alphabet and the Lord's Prayer. Wernicke failed to recognise the wide-spread nature of the affection owing to the fixed preconceptions with which it was approached; in the solemn discussion that follows the report we can only wonder at his clinical obtuseness and want of scientific insight.

It is a pleasure to turn from this work to the monograph of Kussmaul, published in 1877 as part of *Ziemssen's Handbuch*. He regards speech as primarily an organised reflex. We become conscious of some thought and are urged by our feelings to express it; we then choose suitable words and say them to ourselves. Finally, we let loose the reflex apparatus, which gives the words an outward form. All verbal expression follows three stages, preparation, internal diction and articulation.

The further development of Kussmaul's exposition shows the influence of a remarkable paper read in 1870 by Finkelnburg before a provincial medical society. Asked to compile a report on the fashionable subject of aphasia, he began by pointing out that these disorders of speech were part of a wider disturbance, which he called lack of symbolic representation. He brought forward five cases to show that the conventional manifestations of amnesia and aphasia were accompanied by other morbid conditions, not directly associated with word-formation. All the disorders of function he united under the term "Asymboly" (Finkelnburg, 1870:461); this consists of inability to express concepts by means of acquired signs, together with want of comprehension of their significance. In fine, it is a more or less profound disturbance of the power to receive or impart knowledge in as far as this depends on sensory symbols. This morbid condition is essentially both motor and sensory and an organic lesion must disturb both aspects of function.

Kussmaul (1877:33; 127) accepts this view and points out that it is incompatible with the existence of a special centre for speech; "we turn away with a smile from all those naive attempts to seek a 'seat of speech' in this or that cerebral convolution". The cerebral organ is composed of a large number of ganglionic mechanisms widely separated from one another, but connected by numerous tracts and fulfilling certain intellectual, sensory and motor functions; no part of this apparatus subserves speech only. Local lesions of the brain must therefore be associated with some partial damage to this complex group of symbolic activities. We must abandon the old view which regards memory as a special storehouse in the brain where images and ideas lie together arranged in separate compartments (Kussmaul 1877:36).

He insists that visual and auditory images may remain unaffected although their symbolic significance can no longer be recognised. Conversely "word-blindness" and "word-deafness" are disorders essentially independent of defects of speech. Unwittingly he adopted exactly Jackson's view of imperception and he gives Bastian full credit for first describing these morbid states.

Unfortunately he was seduced into constructing a diagram (Kussmaul 1877:182); but his views were not susceptible of schematic formulation and the figure was of such complexity that it failed to make a general appeal. It lacked that definite localisation of centres and paths demanded by the popular taste; but Kussmaul's monograph can be read with profit to-day for its shrewd insight into the problems of disorders of speech.

On the other hand, Lichtheim's paper, which was greeted with enthusiasm and issued simultaneously in German and English, reads like a parody of the tendencies of the time (Lichtheim, 1885a; 1885b). It was definite and precise; his famous diagram was easily reproduced and every form of aphasia could be anticipated by postulating destruction of one of its centres or commissural paths. Even a dominant centre for consciousness was not forgotten. Seven forms of disordered speech were built up categorically from this figure. But, when the actual records of cases were examined, lamentable deficiencies were discovered; sometimes the clinical manifestations can counter to those expected. "In a large number of instances, however, the probability is that they do really belong to one of two forms. But one readily obtains examples in which this is not the case; they seem to differ in one point or another from these morbid types. Do they constitute a serious objection to my theory? I do not think so; most of them can be shown to be reducible to the schema" (Lichtheim 1885a:464).

Here we have the high-water mark of this school of thought. It enabled teachers of medicine to assume an easy dogmatism at the bedside and candidates for examination rejoiced in so perfect a clue to all their difficulties. But serious students could not fit these conceptions of aphasia to the clinical phenomena; incredulous of such scholastic interpretations, they lost interest in a problem of so little practical importance.

Most of the observers mentioned in this chapter failed to contribute anything of permanent value to the solution of the problems of aphasia, because they were dominated by a philosophical fallacy of their day, which can still count its victims amongst writers on the subject. They imagined that all vital processes could be explained by some simple formula. With the help of a few carefully selected assumptions, they deduced the mechanism of speech and embodied it in a schematic form. For every mental act there was a neural element, either identical with it or in exact correspondence. From diagrams, based on a priori principles, they deduced in turn the defects of function which must follow destruction of each "centre" or inter-nuncial path. They never doubted the validity of their postulates, based as they were on the rules of human reason.

They failed to appreciate that the logical formulae of the intellect do not correspond absolutely to physical events and that the universe does not exist as an exercise for the human mind. To them an explanation that appealed directly to reason must of necessity correspond to the facts of observation; the form assumed by the manifestations of organic disease could be therefore confidently anticipated from study of a well considered diagram. They believed that a simple explanation must conform more closely to reality than one so complex that it defies the ordinary means of human expression. Lip service was paid to the theory of evolution; but they could not conceive that the intellect of man was not a paramount and all sufficing instrument for resolving the riddle of the universe.

These observers used analysis as their instrument. So far they were right; but most of them fell into the subtle error of assuming that the elements reached by analysis could be treated as independent entities, which had entered into combination. They thought they had got hold of the sole and ultimate factors in mind and life, and all that happens must be capable of statement in these terms. They did not doubt the completeness of the analysis or its finality.

Hence all psychological problems were stated in terms of sensory processes or laws of association. When difficulty was found in applying these conceptions to action, "kinaesthesis" and "motor" presentations were invented to fill the logical gap.

Most of the English school, accustomed to the positive philosophy of the day, started axiomatically with the idea that we think in words. When the Germans entered the field they found it thickly strewn with theoretical assumptions, both positive and negative. Diagrams were multiplied until the subject of aphasia became the despair of the clinician, especially if he had been trained in the vigorous physiological atmosphere of the eighties. The time was ripe for a ruthless destruction of false gods and a return to systematic empirical observation of the crude manifestations of disease.

Notes

1.   The first diagram seems to have been that of Baginski (1871).

2.   The sole dissenting voice was Maudsley (1868).

3.   In order to understand how the temporal lobe is included in the "posterior" part of the brain, vide Wernicke's diagram (Wernicke 1874:19).

4.   Wernicke (1881:206). He will have nothing to do with word-deafness ("Worttaubheit") suggested by Kussmaul (1877:174).

References

Baginsky. B. 1871. "Aphasie in Folge schwerer Nierenerkrankungen". *Berliner Klinischer Wochenschrift* 8: 428-431; 439-443.

Bastian, H.C. 1869a. "On the various forms of loss of speech in cerebral disease". *British and Foreign Medical and Chirurgical Review* 43: 209-236; 470-492.

———. 1869b. "The physiology of thinking". *Fortnightly Review* 5: 57-71.

———. 1880. *The Brain as an Organ of Mind*. London: Kegan Paul.

———. 1897a. "On some problems in connexion with aphasia and other speech defects". *The Lancet* 1: 933-942; 1005-1017; 1131-1137; 1187-1194.

———. 1897b. "On a case of amnesia and other speech defects of eighteen years' duration with autopsy". *Medical and Chirurgical Transactions* 80: 61-86.

Broadbent, W.H. 1872. "On the cerbral mechanism of speech and thought". *Medical and Chirurgical Transactions* 55: 145-194.

———. 1879. "A case of peculiar affection of speech, with commentary". *Brain* 1:484-503.

Ferrier, David. 1873. "Experimental researches in cerebral physiology and pathology". *West Riding Asylum Reports* 3: 30-96.

———. 1875. "Experiments on the brain of monkeys. (Second series)" *Philosophical Transactions of the Royal Society* 165: 433-488.

Finkelnburg. F.C. 1870. "Niederrheinische Gesellschaft, Sitzung vom 21. März 1870 in Bonn". *Berliner Klinischer Wochenschrift* 7: 449-450; 460-462.

Gardiner, A.H. 1922. "The definition of the word and the sentence". *British Journal of Psychology* 12: 352-361.

Kussmaul, A. 1876. *Die Störungen der Sprache*. Ziemssen Handbuch d. speciellen Pathologie und Therapie 12: Anhang, 1-300. (Also separately published as : Kussmaul; A. 1876. *Die Störungen der Sprache*. Leipzig: Vogel).

Lichtheim, L. 1885a. "On Aphasia". *Brain* 7: 433-484.

———. 1885. "Uber Aphasie". *Deutsches Archiv für Klinische Medizin* 36: 204- 268.

Maudsley, H. 1868. "Concerning aphasia". *Lancet* 2: 690-692; 721-723.

Ogle, W. 1867. "Aphasia and agraphia". *St. George's Hospital Reports* 2: 83-122.

Wernicke, C. 1874. *Der aphasische Symptomencomplex*. Breslau: Cohn & Weigert.

———. 1881. *Lehrbuch der Gehirnkrankheiten*. Berlin: Fischer.

———. 1903. "Ein Fall von isolierter Agraphie". *Monatschrift für Psychiatrie und Neurologie* 12: 241-265.

Kurt Goldstein

Introduced by

RIA DE BLESER*
Research Group for Aphasia and Cognitive Disorders
Department of Neurology
Aachen, Germany

* This work was supported by the Deutsche Forschungsgemeinschaft grant no. PO41/16-1.

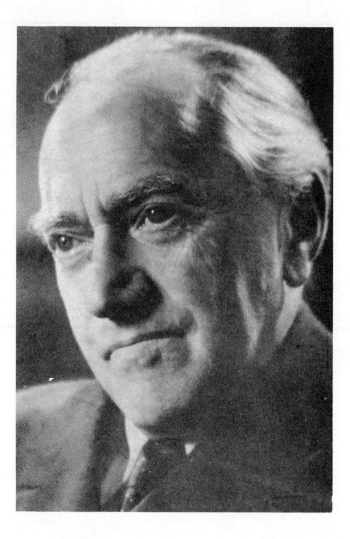

Kurt Goldstein
1878-1965

Biography

Kurt Goldstein was born on 6 November 1878 in Kattowicz, upper Silesia, Poland, which formed at that time a part of Germany. After attending the local public school, he went to the humanistic Gymnasium *in Breslau. At the universities of Breslau and Heidelberg, he studied philosophy and literature. He developed a lifelong admiration for Goethe and a close friendship with his cousin Ernst Cassirer, the Neo-Kantian philosopher. He studied medicine under Carl Wernicke, who stimulated his interest in aphasia, graduating M.D. in 1903. He then became a post-doctoral assistant at the Frankfurt neurological institute, where he practiced comparative neurology in the neuropathological laboratory under Ludwig Edinger. In 1906, he moved to Königsberg, where he worked in psychiatry and neurology, and became acquainted with the Würzburg school of experimental psychology, which emphasizes "imageless thought".*

*In 1914, Goldstein returned to Frankfurt as Edinger's first assistant. He soon established his own Institute for Research on the After-Effects of Brain Injury (*Institut zur Erforschung der Folgeerscheinungen von Hirnverletzungen*). His very productive collaboration with Adhémar Gelb, an experimental psychologist whose strong point was visual perception, also started here. Goldstein succeeded Edinger in the Neurology chair at Frankfurt. In 1930, he left Frankfurt for Berlin, where he became director of a large neuropsychiatric clinic and a professor at the university in the department of Neurology and Psychiatry.*

In 1933, Goldstein was denounced to the Nazis by an assistant and charged with leftist sympathies and Jewishness. Together with Eva Rothmann, a former student who was to become his wife, Goldstein went to The United States in 1935, at the age of 56. He started a new career in New York at Columbia University, the New York Psychiatric Institute, and the Montefiori Hospital. In 1938, he traveled to Boston to deliver the William James Lectures and from 1940 to 1945, he served as clinical professor of Neurology at Tufts University, Medford, Mass. He then returned to New York because of his wife's illness. In 1965, Goldstein suffered a stroke with right hemiplegia and global aphasia. He died on September 19, three weeks post onset, leaving over 200 publications, mostly in German and English and spanning six decades. They include work on the relationship between circumscribed cortical injuries and sensory and motor defects, problems of perceptual disturbances and agnosia, cerebellar function and its relation to tonus, localization on the cerebral cortex, and the problem of aphasia.

Selected Bibliography

Goldstein, K. 1906. "Ein Beitrag zur Lehre von der Aphasie". *Journal für Psychologie und Neurologie* 7: 172-188.
———. 1910. "Uber Aphasie". *Beihefte zur medizinischen Klinik* 6: 1-32.
———. 1911. "Die amnestische und die zentrale Aphasie (Leitingsaphaie)". *Archiv für Psychiatrie und Nervenkrankheiten* 48: 314-343.
———. 1913. "Uber die Störungen der Grammatik bei Gehirnkrankheiten". *Monatschrift für Psychiatrie und Nervenkrankheiten* 36: 540-568.
———. 1914. "Ein Beitrag zur Lehre von der Bedeutung der Insel für die Sprache und der linken Hemisphäre für das linksseitige Tasten". *Archiv für Psychiatrie und Nervenkrankheiten* 55: 158-173.
———. 1917. "Die Transkortikalen Aphasien". *Ergebnisse der Neurologie und Psychiatrie* 2: 349-629.
———. 1924. "Das Wesen der amnestischen Aphasie (Vorläufige Mitteilung gemeinsemaer Untersuchungen mit A. Gelb.)". *Schweizer Archiv für Neurologie and Psychiatrie* 15: 163-175.
———. 1927. "Uber Aphasie". *Schweizer Archiv für Neurologie and Psychiatrie* 6: 1-68.
———. 1934. *Der Aufbau des Organismus. Einführung in die Biologie unter besonderer Berücksichigung der erfahrungen am kranken Meschen.* Den Haag: Martinus Nijhoff. (English translation 1963. *The Organism. A Holistic Appraoch to Biology derived from Pathological Data in Man.* Boston, Massachusetts: Beacon Press).
——— and M. Scheerer. 1941. "Abstract and concrete behavior: an experimental study with special tests". *Psychological Monographs* 53: 2.
——— and M. Scheerer. 1945. *The Goldstein-Scheerer Test of Abstract and Concrete Thinking.* New York, N.Y.: The Psychological Corporation.
———. 1946. "On naming and pseudo-naming". *Word* 2: 1-7.
———. 1948. *Language and Language Disturbances: Aphasic Symptom Complexes and their Significance for Medecine and theory of Language.* New York: Grune & Stratton.

Introduction

Chaos

In his work *Aphasia and kindred disorders of speech* (1926), Henry Head subsumes his contempories including Henschen, Liepmann, Von Monakow, Pick, and Goldstein under the title *Chaos*. "The whole problem of disorders of speech was thrown into the melting pot and each worker was free to take up an individual position. This state of chaos was emphasized by the fact that the leaders in this field of research held views which were mutually incompatible" (Head, 1926, p. 75).

This is a caricature of a very productive liberation movement in the field. If this was chaos, one could only wish there had been more of it sooner. Actually, the differences of opinion had already been foreshadowed in the late 19th century Bismarck era in Germany. In line with different political thinking; there was a sharp division between localizers of the Fritsch and Hitzig creed, and antilocalizers who followed Goltz.

On the basis of his ablation studies with dogs, Hitzig developed a law-and-order model of the human nervous system. He compared the brain to the highly structured bureaucracy of the new Prussian Reich and held that the different "provinces" or brain centers had a strict division of authority for specific psychological functions, without the possibility of responsibility being shared by several centers nor of compensation after damage to one center. Goltz's studies on the adaptive behavior of decerebrated frogs contradicted such simple physical reductionism of psychological functions. An advocate of "Kultur", the ideal of pre-Prussian Germany, he did not want the complexity of the brain nor that of life to be oversimplified (Pauly, 1983).

Localization held the field in the 19th century, but the "geisteswissenschaftliche" antilocalizationists raised their heads again in the 20th century, with Kurt Goldstein as one of their main representatives. The alternative Goltzian view re-emerged, stressing compensation, adaptation, cooperation, and the activity of the organism as a whole, rather than boundaries, order, and regularity of brain functions.

Dropping the localizationist straitjacket naturally led to some extravagances but also to some non-trivial innovations. Both aspects are exemplified in the work of the prolific Kurt Goldstein, who in the best of his papers remains a "classical" author.

Analysis of Aphasic Symptoms

Out of a dissatisfaction with the 19th century concepts of aphasia and the underlying associationist psychology, as represented in Wernicke's work (see elsewhere in this book), Goldstein developed an alternative explanation of aphasic phenomena. The introduction of a specifically linguistic module was a major innovation, which would be disturbed in the true or central aphasia. His organismic doctrine with Gestalt sympathies may be a quirk from a historical point of view even though some very positive points were made, above all on the importance of in-depth single case studies examining different performances. We will take up these points one by one.

The Language Module

Goldstein's early papers on aphasia contain all the ingredients for his later works without the starch of Gestalt theory. The 1910 paper provides a detailed criticism of his teacher Wernicke's model of aphasia (Wernicke, 1874, 1885) based on separate cortical centers containing acoustic, motor, optical, and writing images for speech. Goldstein argued that it is empirically inadequate, because it cannot account for various aphasic phenomena such as literal paraphasias or disturbances of reading comprehension and of writing. It is theoretically insufficient, since the concept of the word is more than an association of auditory and motor images. The experimental psychologists of the Würzburg school (e.g., Bühler, Külpe, Ach) had gathered evidence for "imageless thought" and had postulated a cognitive perceptual and a cognitive language module, which are neither identical to nor analyzable into sensory images on the one hand, nor acoustico-motor images on the other (Mandler and Mandler, 1964). For Goldstein, it is a disturbance of the language module, the "Sprachfeld", which gives rise to true aphasia. This "Sprachfeld" contains "Sprachvorstellungen" or "inner speech". It is central to language and specifically linguistic, "something undefinable, which is not more mysterious than sensation" (1919, p. 17); "its specific nature is as clear to us as it is difficult to characterize more closely" (1927, p. 40).

Accordingly, Goldstein reclassified aphasic phenomena using the following main criteria:

a. Disturbance of peripheral language mechanisms or of the instrumentalities of speech = pure motor and sensory aphasia. Inner speech and the periphery (motor focus and acoustic perception) are intact but interrupted from each other.

b. Disturbance of the central language system or inner speech = central aphasia. The "Sprachfeld" itself is disturbed. This is aphasia proper.

c. Disturbance of non-linguistic cognitive abilities = the transcortical aphasias. Either the conceptual field itself or its connection to the Sprachfeld is disturbed.

Goldstein noticed that pure motor or sensory cases, that is, those cases Wernicke wanted to account for, rarely occur. Also, central aphasia is rare in a pure form. If, however, one subtracts the pure features from the more frequent complex cases, what remains is a disturbance of inner speech or of the central language system. As a first approximation to language and language disturbances, Goldstein's model is certainly superior to that of his predecessors. The introduction of a specifically linguistic module leaves room for the elaboration of formal grammar, including semantics, syntax, and phonology, which was impossible in the previous associationist models. This direction was taken by, among others, Pick (1913). Goldstein accepted Pick's results but did not himself show any particular interest in looking for dissociations within inner speech or between inner speech and non-verbal faculties. Such a research strategy would assume an autonomous language module operating independently from other cognitive faculties, and further autonomous modules within the language system such as syntax, phonology, and morphology, which could be disturbed independent of each other. This line of research is known as the vertical faculty approach in psychology (Marshall, 1984). However, in the organismic theory he develops, Goldstein emphasized horizontal interactions among disturbances of apparently different types, the common disturbance (*"Grundstörung"*) underlying them, and the various inhibitory and compensatory mechanisms covering it up. Critics of the newly revived vertical faculty approach rightly acknowledge their allegiance to Goldstein's horizontalism.

The Organismic Approach

The basic idea behind this approach is that an organism does not consist *of* eyes, legs, a brain, etc. but that it is an organism *with* eyes, legs, etc. When anything happens to a part, it affects the whole, which reacts in its entirety to the changed situation. The same, Goldstein thought, applies to language and language disturbances. "The individual speech performance is understandable only from the aspect of its relation to the function of the total organism in its endeavor to realize itself as much as possible in the given situation" (Goldstein, 1948, p. 21).

The more linguistically minded of Goldstein's contemporaries, such as Isserlin, made the criticism that, indeed, "A corn on the foot causes a general disturbance. As subjective experience teaches us, this disturbance can even be quite severe and also clearly show itself objectively in external stature and behavior. This undoubtedly changed totality notwithstanding, the inquisitive observer will correctly concentrate with special energy on this important circumscribed locus" (Isserlin, 1929, p. 139-140). Goldstein operationalized his holistic approach by means of the *"Grundstörung"*, the pervasive alteration in the mode of functioning after brain damage, which consists of a change in the relation between figure and ground (see Text 2). This leads to a more primitive, concrete type of behavior, with loss of the abstract categorical attitude: reactions are tied more to external situations than is normally the case. It occurs in almost all aphasics. Amnesic aphasia is wholly explained by such impairment of abstract attitude, so that the language disturbance becomes a mere epiphenomenon (see Text 3). Linguistically inclined contemporaries of Goldstein questioned this explanation. Lotmar, for example, remarked that, if one looks at a comparable conceptual and linguistic level of concreteness, naming by patients with amnesic aphasia is possible for some objects but not for others. Furthermore, the amnesic aphasic's difficulties with proper names cannot be explained in this framework. Given that normals, too, are often forgetful in this respect, it is impossible to reduce the underlying defect to a disturbance of categorical attitude, by which the hic et nunc person would not be identified with other possible perceptions of the same person in different contexts (Lotmar, 1936, pp. 117-118).

This criticism was to the point as far as it rejected the total identification of a particular aphasic disturbance with a non-verbal impairment. The more general issue, whether aphasic patients are impaired in non-verbal tasks as well as in verbal ones, still receives the attention of experts. As with Goldstein, the significance of such experiments for a general conceptual defect underlying aphasia remains controversial, since non-verbal tasks such as sorting might require "verbal mediation" or inner speech (Cohen, Kelter, and Woll, 1980). On the other hand, it is probably true that lexical semantics is the least modular of all linguistic components. The interface between the sense and reference of a word is vague, as studies within the recent prototypicality paradigm tend to show (Whitehouse, Caramazza and Zurif, 1979).

The line between linguistic and cognitive disturbances in aphasia will have to be drawn by looking at clearer instances of discrepancies between formal grammar versus cognition, such as in syntactic, morphological, or phonological operations. Goldstein did not do this. In his theory, the horizontalization of faculties not only holds for cognitive and linguistic modules, but also within the linguistic module itself (see Text 5). The subdivision of language into concrete and abstract is reminiscent of Jackson's emotional and propositional language (Head, 1915). It is a division according to linguistic performances rather than to formal characteristics of grammar.

Single Case Study

Goldstein's breach with the classical reduction of schematic psychological functions to specific brain centers led him away from an easy and rigid classification of patients into aphasic syndromes. He recognized the danger of examining the patient through the filter of one's particular brain-and-language diagram and of neglecting to ask a wider variety of questions including the right ones for the patient and for a more adequate theory. This, together with his organismic approach — for all the esoteric subjectivism it may contain — led him to pay close attention to the individual patient in very many performances and situations. Even though he was certainly no enemy of tests, he realized their limits. Goldstein's plea for in-depth single case studies, his comments on their superiority over large but shallow group studies, could have been written today (see Text 5). He exemplified this himself in repeated studies of one patient with visual agnosia over a period of 10 years, in cooperation with Gelb (Gelb and Goldstein, 1924). These papers are undisputed classics. It may be the controversial aspects of his work, the horizontalism, the organismic approach, which make him into a "modern" author, important again for some researchers at the moment.

References

Cohen, R. S. Kelter and G. Woll. 1980. "Analytical competence and languge impairment in aphasia". *Brain and Language* 10: 331-347.

Gelb, A. and K. Goldstein. 1924. "Uber Farbenamnesie". *Psychologische Forschung* 6: 127-186.

Goldstein, K. 1910. "Uber Aphasie". *Beihefte zur medizinischen Klinik* Heft 1: 1-32.

———. 1927. "Uber Aphasie". *Schweizer Archiv für Neurologie and Psychiatrie* Heft 6: 1-68.

———. 1948. *Language and Language Disturbances: Aphasic Symptom Complexes and their Significance for Medecine and theory of Language*. New York: Grune & Stratton.

Head, H. 1915. "Hughlings Jackson on aphasia and kindred affections of speech". *Brain* 38: 1-190.

———. 1926. *Aphasia and Kindred Disorders of Speech*. Vol. I, Cambridge: Cambridge University Press.

Isserlin, M. 1929. "Die pathologischen Physiologie der Sprache". Erster Teil. *Ergebnisse der Physiologie* 29: 129-249.

Lotmar, F. 1936. "Neuere Kämpfe um die Auffassung aphasischer Störungen". *Schweizer Archiv für Neurologie and Psychiatrie* 38:97-149.

Mandler, J.M. and G. Mandler. 1964. *Thinking: From Association to Gestalt*. New York: John Wiley.

Marshall, J.C. 1984. "Multiple perpectives on modularity". *Cognition* 17:209-242.

Pauly, P.J. 1983. "The political structure of the brain: Cerebral localization in Bismarckian Germany". *International Journal for Neuroscience* 17: 145-149.

Pick, A. 1913. *Die agrammatischen Sprachstörungen*. Studien zur psychologischen Grundlegung der Aphasielehre. Teil 1. Berlin: Springer.

Wernicke, C. 1874. *Der aphasische Symptomencomplex*. Breslau: Cohn & Weigert.

Whitehouse, P., A. Caramazza and E. Zurif. 1979. "Naming in aphasia: interacting effects of form and function". *Brain and Language* 6:63-74.

Selections from the work of
Kurt Goldstein

On Aphasia*

I myself have tried to build upon Storch's explanations, which, like Wernicke's teachings are based on psychological grounds. Wernicke's analysis of the psychic elements certainly represented an extraordinary refinement over Gall's yet from the point of view of psychology it cannot be maintained. Storch (1902) is right to ask whether we are actually dealing with psychic elements, whether it is justified to speak of images of sound and of speech movement as if they were elementary psychic images. In order to answer this question, we must ask first: What are they anyway, these so-called images? Since we cannot acknowledge the existence of inborn images, in our conception the image can only be the residue of an earlier perception. Taking a closer look at perception, we can distinguish two aspects: one where perception is based on a sensation, and one where perception did not come about by any sensory stimulation at all. The sensory component, which Storch has called the pathopsychic, is composed of the specific quality of the sense and the sensations which are brought about by muscle contractions that correspond to their site of stimulation and by other stimulations in the same area (the so-called organic sensations). Simultaneously with the sensory component, different indirect images awaken in us with each perception: the image of spatiality, of time, of identity, similarity, difference, etc. These images are produced by means of the assimilation of the sensory factor on the part of the intellect. Where the non-sensory aspect is concerned, it is — at least for the optical-tactile perceptions, which we, for

* Translated from "Über Aphasie" Beihefte zur Medizinische Klinik 1: pp. 13-15 (1910)

the sake of simplicity, will discuss first — spatiality that is of special importance. We can only perceive in space. For the understanding of normal and
of many pathological phenomena, it is of the utmost importance to be
clearly aware of the fact that an object, notwithstanding with which sense
organ we perceive it, always gives us the same spatial image. This uniform
character of the spatial image demands that the image be located at only
one spot, and that this spot cannot coincide with the centers of the pathopsychic components, the sensory fields that are located at different spots.
This field of spatial images, which exists as a single unit vis à vis the different sensory centers and extends between these sensory centers, is called a
conceptual field (Storch's stereopsychic field). The same thing that can be
said for the spatial aspect of perception is true for the other non-sensory
components. They too do not change, whether the sensory qualities differ
or not, and they too can, as little as we know about this, be regarded as a
manifestation of the conceptual field.

Furthermore, the non-sensory part of perception, especially its spatial
aspect, is the essence that stays behind in us as a memory image (while of
the qualitative sensation, only an individual, more or less vivid residue can
be aroused), and upon which the recognition of objects, for example, is
almost exclusively based. Thus we can recognize an object in an incomplete
sketch as well as if we were to see the object itself. Accordingly a concept
is not the sum of its separate parts, but a unity with a more or less large
number of components; it exists in the combination of its parts under such
a point of view as is represented in every concrete concept essentially by the
spatial aspect. Therefore it is not justified to speak of optical or tactile
images, but only of spatial images that are accompanied by a more or less
clear optical or tactical memory image. These sensory memory images of
course, cannot be disavowed completely. They are the basis of purely sensory recognition and can be regarded as the combination of stimulating
forms of the elementary energies deposited in the sensory field. Psychically
they never exist for us in an isolated way, but only in their relation to the
non-sensory part, especially the spatial aspect.

(Same text, pp. 17-18)

This interval image becomes the first step for the articulation of the
sound just as the spatial image does for the performance of some other
movement. Each image of speech corresponds to a certain muscle innerva-

tion, which owes its formation to the endless practicing of the child learning to speak, and which arouses in us the same interval image as does the sound that is being heard. This interval image is the essence of what remains of the motor act as a residue in the conscious mind. Therefore, as Storch says, in speaking and hearing we experience no difference whatsoever with respect to that part in consciousness that is called on for an image. Therefore the distinction between memory images of sound and images of speech movement can be discarded as unpsychological. Certainly, however, of both the motor act as well as the acoustic stimulation, a certain residue stays behind in us, a residue that differs in the strength with which it can be aroused in different individuals. But that does not mean that it is justifiable to speak of acoustic or motor images of speech; on the contrary, it is only a matter of complicated acoustic or motor residues that differ from other acoustic or motor memory images at most in their complexity. Where speech is concerned, they gain importance only by way of their relation to the speech images they accompany. That which belongs to speech images that is common and essential for all human beings is particularly different from the acoustic-motor aspect. We are as clearly aware of its peculiarity as we are incapable of defining it any further. It shares this peculiarity with all other specific elements of the conscious mind, and therefore with the spatial image as well, and is in my opinion no more puzzling than the fact of simple experience.

Because the image of speech can exist in my mind without the acoustic or motor areas of the cerebral cortex being in action, and because this image is the same whether we hear or speak, therefore it is impossible that it be localized either acoustically or sensorially, but instead we must consider its representation in the cortex also to be a cortical area separate from both. This area has been designated by Storch as the glosso-psychic field; I would like to call it simply *speech field*. This central speech field is on the one hand connected to the acoustic perception field and the motor area of the speech muscles, and on the other hand to the whole rest of the cortex, the representation of the "concepts".

(Same text, pp. 18-19)

With respect to the diagram, I hardly need to emphasize that it gives only a very general idea of underlying principles, in order to achieve a better understanding. Indeed, the relations are much more complicated than they would appear from this diagram.

Model of the language apparatus

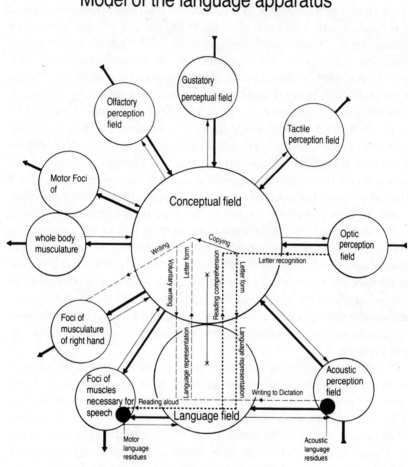

K. Goldstein, 1910: "über Aphasie"

Figure 1.

The principal pathways that are responsible for perception and movement (especially the hearing of speech and speech itself) are represented by the heavy lines. Parallel to them, but in the opposite direction, run thin lines: on the one hand the centrifugal connection between the conceptual field and the perceptual fields which yield the foundation of the so-called sensory flavor of the images, on the other hand the centripetal connection between the conceptual field and the motor foci that supply the conceptual field with the motor stimulation necessary for the development of motor images. The dotted lines represent the pathways used in reading, the dashed lines those used in writing. In reading, the optically perceived letters are recognized in the conceptual field as a spatial structure. From there, they arouse the speech images of the letters in the speech area. These speech images become connected to word images that are transmitted onto the motor foci when reading aloud; when reading for comprehension they arouse the concepts that belong to the speech images. Volitional writing originates from the object concept in the conceptual field; this object concept rouses the image of speech in the speech area, where, at the same time, the latter is analyzed into those letters that call upon the match images of letter forms in the conceptual field. The latter are finally transmitted onto the motor foci. In writing from dictation, the process starts with the acoustic perception arousing the image of speech. From there it follows the same pathway as it followed earlier to the motor foci. In copying, the optically perceived letter calls upon the image of letters in the conceptual field, which is transmitted from there onto the motor foci.

The Problem of the Origin of Symptoms in Brain Damage*

Modification of the patient's performance shows the effects of a blurring of the sharp boundaries between "figure" and "ground". When we look at a picture we see and understand at once what is figure and what is background. The terms figure and ground can be applied not only to visual but to all performances. Figure and background can be discriminated as readily in speaking, thinking, feeling, etc. As examples of this figure-ground phenomenon, if one raises an arm vertically, the execution of this movement requires, as one can feel in oneself and observe in others, a rather definite position of the rest of the body. The raised arm is the figure, the rest of the body is the background. A word becomes meaningful from the context in which it appears; the meaning of a thought is conditioned by a vast contextual background — the individual's educational experience, social status, and so on.

Habitually we ignore the background of a performance and pay attention only to the figure. But figure and background are intimately interconnected. Neither of them can be properly evaluated without the other. Correspondingly, every change of background will produce a change of figure. Figure-ground performances have their counterpart in processes of the nervous system. In any function of the organism the excitation in the nervous system is distributed in such a way that the process in a circumscribed area differs as to form and intensity from the state prevailing in the rest of the nervous system. The process in the circumscribed area corresponds to what we call performance, designated by the term "figure"; the process in the rest of the nervous system we term the "background", or, more briefly, "ground". In normal performances the figure and ground processes are in a definite relation. All damage in the nervous system, especially in the brain cortex, disturbs the normal relation. The sharp differentiation of figure from background suffers, inducing a general leveling or intermingling of figure and background. This is sometimes carried to the point of inversion, where the figure becomes background and the background figure. Many symptoms become understandable from this point of view. We expect the

---

* From *Language and Language Disturbances*. New York: Grune & Stratton, 1948. p. 5.

"figure" as reaction to a definite stimulus, and the patient may answer with the "background": instead of yes, the patient may say no; instead of black, white; instead of the demanded series of numbers, the series of the days of the week, etc.

On Naming and Pseudonaming*

The purpose of this paper is to acquaint the linguist with material that will help elucidate the much discussed phenomenon of naming, and to demonstrate the paramount position of meaning in language. The material concerns patients having speech disturbances due to brain damage, particularly those suffering from so-called amnesic aphasia.

The most striking symptom these patients manifest is a defect in the capacity to name objects, even the most familiar ones occurring in everyday life. Usually this symptom is understood as a dissociation between so-called brain centers for "thing ideas" and a center of "word images", or of a difficulty to evoke the latter. There is no doubt that the inability of the patients to name objects is not due to a disturbance of recognition. This becomes evident by the circumlocutions by which the patients react to the request to name an object, for instance, when a patient — unable to name a pencil, a glass or an umbrella — will say "that is something to write with, to drink with, or a thing for the rain!" Surprisingly the patient sometimes uses words in these circumlocutions that he cannot find for naming, even immediately after having used them in the circumlocution. This proves that the inability is not due to a loss of words.

What then makes the patient incapable of naming the object? The answer to this question and a general clarification of the nature of naming came from a careful consideration of the total behavior of the patients. The patient, in his behavior and thought, is concentrated to an unusual degree on his own personality and his relationship to the world. He is a person acting in the world rather than thinking and speaking about the world. His speech is accompanied by an excessive use of expressive gestures. Often he seems incapable of expressing himself through words, but can do so quite well with the help of gestures. This general change of behaviour shows up very clearly in special tests which we developed in order to study the attitude with which the patient faces the world. Some sorting tests proved to be particularly useful for this purpose. For instance, we place before the patient a pile of skeins of yarn of different colors in the same way as in

* From K. Goldstein, 1946. *Word* 2, no. 1, 1-7.

Holmgren's test for color vision. We ask the patient to select out all the red skeins, including the various shades of red. Or we pick out one skein of, say, a dark red, and ask him to find skeins of the same or similar color. A normal person with good color response usually selects a great number of different shades of the same basic color disregarding differences of intensity, purity, brightness, etc. According to the task, the subject's attention may be directed to the basic color, and he chooses all skeins which he recognizes as belonging to the given type. When the test is given to a patient with amnesic aphasia, the results are quite different. In fact, several types of behavior are observed. For example, in following the instruction to take all skeins similar to a given one, the patient may choose only skeins of the identical or at least of a closely similar shade. Though urged on he limits himself to a small number because there are only a few very similar ones in the heap. Another patient matches a given bright shade of red with a blue skein of great brightness. At first, one might think the patient is colorblind, but it can be demonstrated beyond doubt by other tests that his colour sense is normal, and that he is able to make very fine differentiations. More precise observations disclose that the choice in any given case is determined by a particular color attribute, for example, brightness. We observe further, that the choice may be decided now by one attribute, now by another one; by brightness, softness, coldness, warmth, etc. Moreover, surprising as it may seem, the patient who follows a given attribute, may be unable to follow this procedure if it is demanded of him, viz., if we ask him to choose all bright skeins. Further, we observe that often he does not carry through with the same procedure. He has chosen, for instance, some bright colors. Suddenly he transfers the selection to another occasion, for instance, to coldness. On another occasion, the patient will arrange the skeins as if guided by another scale of brightness. He will begin with a very bright red, then add one less bright and so on to a dull one. But if we ask him to place the skeins in a succession according to their brightness, he shows himself incapable of the performance, even after it is demonstrated to him.

To understand the behaviour of these patients, we must compare the procedure of normal persons in such tasks. If required to choose all red colors, we group various nuances, even though we see that they are not identical. We do so because they belong together in respect to the chosen quality. The several shades are to us only examples of this quality. We treat the skeins not as things in themselves, but as representatives of the given quality. For the moment we ignore all but the specific character requested; we

inhibit or disregard all other attributes which may enter attentive consciousness. We are able to do this because we can abstract and hold fast the direction of procedure once initiated.

There is another approach open to the normal person. If we start with
one particular skein and pass it over the heap, passively surrendering ourselves to the impression emerging as we do so, one of two things will take
place. If skeins in all attributes like our sample are present, all these
immediately cohere in a unitary sensory experience. If, however, they
match our sample in some respects but not in all, we experience a characteristic unrest concerning the heap and a rivalry between groupings according to the different attributes. In either case, we see that the coherence or
conflict results from the sense data. There is an essential difference
between the two kinds of approach. In the first, a definite active ordering
principle determines our action; in the second, this principle fails to work,
and our action is passively determined by the outer impressions. We may
designate the two as the abstract and the concrete attitude. These two
attitudes are merely instances of man's twofold orientation toward the
world. In this connection, let me stress that in the abstract attitude we are
not directed toward an individual object but toward the category, of which
it is an accidental example and representative. Therefore, we call this
attitude also the categorical attitude.

In the concrete attitude, we are directed more toward the actual thing
in its particular uniqueness. To these different orientations correspond two
types of behaviour. In brief we may say that in the first approach we are
mainly thinking about things. Our reaction is determined not by the
demands of the given object, but by the demands of the category which it
represents for us. In the second approach we are manipulating the object
more than thinking about it. Our thinking and acting are determined by the
individual claims of the given object.

The patient's behavior is similar to the concrete approach of the normal person. Because he can act only in this way, we conclude that he is
impaired in his abstract attitude and has become a being dominated to an
abnormal degree by concrete promptings. Returning to the problem of
naming, it is important to recognize that language is related to each type of
behavior in a particular way. In the abstract approach, it is the word which
induces us to take the abstract attitude, to organize the world in a conceptual way. In concrete behavior, language does not play a primary role, and
words merely accompany our acts. The word is not much more than one

property of the object itself, in addition to the physical properties such as color, size, etc. This difference finds its expression in the use of different words in the two attitudes. In the first, the tendency is to use more generic words like flower, colors, etc.; in the latter, words which are especially adapted to the individuality of objects, such as rose, violet, rose-red, strawberry red. In the concrete approach, one does not say simply green, but grass-green, etc.; the words in this situation are "individual" words closely fitting the definite object. They do not designate a group, they do not "represent" things.

We perform the task of naming usually in the abstract attitude. When we name an object such as a table, we do not mean the special table with all its accidental properties, but "table" in general. The word is used as representative of the category "table", as a symbol for the "idea". The patient, we conclude, cannot use words in this sense because he cannot assume the abstract attitude. Since the patient faces the world with the particular attitude to which speech is not relevant (or which we could accompany only with very "individual" words), the nominal words do not even occur to him. He does not find the words because he cannot understand what we mean by "naming", and he cannot understand it because it presupposes the abstract attitude which he cannot assume. He can use words in connection with objects only if he has some which fit the concrete situation in the same way as we use "individual words". The patient who cannot apply or accept the presented word red as fitting all different nuances of red, still uses words like strawberry red, sky blue, etc., immediately in relation to corresponding colors. He has such "individual" words at his disposal. He may not utter the word green — because for him it belongs only to a definite green — but he may designate different greens with words which fit well the individual nuances. The more his premorbid language has developed, the more he utters such words. The language of the patient consists — besides speech automatisms with which we shall deal later and which belong to "concrete" language — only of such individual words. The words are no longer representative beyond their immediate application. One might say that they have lost the character of symbols, they have lost meaning.

The fact that naming becomes impossible with this change in the character of language reveals the nature of naming. It is not based on a simple association between an object and a sound, but presupposes a special attitude toward the object. The name is an expression of the conceptual attitude. Words used as names are not simply tools which may be handled like concrete objects, but a means to detach man from an external world and to help him organize it in a conceptual way. Words are fitted to be used in this way because they correspond to and evoke the abstract attitude. Thus *naming becomes a prototype of human language* and of the behavior characteristic of the human being.

The paramount importance of the abstract attitude for human language becomes evident by another characteristic modification of the language of the patients. We have stressed the fact that patients with impairment of the abstract attitude show changes of behavior in general: they lack initiative, they have difficulty in starting anything voluntarily, they find it difficult to shift voluntarily from one aspect of a situation to another. Their language shows the same deviation from the norm. Their language, reduced in general, has changed from an active, spontaneous, productive means for expressing ideas, feelings, etc., to a passive, more or less compulsive stereotyped and unproductive reaction to definite stimuli. The qualitative difference between the speech of patients and normal speech becomes evident in the fact that the patients are not able to use a word which has normally several meanings, now with one meaning, now with another, and they cannot understand such a shift. They cannot grasp metaphoric use of words, etc.

However, the patients are not without speech. They are able, with the help of speech, to come to terms with the demands of the environment to a certain degree. Some patients even learn again to find the right word for an object, they become able to "name" objects. The following example may illustrate this: A patient of mine behaved in the beginning like other amnesic aphasic cases. In time she was able to give names to some familiar objects. But further examination showed clearly that we were not dealing with real naming. The words could be used only in connection with a definite appearance of the objects. This became particularly clear in connection with colors. She declined to extend the same "name" which she had given to a definite color to the several shades of the given color on the ground that it would not be correct to call these red, blue, etc. However, in the course of time, after repeated examination, the patient came to call various shades by the same name, for instance, she would use the word red for all shades of red. Superficially she seemed to behave like a normal person; one might have thought she had improved. But it was not so. Asked why she now called all these different shades by the same word, she answered, "The doctors have told me that all these colors are named red. Therefore I call them all red". Asked if this was not correct, she laughed and said: "Not one of these colors is red, but I am told to call them by this word". It is clear that she had not used the word as a symbol, but had learned to build quite a superficial connection between a diversity of things and one word, a rather meaningless connection, which, however, helped her to carry out a task, if only in a quite external way. Her good memory helped her in this task. It is very important to bear in mind that words can be used in this way by patients, otherwise we may be easily deceived.

We may illustrate with more examples that the words used by the patient in an apparently normal way are nevertheless of a totally concrete character. Asked to mention the names of some animals, the same patient was at first unable to do so. Then suddenly she said: "A polar bear, a brown bear, a lion, a tiger". Asked why she named just these animals, she said: "If we enter the Zoological Gardens we come first to the polar bear and then to the other animals". Apparently she had remembered the names of the animals in the order in which they were located in the Zoological Gardens of her home town, and she used the words as they belonged to the concrete situation. In this connection it was very characteristic that she did not say "bears" — a word which expresses the category of all different kinds of bears and which we would use when asked to name animals — but that she used the more specific "polar bear, brown bear".

We found the same thing when the patient was asked to mention different female names. She said: "Grete, Paul, Clara, Martha". When we asked why she had given just these names, she answered: "those are all G's" (G was her family name), and went on, "one sister died of a heart neurosis". This example demonstrates very clearly that the patient did not think of names, but only of words which belonged to the particular situation. How very concrete such words are taken may be demonstrated by the following example. When a knife was offered to a patient of this type, together with a pencil, she called the knife a "pencil sharpener", when the knife was offered to her together with an apple it was an "apple parer", in company with a piece of bread it became a "bread knife", and together with a fork it was "knife and fork". She never uttered spontaneously the word knife alone and when she was asked, "Could we not call all these simply knife"? she replied promptly, "No". The words the patient utters apparently do not have the character of names; they indicate external associations which the patient has learned. One should not call this naming, but should differentiate such use of words as pseudonaming. This distinction is important, for various reasons. If we do not distinguish between these two forms of applying words to objects, we may overlook the failure of the patient and make a wrong diagnosis of his defect in naming. The opposite error is also possible. Another type of patient is hampered in evoking words because of a memory defect. From his incapacity to name objects, we might assume that he has an impairment of the abstract attitude, which is not the case. Only by careful study can we decide which is the cause of the inability. But our conclusion is also of significance for the interpretation of speech performance in normals. It is impossible to evaluate any utterance on its face value without a careful analysis of the attitude that accompanies it.

Individuals, normal as well as abnormal, possess a varying number of speech-automatisms. They are acquired like other learned activities, and once set going, they run off as wholes without further stimulation and without the performer's cognizance of the components. We are not necessarily aware of their meaning while bringing them forth. Nevertheless, they are not independent of the attitude of meaning, but are essentially embedded in it. This becomes evident in some observations on patients: Mentally defective children may learn a great number of such automatisms with the help of adults, but they may lose them later because they do not develop the abstract attitude. Adult patients with an impairment of the abstract attitude forget automatisms, for example, the multiplication table, well fixed as it may appear, when they have lost the value of numbers.

A good example to illustrate the difference between automatisms and meaningful language is the learning of vocabulary in a foreign language. So long as we have no real understanding of the foreign language we acquire the words only in their superficial connection with the words of our own language. We know that these words belong to a definite situation and are able to use them correctly without having a real understanding of their meaning. However, this covers only these given situations. We make many a mistake of using words in situations where they do not fit, because we have no real insight into their meaning. The situation changes when we have acquired a real conception of the foreign language, so that we understand the fundamental meaning of its words. Then the words achieve an absolutely different character. They become representatives of the categorical approach to the surrounding world, and only then can one speak of having mastered the language.

The following, then, are the main conclusions derived from our experiences with patients having speech disturbances due to brain damage:

1) The seemingly simple function of naming objects does not present a simple connection between a thing and a word. Naming presupposes a special attitude toward the object; that attitude in which the individual is detached from a given condition, the conceptual or abstract attitude characteristic of human beings.

2) We have to distinguish naming from pseudonaming, which is based on simple associations, speech automatisms which play a great role in normal language. Pathology teaches us that they are not independent from the abstract attitude. The use of these "tools" in language is not quite true language, but they become part of language by their association with meaning. Their conditional background is the abstract attitude.

3) Naming is only one example of human language which is characterized by the phenomenon of meaning; language is a means for building up the world in a particular way, i.e. the conceptual way. Pathology confirms the ideas of W. von Humboldt, who wrote: "Language does not represent objects themselves but the concepts which the mind has formed of them in that autonomous activity by which it creates language".

The significance of this autonomous activity which we will call the abstract attitude can be grasped nowhere as clearly as in the changes of the behaviour of mental patients under observation: in the change of their total personality, in their lack of activity, of creativeness, freedom, and social adaption, and in the changes of their language that we have described.

The Organismic Approach to Aphasia*

There should be distinguished — indeed somewhat abstractly — two types of language and correspondingly two groups of aphasic symptom complexes:

1. Concrete language which belongs to concrete behavior. It consists of speech automatisms, of the "instrumentalities of speech": of sounds, words, series of words, sentences, one form of naming and of understanding of language in familiar situations for which it has been conditioned, and finally of emotional utterances. In pathology, it presents itself in somewhat isolated defects of speaking, understanding, etc. of so-called pure forms of aphasia and central aphasia. Because of the difference of the relationship of emotional and nonemotional language to the personality, there is a difference of impairment of both in aphasia.

2. Abstract language which belongs to the abstract attitude: volitional, propositional, relational language. It is disturbed somewhat isolatedly if abstract attitude is impaired; further, in slight damage of instrumentalities which may leave intact other speech functions but disturbs the highly complex performance of voluntary actions. Because the various speech performances as voluntary speech, conversational speech, speaking of isolated words or of series, repetition, naming of objects, reading, etc. are in a different degree dependent on the abstract attitude, the various performances may be damaged in different degrees.

Everyday language is a combination of both types of language; in a conversation, first automatisms may occur, then appearance of words may be determined by abstract attitude. That form of language is used which permits the individual best to come to terms with the given situation in the trend to realize himself, particularly to express what he wants to express in the moment. If one of the two forms of language is particularly disturbed by pathology, the individual tries to overcome the defect by increased use of the other form. Thus, a complex clinical picture may appear in a damage of

---

* From K. Goldstein, 1948. *Language and Language Disturbances*. Grune and Stratton, New York, pp. 25-26.

the first or second type which can be understood only by careful analysis of each utterance and the circumstances in which it occurs.

The distinction of different forms of speech disturbances does not correspond to the different symptom complexes which usually are distinguished and according to which aphasic patients are examined. One speaks of disturbances of understanding, speaking, repetition, finding words, etc. Performances belonging to one or the other of these categories may represent — considered from the before-mentioned point of view — quite different performances under different circumstances. Therefore, in most cases, the usual terminology does not fit the actual findings based on such an analysis.

On Aphasia

Our methodological demands present us with a problem which we do no wish to obscure. The point is that our demands cannot ever be met completely, just because they require a full single case analysis which, apart from being very painstaking, cannot always be accomplished.

In particular, the question arises as to when an analysis can be considered complete. In practice, this objection is not so important as it might seem at first glance. One shoud not push the principle too far. Certainly an analysis of a case is never fully closed, but nevertheless there is quite a difference between the usual description of singular disturbances of visual or speech capacities, and so on, on the one hand, and an analysis which, albeit not complete, encompasses as many capacities as possible on the other hand. The latter procedure will certainly prevent us from making the worst mistakes, even if it does not yield results which are impeccable. The expert, who is well able to dig into the personality of a patient, will know well enough when to end an analysis without risking major mistakes in his interpretation. We will have to proceed to the point where all phenomena can be explained from the theory that has been built upon previously established facts, or to the point that with each new forthcoming question we can predict with strong probability the way in which the patient will behave. Only then is the analysis complete, as is the case for example with the patient suffering from mind-blindness whom Gelb and I have described. On the basis of our initial examinations, which were not completely exhaustive, we constructed a preliminary theory, which was not altogether satisfactory. The more we proceeded in examining the patient, the more it became clear to us from which functional disorder he was suffering. Today we have reached a point where we are indeed able to predict from the theory we have constructed how the patient will behave in any situation, even with activities we have never examined with him. Only cases that have been examined this thoroughly should actually be used in theory formation. To me, such a single case analysis carried through as far as possible is much

* Translated from "Über aphasie", *Schweizer Archiv für Neurologie und Psychiatrie*, 6, Reprinted in "*K. Goldstein Selected Papers*", edited by A. Gurwitsch, E.M. Goldstein, Handel, W. Handel, The Hague: Martinus Nijhoff, pp. 168-170 (1971)

more valuable that a large number of examinations with patients yielding imperfect results. Whatever enormous accumulation of inadequately established facts there may be, they will never lead to knowledge of the real state of affairs. Our discipline is dominated by the magic of numbers. Important as it is to find that once established facts are confirmed in new material again and again, this confirmation scarcely helps us to a better understanding of the essential points.

A theory becomes more significant to the extent that it succeeds in explaining all the demonstrable phenomena. Therefore, in constructing the theory, it is important that we consider all possible facts which are related to the problem under investigation. In this sense, consideration of linguistic, anthropological, and child-development experiences, as proposed especially by Pick, is to be regarded as a very valuable contribution to our problem. However, here too I would object to applying the results of these research areas to the evaluation of our facts just like that; in view of the instability of all empirical results, this is as objectionable as using arguments from the field of normal psychology. The results of other scientific disciplines should be used only to stimulate the use of certain procedures in investigating our own materials and to check our results, whereby the distinctions between the different materials deserve our utmost attention, to a larger extent that has been the case when child psychology or anthropology has been considered in explaining pathological facts. The comparison of our findings with the findings of the disciplines mentioned above will only be profitable to those disciplines as well if they are handled this carefully.

Norman Geschwind

Introduced by

MARY-LOUISE KEAN
Department of Cognitive Sciences
University of California, Irvine

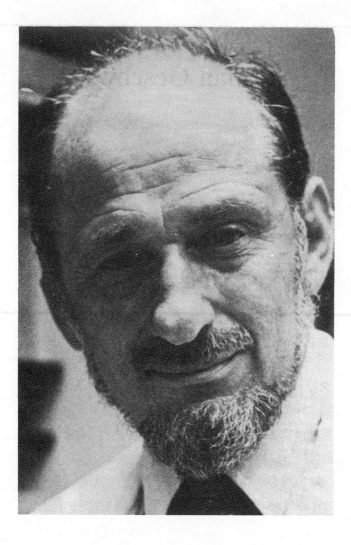

Norman Geschwind
1926-1984

Biography

Norman Geschwind was born in New York City on 8 January 1926. Neither medicine nor science more generally was a major focus of his early intellectual attention. As a student at Boy's High School in Brooklyn, New York, his primary interests were literary; at that time he also became attracted to mathematics, which became his chosen subject when he entered Harvard University in 1942. During his first two years at Harvard Geschwind began to think about entering medicine and precociously applied to Harvard Medical School, only to be turned down. His undergraduate education was interrupted when he was drafted into the Army in 1942. Returning to Harvard in 1944, Geschwind changed his major, moving to the Department of Social Relations, which was an amalgam of social and personality psychology, sociology, and cultural anthropology. Because of a belief that the understanding of behavior lay in the understanding of life experience and culture, Geschwind again applied to Harvard Medical School, and was accepted. He was bent on becoming a psychiatrist. At that time it seemed obvious to him that a knowledge of physiology, anatomy, and biochemistry was totally irrelevant to the study of human behavior. This conviction began to erode when he took neuroanatomy from Dr. Marcus Singer; two topics Singer dealt with struck him and were later to become significant areas in his research: epilepsy and aphasia.

Following his graduation from Harvard Medical School in 1951, Geschwind went to the National Hospital in London, first as a Mosley Travelling Fellow (1952-53) and then on a United States Public Health Service fellowship (1953-55). During his stay he was greatly influenced by Sir Charles Symonds, who made him see the importance of neurological mechanisms in the study of disorders. Geschwind became Chief Resident in neurology at the Boston City Hospital in 1955, under Dr. Derek Denny-Brown, who reinforced the anti-localization biases that he had acquired in England. Geschind's main interest had yet to focus on the neurological study of behavioral systems, and he began his two years (1956-58) as a research fellow in the Department of Biology at the Massachusetts Institute of Technology with the intent of studying muscle disease.

In 1958, Geschwind became a staff neurologist at the Boston Veterans Administration Hospital, where Dr. Fred Quadfasel was Chief of Neurology. The VA offered Geschwind his first opportunity to see a large number of aphasics, including the chronically aphasic. It was in this context that his clinical interest developed into his life-long scientific interest in the study of the neurological foundations of language functions and other higher mental processes. Encouraged by Quadfasel, Geschwind began his scholarly study of the classic texts of neurology at this time. From 1962 until 1966, he was Chief of Neurology at the Boston VA Hospital and Associate Professor of Neurology at Boston University, where he was Professor and Chair of the Department of Neurology from 1966 to 1968. In the early 1960s Geschwind played a central role in establishing the Boston University Aphasia Research Center at the VA Hospital. The Aphasia Research Center was unique in its inception and has been the focal point of interdisciplinary aphasia research in the United States since its foundation.

Geschwind was appointed James Jackson Putnam Professor of Neurology at Harvard Medical School in 1969, succeeding his teacher Denny-Brown. Geschwind occupied that chair until his death on 4 November 1984. During his years at Harvard he continued to pursue his research on aphasia. Throughout his career his research interests were not, however, restricted to the study of aphasia. He made major contributions to the study of epilepsy, anatomy, notably in the domain of lateral asymmetries, and dyslexia, among other areas. Geschwind's contributions to the study of neural mechanisms of higher mental processes reside not only in his extensive research but also in his inspired teaching of medical students and training of residents. Beyond this, throughout his career, he actively encouraged and supported interdisciplinary research involving linguists and cognitive psychologists. He significantly shaped the neurological climate in the United States and Europe during his life, an influence which lives on in his students.

Selected Bibliography

Geschwind, N. 1963. "Carl Wernicke, the Breslau School and the History of Aphasia." *Speech, Language and Communication.* Brain Function, Vol III, ed. by E.C. Carterette. Berkeley: University of California Press.

——. 1964. "The development of the brain and the evolution of language". *Monographic Series on Language and Linguistics*, Vol. 17, ed. by C. Stuart. Washington: Georgetown University Press.

——. 1965. "Disconnexion syndromes in animals and man." *Brain* 88: 237-294, 585-644.

—— and M. Fusillo. 1966. "Color-naming defects in association with alexia". *Archives of Neurology* 15: 137-146.

——. 1967. "The varieties of naming errors". *Cortex* 3: 97-112.

—— and W. Levitsky. 1968. "Human Brain: left–right asymmetries in temporal speech region." *Science* 161: 186-187.

——, F.A. Quadfasel and J.M. Segarra. 1968. "Isolation of the speech area". *Neuropsychologia* 6: 327-340.

Benson, D.F. and N. Geschwind. 1969. "The Alexias". *Handbook of Clinical Neurology* Vol 4, ed. by P.J. Vinken and G.W. Bruyn. Amsterdam: North Holland.

——. 1974. *Selected Papers on Language and the Brain*. Dordrecht: D. Reidel.

—— and A. Galaburda. 1987. *Cerebral Lateralization: Biological Mechanisms, Associations, and Pathology*. Cambridge, Mass.: M.I.T. Press.

Introduction

In the mid-20th century anti-localizationism dominated neurological thinking about the aphasias and other disorders of higher mental processes. The
"classical" localizationist works of such people as Wernicke and Dejerine
were typically dismissed out of hand or, as was only later realized, misrep-
resented in the literature. When Norman Geschwind joined the Neurology
service at the Boston Veterans Administration Hospital in 1958, he shared
the anti-localizationist biases of the day. He had come to this tradition
through his years of study in England (1952-55) and during his residency
under Dr. Derek Denny-Brown at Boston City Hospital. After he had been
at the VA for some time, he began to feel uncomfortable with what he
had been taught. The VA Hospital had an aphasia unit which afforded
Geschwind the opportunity to see many patients. It became increasingly
obvious to him that aphasic patients differed from each other in their clinical pictures and that these differences clearly appeared to be associated
with the location of the responsible lesion.

Dr. Fred Quadfasel was Chief of the Neurology service at the VA Hospital when Geschwind went there. Quadfasel had worked under Goldstein
in Germany and, prior to coming to the United States in the 1930s, had
served as an assistant to Bonhoeffer, who had been one of Wernicke's first
assistants. Despite his lineage, Quadfasel generally shared the anti-
localizationist sentiment of the day. However, he was familiar with the
older literature and possessed a large library which contained many of the
original neurological texts from the 19th and early 20th centuries. Quadfasel made his library available to Geschwind, who effectively devoured it,
finding in the earlier works views which comported with those which he had
been developing in the context of his practice of neurology. In particular,
he was drawn to Wernicke's model. In brief, Wernicke pointed out that at
the simplest level one must make a distinction between lesions which
destroy groups of cells which may be involved in processing and lesions

which destroy fiber connections between different parts of the nervous system.

Early in 1961, Geschwind encountered the work of R.E. Myers on the effects of lesions of the corpus callosum in animals (Myers, 1962a, 1962b). At the time, in common with the standard belief, Geschwind assumed that lesions to the corpus callosum had no effects in humans. By chance, about this time, Quadfasel gave Geschwind a copy of Dejerine's (1892) paper on pure alexia without agraphia in which a lesion of the posterior portion of the corpus callosum in conjunction with a lesion of left visual cortex was seen as responsible for the disorder. To Geschwind the paper was a masterpiece. Within a few weeks of reading Dejerine's paper, Geschwind saw his first patient with this syndrome; over the years he was to see many more such patients. Just a few weeks later Edith Kaplan, a clinical neuropsychologist at the VA, showed Geschwind a patient she had tested who wrote aphasically with his left hand but nonaphasically (normally) with his right. Geschwind immediately realized that this patient must have a callosal syndrome, a prediction subsequently confirmed by post-mortem findings. Geschwind and Kaplan studied this patient extensively. Not long after encountering this patient, Geschwind, pursuing his review of the older literature, discovered that Liepmann had discussed callosal syndromes in man (Liepmann, 1898, 1900; Liepmann and Storch, 1902). Geschwind and Kaplan's case, the first modern callosal syndrome, was originally reported in late 1961, at the Boston Society for Neurology and Psychiatry (Geschwind and Kaplan, 1962). The first surgical division of the cerebral commissures was carried out some months later in California by a group familiar with Geschwind and Kaplan's research (Gazzaniga, Bogen, and Sperry, 1962).

Geschwind attended a meeting on dyslexia in Baltimore in 1961 where he had occasion to discuss his ideas about cortico-cortico connections with the eminent neuropsychologist Oliver Zangwill. Zangwill urged him to write up an extended account of his views. That account was published in *Brain* in two parts in 1965, as "Disconnexion Syndromes in Animals and Man". Geschwind credited Zangwill with "having brought me to a more careful review of the older literature and a more precise account of my own ideas" (Geschwind, 1974). Few works in the history of neurology match the intellectual robustness and scope of "Disconnexion Syndromes" or have had so profound an impact. Bolstering his arguments on the basis of the older literature, animal research, and his own clinical experience, Geschwind developed a connectionist model, exploring its implications not only in the domain of aphasia but also for the apraxias and agnosias. Over the years he wrote numerous articles clarifying and refining the model put forth in "Disconnexion Syndromes". It had been his intention, one day, to write a book-length revision of the paper elaborating the analysis; at the time of his death in 1984, he had not published the extended revised version.

With the publication of "Disconnexion Syndromes", it was no longer possible to dismiss the older literature on aphasia and simply to deny the thesis of localization and connectionism. Largely in consequence of this, it has become the standard practice in aphasia research pursued in a neurological context to cite the earlier literature. This practice is found both in the work of those who would espouse the connectionist framework and those who would quarrel with it. It is a practice which is more than a mere historical nicety. As Geschwind demonstrated in "Disconnexion Syndromes" and a number of historical papers, the earlier literature is filled with well-documented cases which must be taken into account in attempting to analyze behavior in a biological context.

The force of Geschwind's argument throughout his life was that behavioral disorders must be analyzed in terms of explicit hypotheses as to the underlying neural mechanisms. He saw cortico-cortico connections as being a highly significant mechanism. These he investigated in a variety of reports on various disorders. He did extensive research on the acquired alexias and the functional neurological distinction between alexia without agraphia and alexia with agraphia (Geschwind, 1962, 1966; Benson and Geschwind, 1969; Heilman et al., 1973). Following Dejerine, he analyzed the former disorder as a disconnection syndrome; the latter disorder he treated as an impairment to a "center" committed to visual language functions. His analysis of the apraxias, frequent concomitants of aphasias, also turned on the notion of a disconnection syndrome, in that case a disconnection between the language system and the pyramidal motor system which precluded the carrying out of acquired (lateralized) movements to commands (Geschwind, 1967). He also appealed to the concept of disconnection in his analyses of the isolation syndrome (Geschwind, Quadfasel and Segarra, 1968), and conduction aphasia (Benson et al., 1973).

Significant in the development of his ideas and research on aphasia were the people he came to work with at the Boston VA hospital, Harold Goodglass, Davis Howes, and Edith Kaplan. In the early 1960s Geschwind and his colleagues established the Boston University Aphasia Research Center at the VA. The Center was original in its inception, a multidisciplinary unit for the neurological, psychological, and linguistic study of the aphasias, and has been a focal point of aphasia research since its founding. The VA aphasia unit attracted a number of young neurologists as fellows whose work was significantly influenced by Geschwind. D. Frank Benson, François Boller, Antonio Damasio, and Alan Rubens were among the VA fellows. In later years at Boston City Hospital and Beth Israel Hospital he also worked with a number of neurologists to whose future research careers in aphasia he gave significant direction; among these were Kenneth Heilman, Elliott Ross, and David Caplan. These people, as well as those who worked with Geschwind in his other areas of interest — epilepsy, neuroanatomy, and developmental dyslexia, primarily — have carried on in the tradition he (re)invigorated, enriching and arguing with his basic approach to the study of behavior in a neurological context. Beyond his inspired teaching of medical students and training of residents and fellows, he actively encouraged and supported interdisciplinary research involving linguists and psychologists. He is, ultimately, largely responsible for the current richness and enthusiasm of aphasia research; the robustness of the field today is his legacy.

References

Benson, D.F. and N. Geschwind. 1969. "The Alexias". *Handbook of Clinical Neurology* Vol 4, ed. by P.J. Vinken and G.W. Bruyn. Amsterdam: North Holland.
——, W.A. Sheremata, R. Bouchard, J.M. Segarra, D. Price and N. Geschwind. 1973. "Conduction aphasia: A clinicopathological study". *Archives of Neurology* 28: 339-346.
Dejerine, J. 1892. "Contribution à l'étude anatomique et clinique des différentes varieties de cécité verbale". *Mémoires de la Société de Biologie* 4: 61-90.
Gazzaniga, M.S., J.E. Bogen and R.W. Sperry. 1962. "Some functional effects of sectioning the cerebral commissures in man". *Proceedings of the National Academy of Science* (USA), 48: 1765-1769.
Geschwind, N. 1962. "The anatomy of acquired disorders of reading". *Reading Disability*, ed. by J. Money. Baltimore: John Hopkins Press.
——. 1965. "Disconnexion syndromes in animals and man." *Brain* 88: 237-294; 585-644.
—— and M. Fusillo. 1966. "Color-naming defects in association with alexia". *Archives of Neurology* 15: 137-146.
——. 1967. "The Apraxias". *Phenomenology of Will and Action*, ed. by E.W. Strauss and R.M. Griffith. Pittsburgh: Duquesne University Press.
——. 1974. *Selected Papers on Language and the Brain*. Dordrecht: D. Reidel.

———— and E. Kaplan. 1962. "A human cerebral disconnection syndrome: A preliminary report". *Neurology* 12: 675-685.

————, F.A. Quadfasel and J.M. Segarra. 1968. "Isolation of the speech area". *Neuropsychologia* 6: 327-340.

Heilman, K.M., J.M. Coyle, E.F. Gonyea and N. Geschwind. 1973. "Apraxia and agraphia in a left-hander". *Brain* 96: 21-28.

Liepmann, H. 1898. "Das Krankheitsbild der Apraxie". *Monatschrift für die Psychiatrie und Neurologie* 18: 15-44, 102-132, 182-197.

———— and E. Storch. 1902. *Monatschrift für die Psychiatrie und Neurologie* 11: 115-120.

Myers, R.E. 1962. "Commissural connections between occipital lobes of the monkey". *Journal of Comparative Neurology* 118: 1-16.

Selection from the work of
Norman Geschwind

Disconnexion Syndromes in Animals and Man*

Summary

A complete summary of all the material presented would be much too extensive and, indeed, much too repetitious. I will therefore try to outline here the major points presented in this chapter. I have attempted to show that many disturbances of the higher functions of the nervous system, such as the aphasias, apraxias, and agnosias may be most fruitfully studied as disturbances produced by anatomical disconnexion of primary receptive and motor areas from one another. For a detailed discussion the reader is referred to the appropriate sections of the paper.

In the lower mammals connexions between regions of the cortex may arise directly from the primary receptive or motor areas. As one moves up the phylogenetic scale, these connexions come to be made between newly developed regions of cortex interspersed between the older zones. These regions are called 'association cortex'. As Flechsig pointed out for the human brain, all intercortical long connexions (whether in or between hemispheres) are made by way of these association areas and not between the primary motor or receptive areas. It follows from this that lesions of association cortex, if extensive enough, act to disconnect primary receptive or motor areas from other regions of the cortex in the same or in the opposite hemisphere.

The connexions of the visual association regions were discussed in

* From *Brain*, 1965, 88, 639-642.

some detail, and it was pointed out that the major outflow of these regions is to the lateral and basal neocortex of the temporal lobe which in turn connects to limbic structures. Lesions of the lateral and basal temporal lobe therefore tend to disconnect the visual region from the limbic system. This leads to a failure of visual stimulation to activate limbic responses, such as fight, flight, and sexual approach. It also leads to difficulties in visual learning. These can be thought of as resulting from the failure of the animal to form visual-limbic associations (such as learning that a visual stimulus equals the food reward given for correct choice) because of the lack of appropriate connexions. They can also be regarded as disturbances in visual recent memory resulting from a disconnexion between the visual region and the hippocampal region. The discussion was then applied to the tactile and auditory systems. Learning difficulties in primates involving these systems also were thought to result from disconnexions from the limbic system. 'Agnosia' in the sense of failure to respond to stimuli within a single modality appropriately in the face of intact perception in that modality is regarded as being a part of the syndrome of disconnexion of primary sensory modalities from the limbic system. Since callosal fibres arise from association cortex, failures of interhemispheric transfer may result from lesions of association cortex. The problem of whether disconnexions of single modalities from the limbic system in man occur was briefly discussed.

While connexions between primary receptive regions and limbic structures are powerful in subhuman forms, intermodal connexions between vision, audition, and somesthesis are probably weak in these animals, a view for which evidence is available both on the basis of experimental behavioural investigations (e.g. studies on intermodal transfer of learning and on higher-order conditioning) and on the basis of anatomical evidence. In man the situation changes with the development of the association areas of the human inferior parietal lobule, situated at the junction of the older association areas attached to the visual, somesthetic, and auditory regions. It is speculated that this new 'association area of association areas' now frees man from the dominant pattern of sensory-limbic associations and permits cross-modal associations involving non-limbic modalities. It is particularly the visual-auditory and tactile-auditory associations which constitute the basis of the development of speech in most humans. In man the speech area (which constitutes the auditory association cortex, particularly that part of it on the convexity of the temporal lobe, also Broca's area and the connexions between these regions) becomes a structure of major importance in the analysis of all the higher functions.

Pure word-blindness without agraphia was then discussed as an excellent, classical example of disconnexion from the speech area; this syndrome results from a combination of lesions, the usual one being destruction of the left visual cortex and of the splenium of the corpus callosum. The association with this syndrome of colour-naming difficulties and inability to read music is noted, along with the relatively strong preservation of the reading of numbers and the naming of objects. Reasons are advanced for these discrepancies. The problem of childhood dyslexia and its associated disturbances and its possible relation to the acquired dyslexia of adults was briefly presented.

Other disorders with similar pathogenesis (isolation of a particular sensory modality from the speech area), i.e. pure word-deafness and tactile aphasia were then briefly discussed.

The problem of the 'agnosias' was then presented. Evidence was presented against the idea that there exist disturbances of 'recognition' regarded as a unitary faculty. It was argued that most of the 'agnosias' are in fact modality-specific naming defects resulting from isolation of the primary sensory cortex from the speech area and associated with marked confabulatory response. A critique was presented of the classical 'aphasic-agnostic' distinction. There was presented some further discussion on the determinants of confabulatory response. The problem of right parietal syndromes was presented in the light of the preceding discussion of the 'agnosias'.

'Apraxic' disturbances were analysed in detail and were regarded as resulting from disconnexions of the posterior speech area from association areas which lie anterior to the primary motor cortex, and from disconnexions of visual association areas from these 'motor association' areas. The problem of left-sided predominance was discussed. In particular apraxic disturbances resulting from callosal lesions, from lesions of 'motor association' cortex and from damage deep to the supramarginal gyrus were discussed. The apraxia of the left side ('sympathetic dyspraxia') of aphasic right hemiplegics was discussed as well as facial apraxia. The sparing of certain types of movement in the apraxias was discussed, particularly whole body movements and was related to the probable preservation of Türck's bundle (whose connexions were presented in some detail) running from the posterior temporal region to the pontine nuclei and then via synapses to the cerebellar vermis.

Finally syndromes resulting from disconnexions within the speech area (conduction aphasia) and the pattern resulting from the isolation of the speech area were presented.

Some classical objections to the disconnexion approach were presented, in particular the results of Akelaitis and reasons for his negative results were discussed. This section closed by pointing out that this type of theory suggests many experiments and anatomical investigations. The dangers of *ad hoc* postulation of connexions were mentioned.

In a short section attention was called to some philosophical implications of these findings, particularly for the notions of 'regarding the patient as a whole man', the unity of consciousness, the uses of introspection and the relations between language and one's view of the world.

(same text, pp. 272-290)

1. The Anatomical Basis of Language

Man was the first species in whom disconnexion syndromes were clearly delineated. The writings of Dejerine and Liepmann mentioned in the introduction constitute the great landmarks of the early period of this type of investigation. I have placed the human material later in this paper later in this paper because I feel it makes more sense to study it from the point of view of the evolution of the nervous system. As I have pointed out earlier, many of the discussions presented in this section can, in fact, be considered independently of the evolutionary hypotheses; despite this fact, I believe that these hypotheses may aid in bringing order into the material and in stimulating the design of specific experiments.

The preceeding parts of this paper have cited the evidence that in lower mammals, the primary projection areas of the cortex subserve certain functions which tend subsequently to be separated in the primates. In keeping with this relatively minor degree of separation of functions, only a few regions of differing cytoarchitectonic structure are distinguishable. As we ascend the phylogenetic scale, the associative activities become separated to a great extent from the receptive. Large association areas more clearly separable from primary projection areas appear, and cytoarchitectonic differentiations increase. In accordance with the principle of Flechsig (which is applicable to man and the other primates but not to subprimate forms), the primary projection areas now send their connexions primarily to the immediately adjacent association cortex (para- konio-cortex); the long connexions (either within a hemisphere or between hemispheres) between different cortical regions take place predominantly between parts of the association cortex. To a great extent the most important connexions of the association cortex are with the neocortex of the temporal lobe (and perhaps also of the insula) which in turn feeds into limbic structures. In keeping with this, connexions involving linkages between any one sensory modality and the limbic system tend to be powerful (these connexions subserve emotional and autonomic responses to sensory stimuli, associations between one sensory modality and gustatory or olfactory stimuli, etc.) while other non-limbic sensory-sensory connexions tend to be weak. I have, in the first part of this paper, discussed in detail the effects of lesions separating the primary sensory modalities from the limbic structures in the primate.

The situation in man is not simply a slightly more complex version of the situation present in the higher primates but depends on the introduction of a new anatomical structure, the human inferior parietal lobule, which includes the angular and supramarginal gyri, to a rough approximation areas 39 and 40 of Brodmann. In keeping with the views of many anatomists Crosby et al. (1962) comment that these areas have not been recognized in the macaque. Critchley (1953), in his review of the anatomy of this region, says that even in the higher apes these areas are present only in rudimentary form. In keeping with the late evolutionary development of this region are certain other findings. The gyral structure of this area tends to be highly variable. In addition this area is one of the late myelinating regions or 'terminal zones' as Flechsig termed them. In fact, this region was in Flechsig's map, one of the last three to myelinate. DeCrinis (cited by Bonin and Bailey, 1961) showed that part of this region is one of the last cortical areas in which dendrites appear. Yakovlev (personal communication) has pointed out that this region matures cytoarchitectonically very late, often in late childhood. In addition, he has pointed out that preliminary studies suggest that this region receives very few thalamic afferents. In this respect it is similar to part of the frontal association area which is also largely athalamic; this part of the frontal lobe is also phylogenetically new, myelinates late and forms dendrites late. The afferent connexions of this new parietal association area may therefore be predominantly from other cortical regions. As an association area, this region is also different from the older association areas in not being essentially concentric with one of the primary projection centres.

The newness of this region is also reflected in another anatomical feature probably unique to the human brain. G. Elliot Smith (1907) studied distinctions of cortical architecture based on naked-eye appearances of the freshly cut brain. He found that his inferior parietal area A (roughly corresponding to the region I have been discussing here) was bounded above and below by thin distinctive bands of cortex. The lower is the so-called 'visuo-auditory band'. As Elliot Smith comments, "This attenuated band is all that is left of the extensive bond of union between these two areas which in the lower mammals have co-extensive borders: in man and to a less extent in the apes the great development of the inferior parietal area above it and the temporal areas below it have pushed these two parts asunder, leaving this narrow connecting bridge. In support of this hypothesis of the primitive nature of the band, I might call attention to the fact (which Flechsig has clearly established) of its early medullation..." The upper band is the 'visuo-sensory band', another thin band of cortex running along the superior lip of the intraparietal sulcus. Flechsig had shown that this strand also undergoes early myelination. Elliot Smith comments, "It is the attenuated fragment of that extensive connexion between the visual and sensory areas of the brain which has remained after these areas have been pushed apart by the great expansion of the parietal areas..." Cytoarchitectural studies such as those of von Economo and Koskinas have confirmed the existence in this band of cortex of structure different from that of the cortex above and below the band.

Some authors (e.g. Konorski recently) have interpreted certain clinical syndromes as disconnexions between visual and other sensory spheres resulting from lesions of these bands. I believe, in fact, that the primitive character of the bands and their small size make these interpretations unlikely; more probable is that the observed phenomena resulted from lesions of the adjacent portions of the inferior parietal lobule.

We thus have this extensive, evolutionarily advanced, parietal association area developing not in apposition to the primary projection areas for vision, somesthetic sensibility, and hearing but rather at the point of junction of these areas as Critchley (1953) has indicated. This region possibly being one of few thalamic connexions may well receive most of its afferents from the adjacent association areas; it is thus an association area of association areas. In more classical terms, it would be called a secondary association area. The probable significance of this anatomical location is heightened by reference to our earlier discussion of subhuman forms. In these it appears as if association areas feed into temporal neocortex relaying in turn to limbic and rhinencephalic structures. As I pointed out in the earlier discussion, cross-connexions between primary nonlimbic sensory modalities are weak in subhuman forms. In man, with the introduction of the angular gyrus region, intermodal associations become powerful. In a sense the parietal association area frees to some extent from the limbic system. This independence is only relative since ultimately learning still depends, even in man, on intact connections with limbic structures. The well-known permanent severe disturbance of new learning resulting from bilateral lesions of the hippocampal region attests to this fact (Scoville and Milner, 1957).

The development of language is probably heavily dependent on the emergence of the parietal association area since at least in what is perhaps its simplest aspect (object naming) language depends on associations between other modalities and audition. Early language experience, at least, most likely depends heavily on the forming of somesthetic-auditory and visual-auditory associations, as well as auditory-auditory associations. Whether this great association area is as powerfully involved in mediating other cross-modal associations (e.g. visual-tactile) is not clear. Situations which demand these other types of cross-modal association appear to be less important than those involving audition, probably because language depends on this latter type of association. Perhaps in the deaf person learning written language tactile-visual associations become important. Critchley (1953) comments that it is tempting to associate the growth of the post-parietal region with the development of speech. I would think that the parietal region is involved in the development of speech because of its importance in enhancing cross-modal associations. As I have noted earlier, it *cannot be argued that the ability to form cross-modal associations depends on already having speech*; rather we must say that *the ability to acquire speech has as a prerequisite the ability to form cross-modal associations*. An important area of research which remains to be studied extensively is that of the course of acquisition of cross-modal learning in childhood before speech is fully developed.

The objection might be raised that in some congenitally deaf people language is learned entirely in the form of visual-visual associations. If we restate the principle stated above in somewhat more precise form it will be seen that this objection is readily met. *In sub-human forms the only readily established sensory-sensory associations are those between a non-limbic (i.e.*

visual, tactile or auditory) stimulus and a limbic stimulus. It is only in man that associations between two non-limbic stimuli are readily formed and it is this ability which underlies the learning of names of objects (Geschwind, 1964b).

It is also not unlikely that the development of cerebral dominance is related to greater development of this new parietal association area. Bonin (1962) has discussed this problem and stressed the smallness of the differences between hemispheres. However, the results which he himself quotes as well as those cited by Connolly (1950) do, in fact, tend to support the view that the left hemisphere is the more developed, at least as far as fissural pattern is concerned, and it is quite possible that Bonin's assessment of the data is much too conservative. I would speculate that left cerebral dominance is based on (or indeed perhaps equivalent to) the ability of the left hemisphere more readily to make cross-modal associations, an ability perhaps based on greater development of the left posterior parietal region. A detailed discussion of dominance would, however, lead us too afar afield.

We will simply assume from here on that the left hemisphere is dominant for speech functions and that this dominance depends on enhanced activity of the left speech area. The most important part of this area is the middle and posterior portions of the superior temporal gyrus which are, of course, part of the auditory association area and form the classical Wernicke's area. Connexions from other sensory modalities, at least vision and somesthetic sensation, are assumed to come to this speech zone by way of the angular gyrus region. Connexions from the speech area to other sensory parts of brain (i.e. connexions which subserve the arousing of tactile and visual associations by auditory stimuli in general and speech in particular) are presumed to go in the reverse direction by way of the angular gyrus region. An important area of research is suggested by these briefly stated assumptions: the detailed pattern of connexions between the angular gyrus and the specified regions of the superior temporal gyrus (roughly area 22 of Brodmann) deserves careful elucidation.

I would like to point out here that although the predominance of the human parietal association areas is generally admitted not all authors would give them as much prominence as I have. Thus Bonin and Bailey (1947) state, "We cannot agree... that the homologues of Brodmann's areas 39 and 40 in man exist in the macaque only as very small patches..." These same authors, however (Bonin and Bailey, 1961), stress that the part of the brain which increases in man most strikingly is not the frontal lobe but "the parietal and temporal lobe in the widest meanings of that term, and it is here that we should look for the substrate of certain functions which are supposed to be characteristic of man". They quote with approval Weidenreich's statement that the growth of the brain in man affects primarily the parietal lobes and the posterior region of the inferior part of the temporal lobe. At any rate, if these authors deny the marked parietal predominance that I have stressed they at least admit a relative predominance of this region in man. The exact degree of the uniqueness of the inferior parietal region in man remains to be determined.

In the preceding paragraphs I have outlined some of the new elements that must be considered in evaluating disturbances of the higher functions in man. In animals I have stressed disconnexions from the limbic system. In man with the development of speech, Wernicke's area becomes of major importance. Disconnexion syndromes will result from lesions which cut off Wernicke's area from primary sensory areas. Some of these lesions will lie in the white matter of the hemispheres while others will involve the cortex of the angular gyrus which probably acts as a way station between the primary sensory modalities and the speech area. In addition lesions which cut off connexions from Wernicke's area to motor portions of the hemispheres will lead to profound effects on behaviour.

In the following sections I will specify in greater depth some of the clinical and anatomical evidence which supports the model I have sketched. I will first consider lesions which lead to modality-specific disturbances by isolating specific sensory projection regions from the speech area. The lesions producing these disconnecting effects may be either in white matter systems such as the corpus callosum or in the association cortex giving rise to these fibre tracts. This discussion of highly specific receptive aphasic disturbances will lead us into a discussion of a related group of impairments, the agnosias. Similarly, I will consider disconnexions of this posterior temporal speech area from the motor systems, which will lead us into a discussion of the apraxias. Finally, I will consider disconnexions of the posterior speech area from the anterior (frontal) speech region.

2. Pure Word-blindness Without Agraphia

This condition must be regarded as of special importance since it is probably the first example of a callosal disconnexion syndrome for which clear anatomical evidence was forthcoming. I have discussed Dejerine's (1891, 1892) classic papers elsewhere in detail (Geschwind, 1962) and will only summarize here. Dejerine developed his analysis of word-blindness on the basis of the findings of two patients reported in consecutive years. The first patient (Dejerine, 1891) showed the clinical picture of pure alexia *with* agraphia in the absence of other significant aphasic disturbances. The second patient had by contrast the syndrome of pure alexia *without* agraphia. The information from the two cases combines to form a simple picture of the mechanisms of disturbances of reading. Before discussing pure word-blindness without agraphia, I will present first the findings in alexia with agraphia.

The first paper (Dejerine, 1891) described a 63-year-old man who developed the sudden onset of inability to read and write in the absence of other significant neurological disabilities except for a right hemianopia. At post-mortem (eight months after the onset) the brain was entirely normal except for a lesion involving the inferior three-quarters of the angular gyrus and penetrating inwards to the occipital horn of the lateral ventricle. The inward extent of the lesion had, of course, involved the optic radiations. Dejerine concluded that the lesion had destroyed a 'visual memory centre for words' with resultant loss of the ability to comprehend written language or to write. Within a year Berkhan and Serieux (cited by Dejerine, 1892) had published similar cases with similar localization.

The second paper (Dejerine, 1892), longer and more detailed than the first, describes a patient followed by Dejerine over a period of more than four years. This patient suffered from the acute loss of the ability to read letters, words or musical notation in association with a right hemianopia. He could copy words correctly but could not transcribe print into script; he could write correctly (in script) either spontaneously or to dictation but could not read what he had written a short time previously. Although he could not read 'visually', he could 'read' by tracing the outlines of letters with his hand and could recognize the letters formed by having the examiner move his hand passively through the air. Although he could not read, he was able to name even extremely complex objects such as pictures of scientific instruments in a catalogue. There was no evidence of any general intellectual disturbance since the patient continued during his illness to operate a highly successful business, to gamble at cards successfully, and to learn vocal and instrumental parts of operas by ear since he could no longer read music. Ten days before death he suddenly developed an agraphia. At post-mortem the brain showed an infarct of the left occipital lobe and of the splenium of the corpus callosum. The occipital infarct was shrunken and yellow and adherent to the overlying meninges, all of which indicated a lesion of considerable age. By contrast the patient showed a fresh infarct of the left angular gyrus which must have led to the new symptomatology ten days before death.

Dejerine interpreted this case as a disconnexion of the visual cortex from the speech area. Since the left occipital cortex was destroyed, this patient could perceive words only in the left visual field, i.e. only in the right occipital cortex. It is, however, not possible to read with the right hemisphere alone since destruction of the left hemisphere produces an alexia as one part of a gross aphasic syndrome. The visual stimuli received in the right visual cortex must therefore be transmitted to some region of the left hemisphere. It would seem reasonable on the basis of the findings of the first case discussed to assume that the relevant region in the left hemisphere is in the angular gyrus. The extensive lesion of the white matter of the left occipital lobe and of the splenium of the corpus callosum, how- ever, cut off the connexions between the right occipital lobe and the left angular gyrus. Dejerine therefore argued that pure word-blindness without agraphia resulted from disconnexion of the intact right visual cortex from the left angular gyrus in a patient in whom the left visual cortex had been destroyed.

The preservation of the left angular gyrus explains several aspects of the syndrome of alexia without agraphia. Thus, the preserved ability to write suggested to Dejerine that the 'visual word-centre' was intact. The ability to 'read' tactilely clearly relies on the fact that the pathway to the angular gyrus via the somesthetic system is intact.

There is one further difference between pure alexia with agraphia and pure alexia without agraphia which supports the Dejerine interpretation of the former syndrome as the result of a lesion of a 'memory centre' and of the latter as a disconnexion from this 'memory centre'. Dr. Davis Howes and I have had the opportunity to observe the spelling performance of a patient with pure alexia with agraphia. This patient had normal spontane- ous speech. He was unable, however, to spell correctly even the simplest word. Similarly, although he understood complex spoken sentences, he could not understand even three- or four-letter words when they were spel- led to him. By contrast the two patients with pure alexia without agraphia whom I have observed (one in collaboration with Dr. Howes and one with

Dr. Michael Fusillo) have been able both to spell and to comprehend simple spelled words. The explanation of this phenomenon derives from the fact that spelling is learned only as part of learning to read and write. In order to comprehend a word spelled out loud, the listener must transform it into written form and then 'read' it. Conversely, to spell orally one must transform the spoken word into its written form and then 'read' the letters one by one. One can state this argument more simply by noting that a loss of visual word-memory returns the patient to the state of being illiterate; lack of reading, writing, and spelling and incomprehension of spelled words are all components of this more primitive state.[1] The patient with pure alexia without agraphia preserves the ability to spell since he still preserves the 'centre' which turns spoken into written language and also carries on the reverse operation.

Parenthetically it should be noted that this disturbance of spelling gives us a particularly useful clue as to the function of the part of the angular gyrus involved in 'visual word memory'. It is a region which turns written language into spoken language and vice versa. It is, in short, a region specifically designed for carrying on visual-auditory cross-modal associations in both directions and indeed for storing the memory of the 'rules of translation' from written to spoken language. I will return to this point later on.

It should be pointed out that Dejerine's paper described only the gross findings in the brain of the patient with pure alexia without agraphia. Vialet (1893) published a year later the detailed description of the central nervous system which had been cut in whole brain sections.[2] The lesion described by Dejerine for pure alexia without agraphia was soon confirmed by other authors. Bastian (1898) only a few years after Dejerine's publication was able to cite several cases where the lesion had involved the left occipital cortex and the splenium of the corpus callosum.

Many facts can be marshalled to show the importance of the lesion of the splenium which acts to disconnect the right visual region from the angular gyrus. Foix and Hillemand (1925) pointed out that one patient who at post-mortem had an infarct of the left visual cortex without involvement of the splenium had had no alexia in life; another patient with an infarct of the left visual cortex and in addition destruction of the splenium had shown the syndrome of alexia without agraphia. As I have pointed out elsewhere (Geschwind, 1962), the lack of this syndrome after penetrating head trauma results from the fact that a missile is very unlikely to destroy the left visual cortex and the splenium of the corpus callosum. The study of Hecaen et al.

(1952) showed that alexia invariably occurred after left occipital lobectomy but was transient in all cases, clearing in a few months. The splenium, of course, was left intact so that there was a path from the right occipital cortex to the left angular gyrus. The case of Trescher and Ford (1937) and the cases of Maspes (1948) who had the splenium cut in the course of removal of a colloid cyst of the third ventricle all developed alexia in the left visual field. By contrast, the patient of Geschwind and Kaplan (1962b) in whom there was no alexia of the left visual field showed at post-mortem an intact splenium although the anterior four-fifths of the callosum was infarcted. The patient of Gazzaniga, Bogen and Sperry (1962) in whom the splenium was cut showed an alexia in the left visual field.

By contrast to the above results, Akelaitis (1941b, 1943, 1944) described six patients in whom the splenium had been cut and who showed no alexia in the left visual field, I will defer a critique of these discrepancies to a later section of the paper where all the Akelaitis results will be discussed.

A further anatomical point deserves discussion. The first is the exact path of the connexions between the right visual cortex and the angular gyrus. Since the visual cortex has no callosal fibres, this pathway must be by way of the association areas, i.e. the pathway goes from the right area 17 to the right-sided area 18 (Myers, 1962a) and from this it eventually crosses the callosum.

I can conceive of three possibilities for the course of this pathway: (1) The pathway proceeds from the right area 17 to the right visual association areas, from there to the right angular gyrus and finally across the corpus callosum to the left angular gyrus. (2) The pathway runs from the right area 17 to the right visual association areas, then crosses the callosum to the left visual association areas and finally runs forward to the left angular gyrus. (3) The third possibility is that both pathways are used. This possibility is the one that would appear most likely under the assumption that we are dealing with an equipotential system in which a part can take over some of the functions of the whole.

Possibility 2 is ruled out as the *exclusive* pathway by the fact that no permanent alexia results from left occipital lobectomies (Hecaen et al., 1952). But that there is some participation of this pathway is made highly likely by the fact that the alexia from left occipital lobectomy does last for several months, too long for the effect to be due to post-operative oedema but long enough for pathway 1 to come to take over the role completely.

There is probably some permanent effect of destroying pathway 2 since as Hecaen et al. (1952) point out, their patients with left occipital lobectomies disliked reading even after their ability to read had returned.

It is likely that pathway 1 also participates normally since patients with right parietal lesions may show a failure to read the left halves of words despite an intact left visual field (Kinsbourne and Warrington, 1962). The localization of the lesions in this latter paper, however, is not certain and more studies will be needed. The conclusions are, however, in keeping with the clinical observations of others on alexias from right parietal lesions.[3] It would thus appear that both pathways are normally used, i.e. possibility 3 is the correct one.

If we refer back to our earlier discussion of the possible functions of the angular gyrus, we can speculate as to the mechanism of its function as a visual memory centre for words. The angular gyrus, as we have noted already, becomes a memory for written words by acting as an area for form-ing — and storing — cross-modal associations between vision and hearing. It seems likely that this store of cross-modal associations involves more than words. An analysis of what is lost and preserved in pure alexia without agraphia may help to clarify this point.

While the reading aloud and comprehension of written words is lost, the ability to name and recognize objects is preserved. We can expand a suggestion by Adolf Meyer (1905) to develop the explanation for this. Objects have rich associations in other modalities, e.g. we can recognize an apple by vision, touch, taste, smell, even by its texture on being bitten. The arousal of such associations permits the finding of an alternative pathway across an uninvolved more anterior portion of the corpus callosum. The reading of numbers is also frequently preserved in these cases — in Dejerine's case number reading was perfect. Other authors, e.g. Symonds (1953), have discussed this striking fact. The learning of numbers is also associated with heavy somesthetic reinforcement (counting on the fingers) which frequently persists for a long time in childhood because the child can use his own fingers for this purpose. By contrast, reading is learned, except in the very earliest stages, as a pure visual-auditory task.

A difficulty with colours is common in these cases. Dr. Michael Fusillo and I (Geschwind and Fusillo, 1964) have recently studied a case of pure word-blindness with persistent difficulty in colours. We were able to show that this was a pure difficulty in colour-*naming*. Thus the patient matched colours by hue without error despite large differences in brightness and saturation. He would without error identify the figures on two different pseudo-isochromatic tests of colour vision. It is obvious that a colour has no smell, taste, or feel — the only association unique to the colour is its name. The loss of colour-naming is thus another example of loss of visual-auditory associations. The loss of ability to read music, as in Dejerine's case, appears to be another example of loss of visual-auditory associations.

I would like to stress the fact that many combinations of lesions may lead to the same syndrome. I recently observed a patient who had suffered a cerebral vascular accident which seemed likely to have been in the left posterior parietal region. A year later he developed a *left* hemianopia and became alexic. I wondered whether his initial lesion had not destroyed the connexions between his *left* visual cortex and his left angular gyrus so that he was reading only with the right occipital cortex until this was destroyed by a subsequent infarct. Unfortunately a post-mortem was not obtained and the above must remain pure speculation. This case illustrates, however, that it is a serious error to reject a case with multiple lesions since some interesting syndromes may result in such situations which could not be the effect of any single lesion.

Another area of speculation is the applicability of these results to failures of acquisition of reading, so-called congenital dyslexia. One possibility is that this syndrome is due to delayed development of the angular gyrus region — probably bilaterally. The results cited earlier that the angular gyrus region typically matures late make it plausible that a significant group will not have achieved adequate development by the time of the usual age of learning to read. The tendency for this condition to disappear in many children with increasing age is compatible with the notion of slow maturation. The smaller proportion of girls showing this disturbance might be related to a more rapid maturation of the angular gyrus region in girls; this would be consistent with the more rapid attainment of most developmental milestones by girls. Study of an adequate number of anatomical specimens should make possible the verification or rejection of this developmental sex difference.

If the hypothesis of slow maturation is correct and if my views as to the possible functions of the angular gyrus region are correct, then certain predictions are possible. The child with congenital dyslexia should also show slower acquisition of colour-naming and music-reading. Reading of numbers should be more rapidly acquired. In fact, tests specifically designed to study cross-modal associations, particularly visual-auditory but also in the other modalities[4] might well be very rewarding. Birch (1962) has actually done preliminary studies on intersensory transfers in children and in particular in dyslexics. It will be most interesting to follow these pioneering studies.

It is probably necessary to study children as early as possible before language development has progressed very far and certainly before the learning of written language. I believe it would be possible to select a group in whom it could be predicted that the development of reading would be delayed on the basis of failures in learning other visual-auditory associations; it is conceivable that even the age of attainment of colour-naming might be a significant clue to the age at which reading can be acquired. Even casual observation among children shows a great variation in the age of acquisition of colour-naming among children in whom non-verbal testing shows colour-perception to be normal.

3. Pure Word-Deafness

Pure word-deafness probably has a similar pathogenesis to that of pure word-blindness without agraphia. Liepmann (1898) in a very carefully studied patient in whom ordinary deafness was clearly excluded showed that this syndrome could be produced by a unilateral lesion. The pathology was described in fuller detail by Liepmann and Storch (1902). The lesion, located subcortically in the left temporal lobe, had destroyed the left auditory radiation as well as the callosal fibres from the opposite auditory region. The lesion therefore had the effect of preventing the speech area (i.e. that part of the auditory association cortex generally called Wernicke's area, which comprises the posterior portion of area 22 and occupies the posterior part of the superior temporal gyrus) from receiving auditory stimulation. The right primary auditory cortex could receive auditory stimuli but could not convey them to the speech area because the callosal connexions from the right side were destroyed in the left temporal lobe. This syndrome is rarer than pure word-blindness without agraphia for the obvious reason that a lesion which involves these structures usually extends into Wernicke's area and produces a more extensive aphasic picture. Some variation in the extent of the lesion causing pure word-blindness without agraphia would not lead to such obscuring symptoms.

The exact anatomy of the auditory cortex and of the callosal pathways between the two auditory regions is still uncertain in primates and man, in contrast to the more advanced state of knowledge of the anatomical arrangements in the cat (Ades, 1959). The primate data are less complete not only because of the smaller number of experiments but also because of the concealment of areas 41 and 42 in the supratemporal plane, i.e. within the depths of the Sylvian fissure. The crowding of structures in the supratemporal plane makes it particularly difficult to study the responses of TB (area 42) which is interspersed between the primary auditory context TC (area 41) and the rather extensive and on the whole readily accessible TA (area 22) on the lateral surface (occupying the first temporal gyrus in its middle and posterior regions). The cat data cannot be applied to the primate with confidence, not only because the anatomical homologies are not obvious but also because the danger would always exist that the distinction of primary receptive and association areas was more sharply defined in the phylogenetically advanced primates. We have already remarked that such a discrepancy between primate and feline anatomy exists in the visual system; while the cat's visual cortex according to some authors gives rise to callosal fibres that of the primate does not (Curtis, 1940; McCulloch and Garol, 1941; Bailey et al., 1950; Myers, 1962a; Krieg, 1963).

The difficulties resulting from anatomical crowding on the supratemporal plane are reflected in the studies on the macaque where a clear-cut correlation between electrical response and cytoarchitecture has not so far been possible. The chimpanzee would probably represent a more suitable subject for this study because of the larger size of the brain. Bailey et al. (1943a) found in both the monkey and chimpanzee that auditory stimuli caused a large response in area 41 (TC) followed by a small one in area 42 (TB). However, in a later publication on the chimpanzee Bailey, Bonin and McCulloch (1950) note, "It is impossible on the basis of our scanty data to separate surely the connexions of the auditory cortex (TC) from those of the para-auditory (TB). The efferent fibres seem to come mainly from the periphery, therefore, probably from TB". Sugar et al. (1948) studied the supratemporal plane in monkeys; they simply divided this region into five strips without regard to cytological differentiations between areas 41 and 42. They found the area of primary auditory response in the posterior third of the supratemporal plane. On strychninization this region fired the remainder of the supratemporal plane and also areas 22, 21 and 37; however, one cannot conclude with certainty that the primary auditory cortex itself fires these regions since the possibility must exist that the stimulated area may also have included part of area 42. These authors like McCulloch and Garol (1941) found a paucity of callosal fibres arising from area 22 or reaching area 22 from any part of the auditory system of the opposite side. Callosal fibres from one supratemporal plane to the other were plentiful but no distinction was made as to whether they arose from area 41 or 42. The data of Sugar and his co-workers suggest that there are more callosal fibres from the anterior portion of the supratemporal plane. This may correspond to the region in which Bailey et al. (1943a) saw small secondary responses and which they regarded as the anterior part of TB.

The suggestion that the main associative outflow of the auditory cortex is in the anterior part of the supratemporal plane receives some support in the work of Pribram et al. (1954). They found in the macaque that the region of short-latency responses to click lay posteriorly in the supratemporal plane; there was an anterior strip in which responses of much longer latency were seen. It would seem likely that these anterior regions are 'secondary' areas which are fired by the primary areas.[5]

We have presented these data in some detail to emphasize the tenuous nature of our knowledge of auditory association areas in the primate, and, obviously, in man. We might summarize roughly by saying that there appears to be general agreement that the centre of the primary auditory cortex lies in the posterior part of the supratemporal plane. Area 22 on the lateral surface of the first temporal gyrus constitutes a large area of auditory association cortex but is probably not the source of the callosal fibres of the auditory system. Callosal fibres probably arise from the supratemporal plane somewhat anterior to the primary auditory cortex. However, more detailed physiological study is needed to confirm even this rough picture. In addition a more careful study of the correlation of the pattern of transmission of impulses with cytoarchitectural differentiations is badly needed.

Clinical data perhaps may aid us in thinking about this problem and in suggesting further experiments in primates. As we noted at the beginning of this section Liepmann (1898) first described pure word-deafness from a *unilateral lesion*. There are, however, many more cases recorded of this syndrome from *bilateral* lesions. In these cases the most common pattern has been that of bilateral often rather symmetrical cortico-subcortical lesions in the *anterior* Part of T1, with Heschl's gyri intact. The subcortical penetration, particularly on the dominant side, is not very profound. These are the findings of Hoff (1961) but they generally coincide with those of other authors. Kurt Goldstein (1927) in his discussion of the localization of pure word-deafness places the lesion in the bilateral cases in the middle portion of T1. I suspect that this is not a difference from Hoff's data since they were probably both emphasizing as the centre of the involved zone roughly the junction of the anterior and middle thirds of T1. This zone is at the junction of area 42 with the anterior part of area 22. The precise mechanism of this lesion is not clear. One possibility is that the outflow from auditory cortex proper (area 41) goes to area 42, that the outflow path then continues from the region of junction of areas 42 and 22 posteriorly in area 22. The left-sided lesion would cut off the left auditory cortex from the left area 22; the right-sided lesion would cut off the origin of the callosal fibres (presumably coming from area 42) from the right auditory region. This interpretation would be in keeping with the findings in primates that area 22 gives rise itself to no callosal fibres. It would also be in keeping with our tentative summary of the experimental data which suggests that the major outflow from the primary auditory cortex is to a region anterior to itself. The correspondence between the two sets of data is at best rough but is close enough to suggest that further research may clarify this problem.

I will close this section with the consideration of a hypothetical problem. Could one develop pure word-deafness in one ear? The extent of duplication in the auditory pathways would almost ensure that the lesions necessary to produce this in a patient could hardly occur as the result of natural causes. With more detailed knowledge of the anatomy of the system one could probably specify what the requirements of such an unlikely lesion would be. Hartmann (1907) thought that one of his patients showed this phenomenon. There are, however, so many difficulties in the interpretation of other data pertaining to this particular case that I prefer to suspend judgment on the possibility of such a unilateral word-deafness.

4. Lesions of Wernicke's Area

Pure word-deafness as the preceding discussion suggests probably results from the disconnexion of Wernicke's area from auditory stimulation. The normalcy of the patient's speech testifies to the intactness of Wernicke's area. With a lesion in Wernicke's area proper not merely is verbal comprehension impaired, but speech is also impaired. I will not present my conception of this type of aphasia extensively here but would only point out that the loss of Wernicke's area can be regarded as the destruction of a memory store — as it was in fact regarded classically. Presumably it functions importantly as the 'storehouse' of auditory associations. I have already suggested the importance of the angular gyrus in acting as a region involved in cross-modal associations, particularly in cross-associations between either vision or touch and hearing. If the angular gyrus is important in the process of associating a heard name to a seen or felt object, it is probably also important for associations in the reverse direction. A 'name' passes through Wernicke's area, then via the angular gyrus arouses associations in the other parts of the brain. It is probably thus that Wernicke's area attains its essential importance in 'comprehension', i.e. the arousal of associations.

I have presented this only cursorily since a more extensive discussion would lead us to a consideration of topics lying beyond the range of our interest at this point. I would like to stress that what is here regarded speculatively as the function of Wernicke's area implies the existence of extensive connexions to the angular gyrus region. Since this latter region is probably so poorly developed in human forms, the fuller knowledge of this aspect of the connexions of Wernicke's area depends on careful study of those rare human cases with small lesions in the first temporal gyrus, particularly in its posterior portion. It is hoped that such studies will be made in the near future.[6]

5. Tactile Aphasia

This term describes a disturbance characterized by an inability to name objects tactilely with preservation of the ability to name on the basis of visual or auditory stimulation and in the presence of intact spontaneous speech. The existence of this condition has been disputed (see for example the discussion in Critchley, 1953). The case of Geschwind and Kaplan (1962b), however, established beyond doubt the existence of this entity and I will therefore present the relevant findings in this patient. I will confine myself to this aspect of the patient's problem and reserve discussion of the patient's 'apraxic' disturbances until a later section of the paper.

This patient had had an excision of a left frontal glioma. We examined him about six weeks later. This patient, when blindfolded, incorrectly named objects placed in the left hand. That this defect was one of *naming* was proved by several facts: (1) the patient would handle the objects correctly in the left hand while he was giving an incorrect name; (2) if the object was taken away and the patient was then instructed to select the object he had held from a group, he always selected the correct object either visually or tactually with his left hand; (3) similarly he could, after holding an object, concealed from vision, draw it correctly with his left hand although he had misnamed it. By contrast, after holding the object while blindfolded in his *left* hand, he could not afterwards select it from a group or draw it with the *right* hand. He correctly named objects held in the right hand and could draw such objects or select them from a group with the *right* hand but failed if he attempted to use the *left* hand for these taks. That the disturbance was not one of transfer between limbs but rather between hemispheres was shown by the fact that he could draw with the left foot a pattern drawn on his left hand but not one drawn on his right hand.

Testing of elementary somesthetic sensation was difficult to carry out in the left hand if verbal responses were demanded but not if nonverbal responses were used. Thus, he demonstrated correct position sense on the left when he was made to respond by pointing up or down with the left hand; verbally his answers were random in this situation. Two-point discrimination on the left was normal when tested by having the patient indicate with one or two fingers the number of points touched. By contrast his verbal responses were random; not only were replies of 'one' and 'two' given incorrectly, but such totally inappropriate responses as 'four' or 'eight'. He could correctly point with his left hand to a place touched on the left side but gave incorrect verbal responses. Pain sensation similarly could be shown to be normal.

In brief this patient responded correctly to somesthetic stimulation if response was demanded from the same hemisphere as the stimulus but not if respose was demanded from the opposite hemisphere. Thus, the patient responded correctly with his left hand to somesthetic stimulation of the left side of the body. By contrast his responses to such stimulation with the right hand were incorrect. In addition his verbal responses, which of course would have had to come from his left hemisphere, were incorrect when he was given somesthetic stimulation to the left side of the body. By contrast he responded correctly with the right hand to somesthetic stimulation of the right side of the body and gave correct verbal responses to such stimulation; in his testing situation he gave incorrect responses with the left hand.

We interpreted these disturbances as reflecting a failure of somesthetic stimulation to cross the opposite hemisphere and though that we would probably find a callosal lesion. The post-mortem confirmed the presence of a callosal infarction, probably secondary to ligation of the left anterior cerebral artery at the time of excision of the left frontal lobe. Tumour was entirely confined to the left hemisphere and did not involve either the callosum or the right hemisphere.

Had similar cases been observed before ours? Liepmann and others of the writers about the turn of the century had already commented on the inability of a patient to imitate with one hand the postures of the other as reflecting a callosal disconnexion. In addition, Liepmann (1900) called attention to the fact that the Regierungsrat who gave poor verbal responses on somesthetic stimulation must have had nearly intact sensation as evidenced by nonverbal manifestations. This disturbance was due to a disconnexion *within* the left hemisphere rather than to a callosal lesion. Goldstein (1908, 1927) on the basis of his own experience thought that a callosal lesion caused astereognosis on the left side of the body. Critchley (1953) mentions several other authors echoing the same opinion. Goldstein thought that this was the result of the fact that the left hemisphere was dominant for sensation. A more likely explanation is that Goldstein misinterpreted the incorrect verbal responses of his patient as representing sensory loss; he did not check whether sensation was intact when nonverbal criteria were used. The case of Trescher and Ford (1937) was regarded as having a 'tactile agnosia' on the left. Their patient showed only an inability to identify letters but not objects placed in the left hand. This more limited disturbance may well have a somewhat different interpretation from the more extensive disturbance in our patient.

The findings and interpretation of Geschwind and Kaplan have been more recently confirmed by Gazzaniga et al. (1962) who were able to demonstrate similar disturbances in a patient with a surgical transection of the corpus callosum.

None of these cases permit a more precise delineation of the pathways involved; one can only conclude that they traverse the midcallosum, a result already likely on anatomical grounds and on the basis of experimental results (Myers, 1962b). My earlier discussion on the somesthetic system in animals makes it likely that Flechsig's principle is followed here and that there are no callosal fibres from the primary somesthetic cortex in primates: the same rule probably holds in man. Ettlinger's (1962) experiments involved so much of parietal lobe posterior to the postcentral gyrus that they do not help us in deciding whether a more or less circumscribed part of the parietal lobe comprises the association cortex from which the callosal fibres which transfer somesthetic stimulation to the opposite side originate. After synapse at the corresponding locus in the left hemisphere the 'message' presumably can be shunted to the speech area (i.e. the auditory association cortex of area 22) or to other parts of the hemisphere.

This simple model which is concordant with the known anatomical facts has certain interesting implications. A lesion of the right parietal lobe which involves the association cortex might produce the same effect as a callosal lesion, i.e. a defect in naming objects held in the left hand and a failure of the right hand to select or draw correctly objects held in the left hand. It is possible that this syndrome exists although the lesion producing it probably must be a large one. It is also likely that such cases have been incorrectly recognized as cases of astereognosis rather than cases of tactile aphasia because of failure of correct examination technique. The problem of the locus of the lesion producing astereognosis has long béen a moot one and many authors have suggested a posterior parietal localization (see discussion in Critchley, 1953). Perhaps those with posterior parietal lesions were in fact cases of tactile naming defect based on the disconnexion of somesthetic regions from the speech area.

A lesion of the somesthetic association cortex on the left might have a more extensive effect. By destroying the connexion between left somesthetic cortex and speech area it should lead to a failure of tactile naming in the right hand. The lesion could also destroy the terminus of callosal fibres from the right hemispheric somesthetic association cortex and could therefore also produce tactile naming defect on the left. The net result should be a bilateral tactile naming effect. There is some evidence for the existence of this condition. My colleague, Mrs. Edith Kaplan, has recently called my attention to a patient who showed a marked difficulty of tactile naming in both hands while naming *visually* was nearly normal. That the disturbance was one of naming was shown by the fact that the patient could handle the object correctly or could select it afterwards from a group without error. This patient showed a further additional feature; he could correctly select from a group with one hand an object held with the other hand. This suggests that the callosal connexions between the two somesthetic association cortices were intact and that the lesion must lie between left somesthetic association cortex and speech area.

This patient exhibited no aphasia in speaking and an occasional mild visual naming difficulty. His chief finding, other than the tactile naming disorder, was pure alexia with agraphia. The evidence appeared good that the lesion was in the left posterior parietal region but in the absence of confirmatory evidence, we must restrict ourselves to the fact that this case illustrates the possibility of a bilateral disturbance of tactile naming in the presence of a much milder visual naming difficulty.

Other cases described in the literature are almost certainly cases of the same disturbance although again comparison is made difficult by the failure of most authors to have tested for evidence of retained stereognostic function by nonverbal means. Cases such as those of Foix (1922) in which a unilateral lesion is said to have led to bilateral astereognosis might well have turned out to be cases of bilateral tactile aphasia had tests for nonverbal recognition been employed. Some others have preferred the term 'tactile agnosia' for such cases as those of Raymond and Egger (1906). I feel, however, unconvinced by Claparède's highly philosophical critique of the use by these authors of the term 'tactile aphasia'. The broader question of the position of the agnosias will be dealt with in the next section.

Notes

1. This mechanism for incomprehension of spelled words appears to Dr. Howes and myself to be more simply and more clearly based physiologically than the classical explanation, which simply invokes a new disturbance, 'word-sound deafness', to account for incomprehension of spelled words. By any standard the term 'word-sound deafness' is a poor one. 'Letter-name deafness' would have been closer to being a correct description. 'Inability to understand words spelled orally' is the best descriptive term.

2. I am indebted to Sir Charles Symonds for having called Vialet's monograph to my attention. It was in fact his paper (Symonds, 1953) which alerted me to this interesting syndrome. I am also grateful to him for having read and criticized an earlier paper of mine on this topic.

3. It may be objected that the alexia in a half-field from a right parietal lesion is the result of 'neglect' of that field. While I do not wish to discuss this problem extensively here, I would like to point out that what I am attempting to show is that one mechanism of 'neglect' of a normal left visual field is disconnexion of the normal right occipital cortex from the speech area.

4. In an illiterate society a lack of visual-auditory associations would not seriously inconvenience anyone except in unusual situations; literacy makes this ability highly important. Other cross-modal association deficits may exist but might never be detected because they cause so little disturbance. It is conceivable that direct visual-tactile associations may be as badly developed in many humans as they appear to be in monkeys (Ettlinger, 1960) but only specific testing will bring this out. It is important, of course, to study children as early as possible in the course of development.

5. These authors also found another group of parietal areas which corresponded to click with only slightly longer latency than the primary auditory region. They presented evidence that the response in these areas depended on collaterals from the medial geniculate body. These areas would not in my terms be 'association' areas. I will not discuss their possible function here.

6. It should be added that the second temporal gyrus of man appears to be a phylogenetically very late region of whose connexions we know very little. It may be a region of great importance and it is conceivable that the view of Wernicke's area presented above is too narrow. I would, however, disagree with those authors who include in Wernicke's area all the posterior regions involved in speech in both the temporal and parietal lobes.

References

Ades, H.W. 1959. "Central Auditory Mechanisms". *Handbook of Physiology*, Vol 1. Washington: American Physiology Society.

Akelaitis, A.J. 1941. "Studies of the corpus callosum II. The higher visual functions in each homonymous field following complete section of the corpus callosum". *Archives of Neurology and Psychiatry* 45: 788-796.

———. 1943. "Studies of the corpus callosum VII. Study of language functions (tactile and visual lexis and graphia) unilaterally following section of the corpus callosum". *Journal of Neuropathology*, 2:226-262.

———. 1944. "A study of gnossis, praxis and language following section of the corpus callosum". *Journal of Neurosurgery* 1:94-102.

Bailey, P., G. von Bonin, H.W. Garal and W.S. McCulloch. 1943. *The Isocortex of Man Journal of Neurophysiology* 6: 121.

———, G. von Bonin and W.S. McCulloch. 1950. *The Isocortex of the Chimpansee*. Urbana: University of Illinois Press.

Bastian, H.C. 1898. *Aphasia and other Speech Defects*. London: H.K. Lewis.

Birch, H.G. 1962. *Reading Disability*, ed. by J. Money. Baltimore: John Hopkins Press.

Bonin, G. von and P. Bailey. 1947. *The Neocortex of Macaca Mulatta*. Urbana: University of Illinois Press.

———. 1961. *Primatologica*, Vol. 2. ed. by H. Hofer, A. Schultz and D. Starck. Basel: Karger.

———. 1962 "Anatomical Asymmetries if the Cerebral Hemispheres". *Interhemispheric Relations and Cerebral Dominance*, ed. by V.B. Mountcastle. Baltimore: John Hopkins Press.

Conolly, C.J. 1950. *External Morphology of the Primate Brain*, Springfield, Ill.: Thomas.

Critchley, M. 1953. *The Parietal Lobes*. London: E. Arnold & Co.

Crosny, E.C., T. Humphrey and E.W. Lauer. 1962. *Correlative Anatomy of the Nervous System*. New York: The Macmillan Company.

Curtis, H.J. 1940. "Intercortical connections of corpus callosum as indicated by evoked potentials". *Journal of Neurophysiology* 3:407-422.

Dejerine, J. 1891. "Sur un cas de cécité verbale avec agraphie suivi d'autopsie". *Mémoires de la Société de Biologie* 3: 197-201.

————. 1892. "Contribution à l'étude anatomique et clinique des différentes varieties de cécité verbale". *Mémoires de la Société de Biologie* 4: 61-90.

Ettlinger, G. 1962. *Interhemispheric Relations and Cerebral Dominance*, ed. by V.B. Mountcastle. Baltimore: John Hopkins Press.

Foix, Ch. 1922. "Sur une variété de troubles bilateraux de la sensibilité par lésion unilaterale du cerveau". *Revue Neurologique* 29:322-331.

———— and P. Hillemand. 1925. "Rôle vraisemblable du splenium dans la pathogenie de l'alexie pure par lésion de la cérébrale postérieure". *Bulletins et Mémoires de Société medicale des Hôspitaux de Paris* 41: 393-395.

Gazzaniga, M.S., J.E. Bogen and R.W. Sperry. 1962. "Some functional effects of sectioning the cerebral commissures in man". *Proceedings of the National Academy of Science* (USA), 48: 1765-1769.

Geschwind, N. 1962. "The anatomy of acquired disorders of reading". *Reading Disability*, ed. by J. Money. Baltimore: John Hopkins Press.

———— and M. Fusillo. 1964. *Transactions of the American Neurological Association* 89: 172.

————. 1964. "The development of the brain and the evolution of language". *Monographic Series on Language and Linguistics*, Vol. 17, ed. by C. Stuart. Washington: Georgetown University Press.

Goldstein, K. 1908. "Zur Lehre von der motorische Apraxie". *Journal für Psychologie und Neurologie* 11: 169; 270.

————. 1927. "Uber Aphasie". *Schweizer Archiv für Neurologie and Psychiatrie* 6: 1-68.

Hartmann, F. 1907. "Beiträge zur Apraxielehre". *Monatschrift für Psychiatrie und Neurologie* 21: 97-118; 248-270.

Hécaen, H., J. De Ajuriaguerra and M. David. 1952. "Les déficits fonctionels après lobectomie occipitale". *Monatschrift für Psychiatrie und Neurologie* 123: 239-290.

Hoff, H. 1961. "Die Lokalisation der Aphasie". *Proceedings of the 7th International Congress of Neurology*, Vol 1. Rome: Societa Grafica Romana.

Kinsbourne, M. and E.K. Warrington. 1962. "A variety of Reading Disabilities Associated with Right Hemisphere Lesions". *Journal of Neurology, Neurosurgery and Psychiatry* 25: 339-344.

Krieg, W.J.S. 1963. *Connections of the Cerebral Cortex*. Evanston: Brain Books.

Liepmann, H. 1898. *Ein Fall von reiner Sprachtaubheit*. Breslau: Cohn & Weigert.

———— and Storch, E. 1902. "Der mikroskopische Gehirnbefund bei dem Fall Gorstelle". *Monatschrift für Psychiatrie und Neurologie* 11:115-120.

Maspes, P.E. 1948. "Le syndrome expérimentale chez l'homme de la section du splénium du corps calleux". *Revue Neurologique* 80: 101-113.

McCulloch, W.S. and H.W. Garol. 1941. "Cortical origin and distribution of corpus callosum and anterior commissure in the monkey (Macaca mulatta)." *Journal of Neurophysiology* 4: 555-563.

Meyer, A. 1905. "Aphasia". *Psychological Bulletin* 2: 261-277.

Myers, R.E. 1962. "Commissural connections between occipital lobes of the monkey". *Journal of Comparative Neurology* 118: 1-16.

Pribram, K.H., B.S. Rosner and W. Rosenblith. 1954. "Electrical responses to acoustic clicks in monkey: extent of neocortex activated". *Journal of Neurophysiology* 17: 336-344.

Raymond, F. and M. Egger. 1906. "Un cas d'aphasie tactile". *Revue Neurologique* 14: 371-375.

Scoville, W.B. and B. Milner. 1957. "Loss of recent memory after bilateral hippocampal lesions". *Journal of Neurology, Neurosurgery and Psychiatry* 20: 11-21.

Smith, G.E. 1906. "New studies on the folding of the visual cortex and the significance of the occipital sulci in the human brain". *Journal of Anatomy* 41: 237.

Sugar, O., J.D. French and J. Chusid. 1948. "Cortical connections of the superior surface of the temporal operculum in the monkey (Maccaca mulatta)". *Journal of Neurophysiology* 11: 175-184.

Symonds, C.P. 1953. "Aphasia". *Journal of Neurology, Neurosurgery and Psychiatry* 16: 1-6.

Trescher, J.H. and F.R. Ford. 1937. "Colloid cyst of the third ventricle". *Archives of Neurology and Psychiatry* 37: 959-973.

Index

In the CLASSICS IN PSYCHOLINGUISTICS (CiPL) series (Series Editor: E.F. Konrad Koerner) the following volumes have been published thus far:

1. THUMB, Albert (1865-1915) & Karl MARBE (1869-1953): *Experimentelle Untersuchungen über die psychologischen Grundlagen der sprachlichen Analogiebildung. New edition, together with an introd. article by David J. Murray, appendix by Erwin A. Esper. (Foreword K. Koerner).* 1978.

2. MERINGER, Rudolf (1859-1931) & Carl MAYER (1862-1936): *Versprechen und Verlesen: Eine psychologisch-linguistische Studie. New edition, together with an introd. article and a select bibliography by Anne Cutler and David Fay.* 1978.

3. BLOOMFIELD, Leonard: *An Introduction to the Study of Language. New edition, with an introduction by Joseph F. Kess.* 1983.

4. ELING, Paul (ed.): *Reader in the History of Aphasia. From Franz Gall to Norman Geschwind.* 1994.

5. WEGENER, Philipp (1848-1916): *Untersuchungen über die Grundfragen des Sprachlebens. Reprint from the 1885 edition. Edited by E.F. Konrad Koerner, with an introduction in English by Clemens Knobloch.* 1991.